LEADERSHIP IN HEALTH CARE

Sara Miller McCune founded SAGE Publishing in 1965 to support the dissemination of usable knowledge and educate a global community. SAGE publishes more than 1000 journals and over 800 new books each year, spanning a wide range of subject areas. Our growing selection of library products includes archives, data, case studies and video. SAGE remains majority owned by our founder and after her lifetime will become owned by a charitable trust that secures the company's continued independence.

Los Angeles | London | New Delhi | Singapore | Washington DC | Melbourne

4TH EDITION

LEADERSHIP IN HEALTH CARE

JILL BARR & LESLEY DOWDING

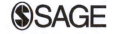

Los Angeles | London | New Delhi
Singapore | Washington DC | Melbourne

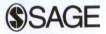

Los Angeles | London | New Delhi
Singapore | Washington DC | Melbourne

SAGE Publications Ltd
1 Oliver's Yard
55 City Road
London EC1Y 1SP

SAGE Publications Inc.
2455 Teller Road
Thousand Oaks, California 91320

SAGE Publications India Pvt Ltd
B 1/I 1 Mohan Cooperative Industrial Area
Mathura Road
New Delhi 110 044

SAGE Publications Asia-Pacific Pte Ltd
3 Church Street
#10-04 Samsung Hub
Singapore 049483

Editor: Alex Clabburn
Editorial assistant: Jade Grogan
Assistant editor, digital: Chloe Statham
Production editor: Victoria Nicholas
Marketing manager: Tamara Navaratnam
Cover design: Wendy Scott
Typeset by: C&M Digitals (P) Ltd, Chennai, India
Printed in the UK

Library of Congress Control Number: 2018955505

British Library Cataloguing in Publication data

A catalogue record for this book is available from
the British Library

ISBN 978-1-5264-5939-8
ISBN 978-1-5264-5940-4 (pbk)

At SAGE we take sustainability seriously. Most of our products are printed in the UK using responsibly sourced papers
and boards. When we print overseas we ensure sustainable papers are used as measured by the PREPS grading
system. We undertake an annual audit to monitor our sustainability.

Lesley would like to dedicate this book to her mother Bunny who has been a great supporter of the 'Leadership in Health Care' journey.

Jill would like to dedicate this book to her brother, John Murray, who was so enthusiastic and encouraging about our healthcare ideas. He sadly died in 2017.

CONTENTS

ABOUT THE AUTHORS

Jill Barr is a lecturer at Coventry University, teaching student nurses and MBA/MSc students in health care. She has worked as a Principal Lecturer at the University of Wolverhampton and also at De Montford University, with a number of awards from pre-registration nursing to Community Specialist Nursing programmes, Non-Medical Prescribing, Physician Assistant/Associate, Advanced Practitioner and Public Health Masters. Her own professional career has been exciting, varied and totally integrated with personal development, including writing with Lesley Dowding for over twenty years. Jill qualified as a nurse, midwife and health visitor, working in all these areas in practice as well as gaining her nurse licence in Michigan, USA. With a breadth of practice experiences in acute, community and industry, the patients, women, families and communities that have been served have been an important tapestry in her personal development.

Lesley Dowding's career has encompassed a number of differing experiences since qualification, as a nurse and midwife, ranging from General Theatres, Midwifery, Gynaecology, nanny in the USA, veterinary assistant, Anaesthetics & Recovery Sister, and as Nurse Tutor within schools of nursing and universities. Lesley teaches a variety of subjects for pre-registration nursing students including Management Studies, and has a passion for effective management techniques, endeavouring to make what might be considered dry theory applicable to clinical practice. To do this Lesley and Jill have written two books related to management theory and practice in health care: *Managing in Health Care: A Guide for Nurses, Midwives and Health Visitors* (2002, Pearson Education) and *Leadership in Health Care* (Sage, first edition 2008).

FOREWORD

In an era of ever-increasing complexity and demand, the emphasis on leadership and developing new leaders has never been greater. The general sentiment is that it is never too soon to begin developing the skills, knowledge and attributes for leadership. Indeed, 'leadership' is now viewed as a core aspect, and differentiator of the health care professional's identity, and an integral part of their role. Developing the skills and capabilities to perform as a leader often requires a process of personal development, beginning with a commitment to self-awareness, and an understanding of personal values, beliefs, attitudes, skills and knowledge. Knowing oneself provides the bedrock to working with others and leading others, to achieve more than can be achieved alone.

I am very pleased to introduce this new and revised 4th edition of *Leadership in Health Care*. Reading this book will support the process of leadership development and provide important knowledge and insight across a range of topics, spanning theories of leadership, ethical and professional influences, the impact of culture and teamwork practices, as well as conflict management. An individual's ability to lead may emerge over time, and with preparation, practise, coaching and support, fulfilling a leadership role can be extremely rewarding. This book provides a valuable companion to the leadership journey, being both a foundation and stimulus to further individual growth.

The notion of personal growth and lifelong learning is an important theme. The health care environment within which so many people work and learn can be described as complex and uncertain, subject to much change and fluctuation. Within this context, the need for leadership has never been clearer, as we strive for excellence in care quality, effective team-working and service improvement within the midst of vast shifts at the socio-cultural, political, technological, ethical, legal and economic level.

Amidst much pressure and frequently, much organisational turmoil, leaders must take time to pause and reflect on their activities and interactions and the environment around them. In challenging contexts, the importance of self-compassion and compassion towards others, and the values of trust and respect cannot be underestimated. Leaders must consider their own wellbeing, in order to maintain the resilience needed to serve those around them. Leaders must also have the capacity for meaning and purpose in life, a capacity for optimism, empathy with others and a base of calm with which to manage and respond to stress.

For aspiring, new and developing leaders, this text will be an invaluable source of information and learning. The authors draw upon a wealth of clinical and educational experiences and in doing, have created a text that I am proud to endorse.

Dr Rosie Kneafsey
Head of School, Nursing, Midwifery and Health,
Coventry University

PREFACE

WHY THIS BOOK?

Effective leadership underpins the efficient and safe running of any clinical practice. Indeed, in everyday life it may be necessary to use leadership skills in our family life in getting children to school on time, managing domestic chores and planning for future holidays. The way in which we do it, and the effects it has on others, is important. Leadership is a topic that concerns policy through to practice in health care. Seventy years since the NHS began and the importance of leadership in clinical practice is gaining momentum. The NHS Leadership Centre exemplifies that importance through a range of initiatives. Being able to give skilled and evidence-based care is important, but it is also about working in a performance-measured health service to meet the expectations of society.

Leadership is a vital part of today's health care practice and the Nursing and Midwifery Council (2018) has recently highlighted it as an important platform for the standard of clinical training and future nurse registration. The emergence of new roles such as the registered Nursing Associate and a commitment from the Department of Health to progress regulation of the Physician Associate in 2018 highlights the changing face of the health care workforce. The NHS Leadership Academy is also actively working with allied health and medical professionals to improve leadership and innovation capability. It is useful for everyone in health care to understand the variety of theories supporting actions and applications to leadership practice not only in the country but also in a more global sense. One view may be that leadership comes from within and is something that is with you from birth. Contrary to this is the idea that leadership skills can be learned or developed. It is our belief that an ability to lead people in delivering a quality, patient-centred health care service relies on developing these skills.

Throughout this book we have used the word 'nursing' to apply to the work of all health care workers irrespective of their role in the delivery of health care; each will have their own distinct professional register and requirements for practice. To that end, this new edition explores the underpinning theories of leadership and applies them to health care situations wherever they are practised. It debates the nature of leadership by examining diversity, individual values, the idea of the team as 'hero', and the variety of skills required to achieve effective and efficient health care delivery. It also reflects the changing health care structures and quality improvement initiatives, and includes a new chapter concerning the ethics, legislation and professional issues that underpin clinical practice and leadership.

WHO IS IT FOR?

This book supports the health care professional (HCP) in identifying the application of leadership theory to their own clinical practice. It is applicable to all professions allied to medicine, including students of adult, mental health, children, and learning disability nursing and midwifery, as well as nursing associates, specialist community public health nurses, physician associates, operating department practitioners, paramedic sciences, and more. Theories offer the 'bones' for exploring the nature of leadership; the difficulty comes in applying those theories to practice.

Recognising the theory–practice gap is important because each informs the other when searching and developing more effective ways of delivering health care to a demanding public. Pre- and post-registration courses usually include aspects of leadership theory, but it has been noted that some students experience difficulty in application; as such this book is for them.

HOW DO I USE IT?

The chapters are designed to direct you as a health care professional through a structured approach, starting with leading as an individual through to team working and on to the organisational perspective, reflecting both the micro and macro levels of health care systems.

Each chapter commences with a list of Learning Outcomes followed by an Introduction outlining the content of the chapter. Within each chapter there will be a variety of activities with questions related to the content, self-knowledge, literature application, review questions, 'stop and think' activities and preferred styles. Every chapter will conclude with a Summary of Key Points, highlighting the ways in which the learning outcomes have been met. The Online Resources for the book will allow you to go deeper into the subject material of the book, providing you with SAGE journal articles, useful weblinks and introductory/explanatory videos per chapter.

Throughout the book, the words 'patient' or 'client' are used interchangeably to indicate the care user, patient or client depending on the context of care.

We hope that you find this new edition – used in conjunction with other texts – a useful tool to aid you in interpreting and using effective leadership skills in your professional and personal life.

PUBLISHER'S ACKNOWLEDGEMENTS

The publishers are grateful to all third-parties for permission to reproduce the following material:

Table 2.1 Indispensable qualities of a leader. Maxwell, J.C. (1999) The 21 Indispensable Qualities of a Leader. Nashville, TN: Thomas Nelson.

Figure 2.2 Johns' Model of Reflection. Johns, C. (1995) 'Framing learning through reflection within Karper's fundamental ways of knowing in nursing', *Journal of Advanced Nursing*, 22 (2): 226–34.

Figure 4.1 Functional needs to be fulfilled for effective team working. Adapted from Adair, J. (1997) *Decision Making and Problem Solving*. London: Institute of Personnel and Development.

Figure 4.3 Vroom-Jago contingency model. Vroom, V.H. and Jago, A.G. (1988) *The New Leadership*. Englewood Cliffs, NJ: Prentice Hall.

Figure 4.4 The level 5 hierarchy model. Collins, J. (2001) 'Level 5 leadership: the triumph of humility and fierce resolve', *Harvard Business Review*, January: 67–76.

Figure 7.2 The basic communications model. Weightman, J. (1999) *Introducing Organisational Behaviour*. Harlow: Addison Wesley Longman.

Figure 8.2 Unbounded problems. Drucker, P.F. (1967) 'The effective executive', in H. Flanagan and P. Spurgeon (1996) *Public Sector Managerial Effectiveness*. Milton Keynes: Open University Press.

Table 8.8 Types of decision makers. Vroom, V.H. and Yetton, P.W. (1973) *Leadership and Decision Making*. Pittsburgh: University of Pittsburgh.

Figure 10.2 Consequences of conflict. Almost, J. (2006) 'Conflict within nursing work environments: concept analysis', *Journal of Advanced Nursing*, 53 (4): 444–53.

Table 11.3 Characteristics of EI people and less EI people. Kite, N. and Kay, F. (2012) *Understanding Emotional Intelligence: Strategies for Boosting your EQ and Using It in the Workplace*. London: Kogan Page.

Table 12.1 Schein's (1985) relationship between leadership and culture formation. Schein, E.H. (1985) *Organizational Culture and Leadership*. San Francisco, CA: Jossey-Bass.

Figure 12.4 Johnson and Scholes' (1989) organisational cultural web. Johnson, G. and Scholes, K. (1989) *Exploring Corporate Strategy*. London: Prentice Hall.

Table 13.2 Dimensions of quality. Berry, L., Zeithaml, V. and Parasuraman, A. (1988) 'The service quality puzzle', Business Horizon, Sept.–Oct.: 35–43, in M. Moullin (2002) *Delivering Excellence in Health and Social Care*. Buckingham: Open University Press.

Figure 13.3 Denison's model of cultural change. Denison's model is reproduced with kind permission of Denison Consulting www.DenisonCulture.com

ONLINE RESOURCES

The 4th edition of *Leadership in Health Care* is supported by a variety of online resources for both students and lecturers. These resources aid both learning and teaching, pointing you in the direction of personality and leadership tests, video introductions, and scenarios encompassing all of the book's topics, along with further reading and multiple choice questions per chapter.

All resources are available at: https://study.sagepub.com/barr4e

RESOURCES FOR LECTURERS AND STUDENTS

FURTHER READING

- **Read more widely!** A selection of **journal articles** that support each chapter to help deepen your knowledge and reinforce your learning of key topics. An ideal place to start for literature reviews/dissertations/assignments. Preceding each article is an annotation from the editors, Jill Barr and Lesley Dowding, introducing its relevance for practice and/or revision.

WEBLINKS

- **Weblinks** direct you to relevant resources to broaden your understanding of chapter topics and expand your knowledge of leadership and character. Preceding all links is an annotation from the editors, Jill Barr and Lesley Dowding, introducing their relevance for practice and or revision.

MCQS

- **Multiple Choice Questions** per chapter, written by the book's editors, test your core knowledge of the topic covered, making sure you understand the material covered, highlighting areas for further revision and reading.

VIDEOS

- **Videos** cover a vast range of sources and guides on all aspects of leadership covered in the book. Whether this be styles of leadership, communication or team-working skills in a health care setting, the editor's choice of 2–4 videos per chapter should supplement your reading of the book and bring the theory to life.

PART 1

THE INDIVIDUAL

1 THE NATURE OF LEADERSHIP

Chapter Contents

Learning Outcomes

By the end of this chapter you will have had the opportunity to:

- Discuss the notions of leadership and followership
- Define leadership
- Discuss the importance of the changing context related to health care
- Compare leadership and management
- Debate the art and science of leadership

INTRODUCTION

The concept of leadership seems to be all-important in health care today; you may have limited experience of health care leadership or no aspirations to be a leader, or perhaps a large amount of leadership experience. Whatever the reason, this chapter will start to make you think about leadership and its role in your life and career.

Florence Nightingale (1820–1910) is famous not only for her work at Scutari (Barrack) Hospital in Turkey during the Crimean War but also, Kopf (1916) noted, for her role in analysing data collected by the War Office. This could be said to mark the beginnings of the use of research in nursing to improve practice. Her impact is still felt today and at the time of writing (2018) the International Council of Nursing and World Health Organization are promoting the Nursing Now! Campaign – a three-year programme of events timed to coincide with the 200th anniversary of Florence Nightingale's birth and a year when nurses will be celebrated worldwide.

Mary Seacole (1805–1881), known as a 'doctress, nurse and mother', also asked to be considered for service during the Crimean War, but was informed that the full complement of nurses had been secured and that her offer of help could not be entertained (Seacole, 2005 [1857]). Such was her belief that there was a real need for her talents in the area that she funded herself to travel to the region where she set up and ran the British Hotel approximately two miles from Balaclava. She provided warm hospitality and care for soldiers and was ultimately known as 'Mother Seacole'. She is now widely seen as one of history's great black female heroes.

Dr E.L.M. Millar highlighted the need for effective training within the Ambulance Service of the 1960s, which ultimately led to today's technician training and paramedic degree (Kilner, 2004). The current framework for paramedic training and career framework goes on to reflect the changes in practice and current expectations (Harris, 2015). These people did much for caring through their pursuit of improved standards and by acting as role models in the health care work they did.

Activity

Who do you see as an effective leader?

John F. Kennedy (1917–1963), Nelson Mandela (1918–2014), Barack Obama (1961–), Benazir Bhutto (1953–2007), Indira Gandhi (1917–1984), Tony Blair (1953–), Donald J. Trump (1946–), Pope Francis (1936–), Adolf Hitler (1889–1945), Kim Jong-un (1983–), Park Geun-hye (1952–), Aung San Suu Kyi (1945–), Angela Merkel (1954–), Abdel Fattah el-Sisi (1954–), Julius Caesar (100BC–44BC), Abraham Lincoln (1809–1865), Mahatma Ghandi (1869–1948), David Cameron (1966–), François Hollande (1954–), Vladimir Putin (1952–) are world leaders, but it is up to you to decide if you think they are excellent or poor in this regard.

Who would fit in the 'Excellent' column and who in 'Poor'? If you discuss your list with someone else you may be surprised at the similarities and/or the differences in your perceptions.

Excellent Leaders	Poor Leaders

As a nurse, I have been lucky to work with some excellent clinical leaders. (I have also worked with some 'shockers', but that's another story!) One of the best I have listened to is Professor Beverley Malone (1948–) who is currently the chief executive officer of the National League for Nursing in the United States; prior to assuming this position in February 2007, she served as general secretary of the Royal College of Nursing for six years. I heard her speak at a National Association of Theatre Nurses conference: she was inspirational, and enthusiastic about nursing today and everyone left with the intention of being that nurse who has the power to strongly advocate for their patients. Indeed one nurse, writing on an American nursing website, stated that 'To hear Beverly Malone speak is to come away with a renewed nursing pride and with a missionary zeal to harvest the "best and the brightest" into the profession now'. Christine Beasley, DBE (CNO for England 2004), also offered an inspirational dialogue regarding nurses' engagement in leading service improvement. Whoever you think of as influential clinical leaders, they must be motivators, love their chosen profession, and command such respect to be able to infuse others with energy and enthusiasm. Leadership involves people being led, so there have to be those who are happy to be followers. We must therefore remember that effective leaders and effective followers may sometimes be the same people playing distinct roles at various times. This book will try to engender this verve for effective leadership. To address the identified learning outcomes, this chapter will introduce the nature of leadership, comparing management and leadership, and the art and science of leadership.

THE IMPORTANCE OF LEADERSHIP IN PATIENT AND CLIENT CARE OUTCOMES

Several high-profile system failures where patient/client care has been affected through poor and ineffective leadership have been highlighted. Following the Francis Report (2013) the then prime minister David Cameron asked Professor Don Berwick, a leading expert in patient safety, to look at what needed to be done 'to make zero harm a reality in our NHS'. The Berwick Report (2013: 4), *A Promise to Learn – a Commitment to Act*, identified a number of existing problems such as a lack of leadership in risk management systems. The executive summary made ten recommendations which were as follows:

1. The NHS should continually and forever reduce patient harm by embracing wholeheartedly an ethic of learning.
2. All leaders concerned with NHS health care – political, regulatory, governance, executive, clinical and advocacy – should place quality of care in general, and patient safety in particular, at the top of their priorities for investment, inquiry, improvement, regular reporting, encouragement and support.
3. Patients and their carers should be present, powerful and involved at all levels of health care organisations from wards to the boards of Trusts.
4. Government, Health Education England and NHS England should assure that sufficient staff are available to meet the NHS's needs now and in the future. Health care organisations should ensure that staff are present in appropriate numbers to provide safe care at all times and are well-supported.
5. Mastery of quality and patient safety sciences and practices should be part of the initial preparation and lifelong education of all health care professionals, including managers and executives.
6. The NHS should become a learning organisation. Its leaders should create and support the capability for learning, and therefore change, at scale, within the NHS.
7. Transparency should be complete, timely and unequivocal. All data on quality and safety, whether assembled by government, organisations, or professional societies, should be shared in a timely fashion with all parties who want it, including, in accessible form, with the public.
8. All organisations should seek out the patient and carer voice as an essential asset in monitoring the safety and quality of care.
9. Supervisory and regulatory systems should be simple and clear. They should avoid diffusion of responsibility. They should be respectful of the goodwill and sound intention of the clear majority of staff. All incentives should point in the same direction.
10. We support responsive regulation of organisations, with a hierarchy of responses. Recourse to criminal sanctions should be extremely rare and should function primarily as a deterrent to wilful or reckless neglect or mistreatment.

The need for quality in the delivery of care is vital, and failings were highlighted where this has clearly not been the case, e.g. the Bristol Royal Infirmary (Kennedy Report, 2001) and Gosport Hospital (Baker, 2003), Baby P in 2007 (The Lord Laming Report, 2009; Department for Education, 2010), the Mid-Staffordshire NHS Foundation Trust scandal (Francis, 2013), and the Heart of England Inquiry (Kennedy Report, 2013) to name but a few. All of these events changed the landscape of how we look at duty of care – in all these situations, the failure of effective leadership and management strategies was shown to be complicit in the failure of care provision and workers seemed to have become complacent about their roles. They have reminded us of the importance of raising concerns and acting on them before it is too late, and of developing a workplace culture which enables staff to have the confidence to speak out (UNISON, 2011). In order to help NHS staff raise concerns in a timely manner, a paper titled 'Freedom to Speak Up: Whistleblowing Policy for the NHS' has encompassed the recommendations highlighted by Sir Robert Francis in his *Freedom to Speak Up – Review* (NHS Improvement, 2016).

Leaders, whatever their background, must demonstrate 'best practice' in their clinical areas and dedicate themselves to supporting, marketing, and 'driving through' an innovation (Greenhalgh et al., 2004: 182). These people are known as 'Champions' and practise at a level that encourages others to better themselves to ensure all patients receive first-class, evidence-based care always. The notion of effective, inspirational leadership is not new: as Markham and Aiman-Smith (2001: 44–50) state, 'A new idea either finds a champion or dies'. Stoddart et al. (2014) highlighted a project that suggested systematic 'Care Comfort Rounds' for all patients/clients whether they were in hospital or care/nursing homes; the project led to proactive rather than reactive nursing care delivery and the number of falls and use of all buzzers was reduced. Active nursing rounds – variously known as 'intentional' or 'care and comfort' rounds – are still relatively new in their present format; what is important is that these are patient (rather than task) focused: every hour a nurse checks in with each patient, not to 'do something' but to find out if they are comfortable and if there is anything they need. Whilst this might be thought to be a regressive move (in that it was commonplace in the 1950s, 1960s and 1970s) it means that the patients' health and welfare are assessed at regular (hourly) intervals during the day, thereby leading to safer, effective, patient-centred practice (The King's Fund, 2012b). The current notion of care comfort rounds started in the United States and has been adopted in some UK hospitals, including some hospital Trusts participating in the Hospital Pathways Programme (The King's Fund, 2012a). In acute settings key aspects that are usually checked during Care Comfort/Active Nursing/Intentional rounds include the 'Four Ps':

1. Positioning, i.e. making sure the patient is comfortable and assessing the risk of pressure ulcers
2. Personal needs, i.e. scheduling patient trips to the bathroom to avoid the risk of falling
3. Pain, i.e. asking patients to describe their pain level on a scale of 0–10
4. Placement, i.e. making sure the items a patient needs are within easy reach.

During each round the following behaviours (which may be summarised on a prompt card) are undertaken by the nurse:

- Using an opening phrase to introduce themselves and put the patient at ease
- Performing scheduled tasks
- Asking about the 'Four Ps' (described above)
- Assessing the care environment (e.g. fall hazards, temperature of the room)
- Using closing key words (e.g. 'Is there anything else I can do for you before I go?')
- Explaining when the patient will be checked on again
- Documenting the round.

The whole concept of intentional rounding is that it is applicable to every patient/client requiring care at whatever level; as time progresses interventions may be limited *but patients/clients in structured settings should be approached on an hourly basis to ascertain care needs*. Clearly with those being cared for in the community, their own home or somewhere that offers informal care this should become a normal part of assessment during each interaction with a care professional. Structured methods of intentional rounding are underpinned by leadership support, e.g. regular staff meetings to review activities and progress. Staff training and accountability structures are used to 'hardwire' the required behaviours and competencies into routine practice (Studer Group, 2007). In the USA it is deemed part of daily care for the registered nurse to conduct a full health assessment on all patients. In 2011 the UK's prime minister called for changes in the way nurses delivered care (NNRU, 2012), recognising the need for hourly nursing rounds, i.e. intentional rounding. To ensure that this is not just a paper exercise, NHS Trusts need to identify suitable registered nurses whose responsibility it will be to implement this systematic care standard as a change in practice. These leaders need to ensure an effective implementation of this strategy (during the day, night, and at weekends, i.e. 24/7) to improve patient outcomes.

Activity

- In your experience, have you observed a similar activity to 'Care Comfort Rounds'?
- Consider your clinical environment and list the pros and cons in implementing a system such as 'Care Comfort Rounds'.

You might have thought of the time-consuming element of filling in yet another form, but Stoddart's project has shown that not only was all-round patient care improved but that staff satisfaction in care delivery was also increased (Stoddart et al., 2014: 22). As with any change the implementation of a 'new' work practice should be considered with a great deal of communication, planning and education for it to succeed (see Chapter 13). The impact of the clinical nurse leader on quality patient outcomes was highlighted by Hodge (2017), when she discussed the need for healthy work environments where clinical nurse leaders were able to assist staff in identifying areas of care that needed improvement and developing strategies to meet care outcomes, so raising standards.

Employees have rights just as patients and patient/clients have rights, and similarly employers have a duty of care (Department of Health (DH), 2005, 2018). Under the *Management of Health and Safety at Work Regulations* (DH, 1999) employers are obliged to assess the nature and scale of risks to health and safety in the workplace and base their control measures on the outcome. We have to accept that as humans we are all able to make mistakes but learning from the failure of others is imperative; the Department of Health's (2000) paper, 'An Organisation with Memory', highlighted that failure is almost always unintentional, and comes about through a variety of small omissions/errors rather than via a single colossal one. It set out to understand what was known about the scale and nature of serious failures in the United Kingdom's National Health Service (NHS) system, examine how the NHS might learn from those failures, and recommend methods to minimise future failures. Despite the valuable information contained within the document the NHS continues to struggle with implementing those recommendations.

RELATIONSHIPS BETWEEN LEADERSHIP AND FOLLOWERSHIP

Consider the decisions you made earlier in the first Activity: what made you think one leader was good, yet another was poor? Whatever your decision, they all managed to acquire followers. The better ones may have been acting as leaders and had the ability to listen when others put forward their opinions. Young (2016) suggests that there is a belief that leadership may be related to seniority. However, leadership is not about position but about behaviour. Think about the following situation in relation to leadership:

> Sue Potter is a third-year student on placement in the clinical area, and notices that a second-year student in the same placement area often comes to ask her for advice related to patient/client care. Sue happily explains the procedure to the other student, highlighting the current research supporting the action. A qualified member of staff also approaches Sue for research information, as it was an area of care he had not been involved with for some time. Sue was happy to tell the qualified person what she knew and then started to reflect on her own abilities in leading and teaching. She then started to question why people felt that they could come to her for information and support.

Although Sue was not yet qualified, she was clearly seen as a leader within that situation. The skills Sue demonstrated – being approachable and teaching others willingly – are those of leadership. Her example of supporting and sharing her knowledge can be applied to any field of health care provision.

It is important then to examine some of the variety of definitions of leadership available. Daft (2017: 4) states that 'scholars and other writers have offered more than 350 definitions of the term leadership', and concludes that leadership 'is one of the most observed and least understood phenomena on earth'.

Tappen et al. (2009 [2004]: 5) suggest that there are several primary tasks involved with being a leader:

1. Set direction: mission, goals, vision and purpose
2. Build commitment: motivation, spirit, teamwork
3. Confront challenges: innovation, change, and turbulence.

So, leadership would appear to be a people activity and occurs within group life; it is not something done to people. Effective leaders are seen to have charisma which allows them to articulate a vision for a given group of followers, and generate enthusiasm for that vision, and are seen by all as members of a team (Haslam et al., 2013: 22). Without followers there cannot be leaders, and without leaders there cannot be followers, so being an effective follower is as important to the health care professional as being an effective leader.

Activity

Can you identify situations when you have been a leader and when you have been a follower?

You might have been a leader during your time at school as a prefect or sports team captain; or outside school as a Girl Guide, Boy Scout, youth club leader; or even as a member of a parent–teacher association. Conversely, you might also have identified those same situations as being times when you were a follower. Similarly, there may be times in your clinical area when you were a follower due to being unsure of yourself, but other times when you were a leader like Sue. 'Followership' is not a passive, unthinking activity. On the contrary, engaged followers are critical to the success of an organisation (Grossman and Valiga, 2016: viii). Tappen et al. (2009 [2004]: 5–6) suggest that there are several things you can do to become a better follower:

1. If you discover a problem, clearly you would inform your team leader of the problem, but you might also offer a suggestion as to how it might be rectified
2. Freely invest your interest and energy in your work
3. Be supportive of new ideas and new directions suggested by others
4. When you disagree with ideas explain why
5. Listen carefully and reflect on what your leader or manager says
6. Continue to learn as much as you can about your speciality area
7. Share what you learn with others.

If you are to be an effective leader, it is vital that you recognise the opportunities for leadership all around you and that in these situations you act like a leader, influencing others to bring about change for a better quality of care provision. Leaders must face some hard decisions in their work, remembering always that managing scarce resources – such as equipment, pharmaceuticals, and transport – may not be easy, and that managing people is much more complex.

DEFINING LEADERSHIP

Leadership can be defined in several ways, but it is still an elusive concept. Indeed, key authors cannot agree on the nature or essential characteristics of leadership but offer a variety of perspectives. This indicates that leadership is thought to be about relationships. Leadership is a discipline that is evolving – indeed Alvesson and Spicer (2010: 4) note that our understanding, interpretation and response to leadership are variable and complex: on the one hand distrust and control are features while on the other hand support and close contact may be dominant. Leadership theory is not a new phenomenon: Burns (2010: 4) has suggested there are two types of leadership, i.e. transformational and transactional approaches. Transformational leaders recognise and possibly exploit an existing need or demand, creating a positive change in the followers, taking care of each other's interests and acting in the interests of the group (this is explored further in Chapter 4). The transactional approach, on the other hand, focuses on established standards and practices with goals to be met (like the 4-hour rule in A&E) and penalties for not meeting that rule; there is usually a system of supervision related to organisation and performance (annual personal development reviews) and the potential for retribution if those goals are not met.

Daft (2017) expands on this by indicating that rather than being a controller, the leader is a facilitator who helps people do their best by removing obstacles to performance; they also provide learning opportunities and offer support and feedback. Sayle (1993, in Sadler, 2003: 33) takes a less dramatic view of leadership, i.e. the working leader. A case for the working leader is presented as the person who makes the organisation work to its maximum effect. Leadership skills are needed to overcome the bureaucratic contradictions of organisational life.

Activity

Can you find a definition that fits in with clinical leadership?

Clinical leadership is a relatively recent term and is seen as being about facilitating evidence-based practice and improved patient outcomes through local care. Fenton (2012) reminds us that Florence Nightingale said 'Let whoever is in charge keep this simple question in her head … How can I provide for the right thing to be always done?' Working with common definitions can lead into concept analysis: a deeper process involving antecedents, attributes and consequences being unpacked (Walker and Avant, 2010). At a deeper level, leadership could be seen from various perspectives as being:

- A characteristic trait – based in trait theory
- A position – based in the functional approach
- A quality – based in trait theory
- A process – based in functional approaches
- A power relationship – style, or the effect on group behaviour.

These perspectives will be developed further in Chapter 4. How you view leadership will influence your clinical beliefs, values and behaviours, and that leadership must be a part of caring. Patients and clients deserve care that is well led at all levels of the NHS or health industry organisations.

HEALTH CARE: A CHANGING CONTEXT

Due to the driving, technological forces and rising expectations, our health service has expanded to encompass a much greater provision than that envisaged when the NHS was set up in 1948. The NHS has its history in a liberal socialist ideology of health being a right for all, regardless of ability to pay. At a time of enormous change in the service, leaders and managers have a crucial role to play. Currently there is great debate related to the general public's expectations, and underfunding of the NHS whilst people are living longer and hence may have multiple pathologies to cope with, but those expectations continue to rise.

The King's Fund (2011) set up a commission on leadership and management in the NHS with a brief to:

- take a view on the current state of management and leadership in the NHS
- establish the nature of management and leadership that will be required to meet the quality and financial challenges now facing the health care system
- recommend what needs to be done to strengthen and develop management and leadership in the NHS.

The Future of Leadership and Management in the NHS: No More Heroes (The King's Fund, 2011) reflects the conclusions of the commission's work that challenge some of the negative attitudes towards managers, and question current plans for major reductions in management and administration costs. The commission believed that the NHS needs to move beyond the outdated model of heroic leadership to recognise the value of leadership that is shared, distributed and adaptive. In the new model, there is recognition that leaders exist at all levels – from the board to the ward – and the increasing importance of leadership feeding information upwards from the ward to the board cannot be denied.

The current Brexit negotiations must consider the impact on recruitment to all health care professions. Following the referendum, The King's Fund (2016) identified five 'Big Issues for Health and Social Care' which were:

1. Staffing
2. Accessing Treatment (both here and abroad)
3. Regulation
4. Cross-Border Cooperation
5. Funding and Finance.

In terms of finance, a study conducted in July 2016 by the Health Foundation estimated that the NHS could be £2.8bn poorer than currently planned in 2019–2020 if the government aimed to balance the books overall (The Health Foundation, 2016). Nevertheless the public, regardless of how they voted, will expect politicians to deliver their promise of a better-funded NHS. In addition, NHS England is now establishing an NHS Europe Transition Team to work with the wider health service, the Department of Health, the Cabinet Office and others.

Storey and Holti (2013: 8) advocated a new NHS leadership model that encouraged high staff involvement and engagement focusing on meeting service user needs. They highlighted the need to manage and improve care with openness to a variety of perspectives including 'soft' intelligence rather than the narrow range of hierarchical imposed targets. In support of this, nurses and health care practitioners today need specific leadership skills and clinical development to help them deal with this rapidly changing situation in clinical care (Barr and Dowding, 2016; Gopee and Galloway, 2017). Indeed, this can relate to all health care professionals as changes are occurring rapidly everywhere. Rippon (2001), however, argued that leadership training per se will not produce the quality of leaders required to bring through change. A more sustainable solution lies with the development of what he terms 'growth cultures' to develop leaders with emotional intelligence (see Chapter 11). It is emphasised that leaders need to focus on inward rather than outward bound experiences, enabling a spiritual growth based on relationships and awareness (Wright, 2000). 'Inward' could mean greater self-awareness and need for learning whereas 'outward' could relate to expected behaviours.

GLOBAL LEADERSHIP

The notion of global leadership is a relatively new term which developed in the 1990s (Lobel, 1990; Kets de Vries and Mead, 1992; Pucik et al., 1992; Rhinesmith, 1993; Moran and Riesenberger, 1994; Brake, 1997). The term 'global' encompasses more than simple *geographic reach* in terms of business operations; it can be about the world but is generally thought to be about having *helicopter vision*, or being *across* several areas, i.e. when a helicopter is on the ground, if the pilot looks down they can see only a small circular surface area below the helicopter and has virtually little or no information about the surroundings. The more it goes up the more surface it covers, meaning that the pilot gradually starts to get a clear picture of the ground and surroundings; they can see every detail of the area they are covering at this stage. By ascending more information can be gained.

Global leadership also includes the notion of *cultural reach* in terms of people and *intellectual reach* in the development of a global mindset (Osland et al., 2006). It could be suggested that it is concerned with the interaction of people and ideas among cultures rather than the efficacy of leadership styles demonstrated by leaders in their home countries. Global leadership differs from domestic leadership in terms of issues related to connectedness: boundary spanning; complexity; ethical challenges; dealing with tensions and paradoxes; pattern recognition; building learning environments in towns and communities; and leading large scale efforts – across diverse cultures (Osland et al., 2006). We could think of the World Health Organisation (WHO) as one organisation that leads on health globally.

Activity

Can you think of any situations where a leader might have had a global effect within healthcare provision?

In terms of world influence you may have thought of Gandhi (political influence), Alexander the Great (military influence), Mother Theresa (spiritual influence), or within health care there are many to consider, e.g. Waterlow (2005) and the development of the pressure sore risk assessment tool that is used globally; Roper, Logan and Tierney (1980; 2000) who identified the activities of daily living used for the basis of assessment within the majority of health care provision in the acute sector; or further back in nursing history Florence Nightingale, who worked so hard to get basic nursing practice recognised for the good it did. Within the ambulance service it could have been Dr Millar who introduced the standardisation of training, which again is the foundation for all training within the service and is an idea used to underpin training throughout the world. Today, global health leaders may not be famous but locally there may be Unit Leaders you can think of who have helped generate better practice by '*borrowing*' ideas from other areas in the world to implement in their own practice. Sharing best practice is a very good global health activity.

Freshwater (2014: 93–7) distinguishes that leaders need to anticipate challenges, contest the status quo, work towards creativity and diversity, make decisions, and learn through reflection and feedback. However, 'a really formidable leader is the person who can balance and integrate the caring heart with the global mind'. This perspective highlights that leaders need to attune or resonate with patients and clients who ultimately will be able to receive the outcome of good leadership.

HOW WE SEE OURSELVES AND HOW OTHERS SEE US

To move forward in considering our readiness for leadership it might be useful to consider how we see ourselves and more importantly how others see us. The 'Johari Window' (Luft and Ingham, 1955) allows us to discover how much the perceptions and knowledge we have about ourselves are also seen by others. The 'Window' has four areas (see Figure 1.1).

Known to self/known to others (Arena)	Not known to self/known to others (Blind Spot)
Known to self/not known to others (Facade)	Not known to self/not known to others (Unknown)

Figure 1.1　Johari Window – the four areas

What is interesting about this is that if you ask your friends or colleagues what they think your characteristics are they will often see differing elements to you. By understanding who we are and how others see us we can begin to adapt our behaviours at work to get the best from our teams. Remember this is about you and so there are no correct answers. As we receive feedback from friends we might be able to change any negative elements and also recognise the positive elements of our personalities and adapt to meet the role of leadership, so improving relationships with others within the team.

Recently I met with a student who displayed a lovely disposition, a keenness to learn, who engaged well with reflection but presented with a constant frown on her face, portraying her anxiety to her team and clients. On discussing this perception, which may be her blind spot, the student thought about it and noted that it had come as no surprise; she relayed that her daughter had commented on her '*scary face*' in the past and thought that the façade could be because she was really shy and worried about talking to strangers. However, often when a person puts on their uniform or work clothes they also 'put on' their altered persona.

COMPARING LEADERSHIP AND MANAGEMENT

There appears to be some ambiguity between the notions of leadership and management. Currently the terms *leadership* and *management* may be used interchangeably because the differences between them may not always be straightforward. Most of us think we can recognise leadership but we may not find it easy to find in ourselves.

Activity

Jot down your ideas of the differences between a manager and leader in healthcare.

Current thinking indicates that managers have formal authority to direct the work of a given set of employees; they are formally responsible for the quality of that work and what it costs to achieve it. Neither of these elements is necessary to be a leader. Leaders are an essential part of management, but the reverse is not true: you do not have to be a manager to be a leader, but you do need to be a good leader to be an effective manager. Table 1.1 reflects some of the differences between leadership and management.

Table 1.1   Differences between leadership and management

Leadership	Management
• Based on influence and sharing	• Based on authority and influence
• An informal role	• A formally designated role

(Continued)

Table 1.1 (Continued)

Leadership	Management
• An achieved position	• An assigned position
• Part of every healthcare professional's responsibility	• Usually responsible for budgets, hiring and firing people
• Initiative	• Improved by the use of effective leadership skills
• Independent thinking	

The amount of time taken up in leadership activities might differ from person to person (Sadler, 2003). Cunningham (1986, in Sadler, 2003) noted that leadership is an 'integral part' of the management role and as such may not be seen as a separate entity (Figure 1.2). However, Bennis and Nanus (2004) indicate that there are two other models to be considered. These are where leadership is half-and-half of the same concept (Figure 1.3) and where there is partial overlap (Figure 1.4).

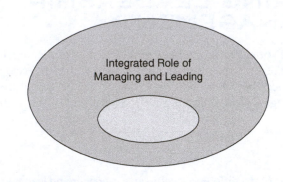

Figure 1.2 Leadership within management

Source: Adapted from Sadler, 2003

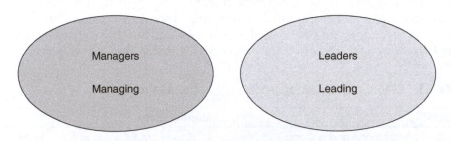

Figure 1.3 Leadership alongside management

Source: Adapted from Sadler, 2003

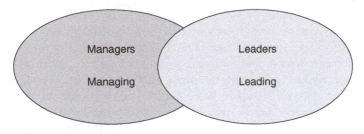

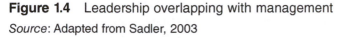

Figure 1.4 Leadership overlapping with management

Source: Adapted from Sadler, 2003

In each case the time taken up by leadership functions will differ. Overall, management is defined in relation to the achievement of organisational goals in an effective and efficient way. This means that planning, vision, staffing, direction, and resources are the main concerns that need to be managed. Managers often seem to have a bad press as *us and them* with the *them* controlling the *us*. It should be remembered that management and leadership should work together to achieve a common aim of effective quality patient care. Dowding and Barr (2002) discuss the potential effects of a wide variety of management approaches on practice. Examining these individually – or in some detail – is not the remit of this book. However, if you consider the history of management approaches, it is evident that the way in which leaders and managers function within the health care system is greatly influenced by the overall management philosophy in place. Miner (2005) suggested that organisational knowledge goes hand in hand with effective management.

Therefore, it is necessary to view the different elements of an organisation to understand why it functions in a specific manner (see Chapter 11). It can also help to clarify or structure how you might be expected to behave in each situation to uphold the reputation of that organisation. Similarly, it may help us to adopt management practices which, while considered 'old', might be the most appropriate for a given situation.

THE ART AND SCIENCE OF LEADERSHIP

Florence Nightingale (1820–1910) once said 'Nursing is an Art', and Max DePree (2004) concurred by stating that 'Leadership is an Art', in his book by that title, so it could be construed that any nurse who leads, in any capacity, is an artist and fosters a passion for creativity and innovation. Nurses who lead have a foundation in caring and nursing science, but together with this bring a wide range of colours, capabilities and creativity. Daft (2017: 27) also reminds us that it is important to bear in mind that leadership is both an art and a science. It is an art because many of the leadership skills and qualities required cannot be learned and a science because there is a growing body of knowledge that describes the leadership process. By keeping this in mind we can understand how a variety of leadership skills can be used to attain the best possible care for our patients whatever our role is within health service provision. In terms of the nursing profession Jeffrey (2013) wrote of the term *nurse leader* as being a misnomer because in the English language we place adjectives in front of nouns (e.g. the blue car, not the car blue); the term 'nurse leader' would therefore imply that this person is a leader who just happens to be a nurse; again, whilst the text is primarily about nursing the theory extends itself to all healthcare provision.

Donahue (2011) indicated that nursing has been called the oldest of the arts and the youngest of the professions. Stewart (1918, in Donahue, 2011) goes further to state that the science, spirit, and skill of nursing were beginning to develop as it became apparent that love and caring alone could not ensure health or overcome disease. Nursing education, in the past, has concentrated on the science element or *medical model*, whereby nurses were told what to learn and when to learn it in relation to the disease and the disease process. More recently, it was recognised that the patient is unique and not just a collection of symptoms. Nursing then became more 'art' focused, concentrating on holism, rather than being medical/science focused, concentrating on the disease process. This has now changed to include a holistic approach, not only to deliver care in relation to a specific condition but also to include the family and regular carers. However, health care professionals need to recognise the strength of their medical knowledge as health technology advances to provide health education to the patients and their families. For leadership, the notion of science and art must go hand in hand to respect the uniqueness of the patient and their health condition.

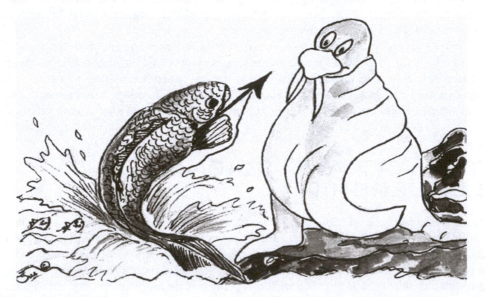

Source: Sue Saillet

As the cartoon depicts, the concept of leadership has evolved over the last century and continues to change, and the hunter can now also be the hunted. That isn't to say that the old ways of doing things are not good, but that in today's health business society there are diverse ways of getting things done, ways that enable 'management' and 'leadership' to work together. Leadership is both an art and a science. It is an art because of the many skills and qualities that cannot be learned via a textbook and a science because of the growing body of knowledge that describes the leadership process, leadership skills and the application of those elements within a given practice area. Knowing about leadership theories allows us to analyse situations from a variety of perspectives, to understand the importance of leading an organisation to success and to suggest well-thought-out alternatives to enhance a quality practice. Studying leadership gives you skills that can be applied not only within the workplace but also in your everyday life. This book will lead you through a variety of situations as an individual and a member of a corporate body.

Summary of Key Points

This chapter has briefly looked at various aspects of leadership to meet the identified learning outcomes. These were:

- **Discuss the notions of leadership and followership** This was achieved by examining how you might already be a leader in some situations and a follower in others. Also, we looked at how a variety of writers have described leadership so that you can select the definition that comes closest to your own perception of the role. The use of the Johari Window will help you recognise your attributes and weaknesses, thereby making you a better leader.
- **Define leadership** By selecting and understanding the multifaceted nature of leadership the benefits of effective leadership were examined: as Daft (2017: 4) said, 'leadership is an emerging discipline that will evolve'. Don't expect to get it right every time but with knowledge of the leadership theory you might get it right some of the time.
- **Discuss the importance of the changing context related to health care** The National Health Service (NHS) emerged due to a socialist ideology of health being a right for all, regardless of ability to pay. Leadership within the health service has always been seen as important because of the size of the NHS and the changing policy and practices. Global leadership as a notion has also been explored.
- **Compare leadership and management** This perennial argument related to the differences (or not) between leaders and managers. Much of the problem in understanding the concepts relates to the fact that the two philosophies are so closely linked, and the words used are interchangeable, hence the possible lack of differentiation when we think and speak of leaders.
- **Debate the art and science of leadership** Stewart (1918) highlighted that the science, spirit and skill of health practice were beginning to develop as it became apparent that love and caring alone could not ensure health or overcome disease.

ONLINE RESOURCES

For online resources, including SAGE journal articles, weblinks and videos, visit the book's website: https://study.sagepub.com/barr4e.

FURTHER READING

Cook, M.J. (2001) The attributes of effective clinical nurse leaders, *Nursing Standard*, *15* (35): 33–6.
Cook, M.J. and Leathard, H. (2004) Learning for clinical leadership, *Journal of Nursing Management*, *12* (6): 436–44.

2 WHAT MAKES A LEADER?

Chapter Contents

Learning Outcomes

By the end of this chapter you will have had the opportunity to:

- Discuss the notions of leadership and followership
- Define leadership
- Discuss the importance of the changing context related to health care
- Compare leadership and management
- Debate the art and science of leadership

INTRODUCTION

In Chapter 1, the concept of leadership was examined. It is now appropriate to scrutinise some of the experiences related to leaders we have met in clinical practice. Highlighting the ideology related to clinical leaders in health care will lead us into the characteristics of a leader. Discussion related to leaders met in practice will direct us to a consideration of the possible reasons for their actions. To investigate your own abilities, various tools are provided which you may use; this can assist in self-evaluation and personal reflection. The notion of practice mastery and the need for evidence-based practice will be addressed as the chapter concludes.

CLINICAL LEADERS IN HEALTH CARE

Globally, health care has the same complex issues whether it is in a developed, developing or underdeveloped country. In Britain, the NHS has been led by a succession of governments, with manifestos which addressed their vision for improving the health service. Private health care has either been led by a group of Board Trustees for large companies specialising in medicine and surgery, nursing homes or an ambulance service, or as a small personal business with a lone lead practitioner such as a physiotherapist, podiatrist or optician. 'General Practice' falls between an NHS service and a personal business led by the practice management team who may be general practitioners but not always.

Historically, health care was built on a system of vocational leaders such as doctors, nurses, midwives and ambulance technicians who used 'care and cure' methods to help people get better. Leadership has more recently been important because of the size of the NHS. A few years ago it was the largest European employer with 1.3 million employees (NHS Jobs, 2014) and hailed as the third largest world industry after the Red Army in China and the Indian Railway. However, it is now in fifth position (with 1.7 million employees) after McDonald's, Walmart/Asda and the Chinese military, with the US Department of Defense at the top (BBC, 2012).

The current economic climate requires public services to be managed more efficiently – especially around staffing and in light of the ongoing burden of pensions in the UK. The context of public service effectiveness, however, is paramount. Clinical leadership, as well as educational and research leadership, are required in the health service to respond to the demands of society for the future. Thompson and Hyrkas (2014) have gone further to promote the need for *global leadership* strategies for high-quality health services in terms of empowerment, competency development and excellent leadership including patient and workforce safety issues in the context of globalisation. Excellent leadership is often perceived in the skills and characteristics of those who lead teams.

CHARACTERISTICS OF A LEADER

Maxwell (1999) maintains that there are 21 indispensable qualities of a leader. These are listed in Table 2.1.

Activity

- Rank these qualities in the order you think most important.
- Justify why you believe in their importance.

Table 2.1   Indispensable qualities of a leader (Maxwell, 1999)

Character	Charisma	Commitment
Communication	Competence	Courage
Discernment	Focus	Generosity
Initiative	Listening	Passion
Positive Attitude	Problem Solving	Relationships
Responsibility	Security	Self-discipline
Servanthood	Teachability	Vision

Although the skills required are far reaching, they need a great deal of thought and discussion from a personal perspective. The following can be highlighted:

- **Character** The disposition, quality or calibre of ability a person has is important. For instance, the way an individual handles a clinical emergency will create either respect or distrust for future events. Maxwell (1999: 5) highlights a saying that states, 'If you think you are leading and no one is following you, then you're only taking a walk.'
- **Charisma** This is about making others feel good about themselves by trying to see the best in them rather than concentrating on their faults. Napoleon Bonaparte called leaders 'dealers in hope' (Maxwell, 1999: 11). Whenever you meet someone new, try to make a good impression by doing things like remembering their name. Do it every day and it will increase your charisma, as people will recognise that you care about their feelings.
- **Communication** This element is vital, as good leaders must be able to share their knowledge and ideas with others to achieve organisational goals. Getting people to work together requires effective communication, so without excellent communication you will travel alone. Be clear in your writing and speaking but also be aware of the need for active listening. Rudy Giuliani (2002) (the mayor of New York at the time of the 9/11 attacks) describes a successful leader as someone who can not only develop and communicate strong beliefs, accept responsibility and surround themself with strong people, but also study, read and learn independently. Sullivan and Garland (2013: 23) concur with this, noting that 'the leader is anyone who uses interpersonal skills to influence others to accomplish a specific goal'. It can be seen then that the

position a member of staff holds in the organisational structure is associated with a pattern of expected behaviour, and may be related to others' expectations of that role.

- **Passion** If, as Nightingale, Seacole and Millar demonstrated, you have a passion for your profession this is usually met with a positive response. The impossible might become possible. Passion is contagious; I recall hearing Beverly Malone, General Secretary of the Royal College of Nursing (2001–2006), speaking about the power to care in nursing at a theatre nurses' conference, and how much power nurses hold even if they think they don't. The passion for nursing she imparted was terrific; I became excited about my profession again (as did most of the audience).

- **Servanthood** Maxwell (1999: 133) asserts that you must love your people more than your position, thus being a servant leader. This is not a low skilled activity – it is about attitude. A true leader serves people by ensuring that their best interests are maintained. Maxwell (1999: 138) further states that effective servanthood will be attained if the leader can:

   o   **stop** lording it over people and **start** listening to them

   o   **stop** role-playing for advancement and **start** risking for others' benefit

   o   **stop** seeking your own way and **start** serving others.

It seems that today you cannot open a journal related to any industry without leadership, in some context, leaping out at you. This is because we are currently in a state of change, which is moving the business of organisations from the 'old style' management approach, emphasising stability and control, to a more rational approach which purports to encourage effective leadership that values change, empowerment and relationships. The King's Fund (2015: 18–20) explored the notion of the skills of an NHS 'systems leader' in the context of change, chaos and complexity as one who:

- does NOT try to take the credit
- demonstrates 'emotional intelligence'
- has the ability to walk in other people's shoes
- works hard to persuade people in different ways
- is able to be an effective whistleblower.

The management of change is another subject area to consider in understanding how effective leadership can be in enhancing the change process (see Chapter 14).

There is more recent debate comparing research from Mann (1959), Stogdill (1974) and Zaccaro et al. (2004) about which leadership characteristics are innate personality traits and which maybe also need to be taken into consideration *along* with situational aspects (Northouse, 2016: 21). The characteristics of a good leader also include the ability to use interpersonal skills to engender trust among the team members as they address and work through change. In an organisation without a clear mindset a leader will not have the ability to be effective; John F. Kennedy intimated that you cannot know you have arrived if you don't know where you are going, which indicates that planning, passion and vision are vital.

EXPERIENCES OF LEADERS IN CLINICAL PRACTICE

West et al. (2017: 3) explore the notion of leadership and innovation in the context of the concept of care and compassion. These ideas therefore relate to all clinicians in their everyday work. When we think about our own clinical experiences in the context of leaders, we may think about role models and people we wish to emulate. Qualitative research through in-depth personal interviews in Canada by Anonson et al. (2014), on perceptions of frontline staff regarding exemplary nurse leadership, found the key common characteristics were:

- a passion for nursing
- a sense of optimism
- the ability to form personal connections with their staff
- excellent role modelling and mentorship
- an ability to manage a crisis while guided by a set of moral principles.

On reflection, we remembered three people in our own professional experience that were all quite different:

1. **Charge Nurse A** 'ran' the medical ward and linked to a CCU. It was my first nursing experience and I had nothing else to compare it with. He was a quiet but very efficient manager. I have to say I do not remember his presence very much, but there was a very happy team spirit, with each part of the hierarchy supporting and teaching others. There was a sense of belonging because individuals were able to contribute their ideas of how tasks might be completed; also, they were able to suggest how things might be 'done better'. From memory, the care on the ward was excellent and he set and monitored the standards. In those days it was task-driven duties. There were constant emergencies, but the team felt a sense of achievement at the end of the long shifts.
2. **Sister B** ran a surgical ward. Again, the mode of working was that of task allocation, but the ward was run with precision, in a military style. Everyone knew their allocated job, what was expected of them and the time frame in which they had to function. I recall being quite scared by Sister and would never dream of speaking to her unless she spoke to me first. Although this placement was very intimidating at times, it was happy and the patients all felt that they were getting the best care possible in a very efficient and effective way; and the staff felt that they had done a 'good' job when they completed their shifts, however difficult they might have been.

3. **Sister C** by comparison was quite disorganised; nobody knew what was going
    on or what they were supposed to be doing, and often there were panic situa-
    tions where something had to be done all of a rush. Sister used to shout a lot
    when things were not done, but unless we were at 'panic stage' didn't tell us
    what we were supposed to be doing. Many people work in a frenzied panicky
    way because that is how their mind works, but in a leadership situation it is
    imperative that all members of the team know what is going on, and so it is vital
    that there is a degree of organisation.

Each of these leaders, in their own way, demonstrated their own style. Two were far
more effective than the third but each presented communication skills at differing
levels. Indeed, Starns (2000) highlights the militarisation policy adopted in early
British nursing history. Dame Katherine Jones, the first Matron-in-Chief, wanted to
link the registered nurse with the military 'officer classes'; she felt that the registered
nurse status would be further secured by imposing the Army framework and style
on civilian nursing. This might reflect the actions and leadership style of Sister B.

Lewin et al. (1939) originally identified three main leadership styles:

*   Laissez-faire: little direction or facilitation approach (Sullivan and Garland,
    2010: 16; Northouse, 2016: 67)
*   Autocratic: directive and controlling (Tappen et al., 2004: 7; Gopee and
    Galloway, 2017: 43)
*   Democratic: participative and encouraging collaborative teamwork (Gopee and
    Galloway, 2017: 43).

The Leadership Foundation for Higher Education (2017) also identify strengths and
weaknesses in various leadership styles (www.lfhe.ac.uk/en/general/lf10/ten-times-
tables/10-leadership-styles.cfm).

Activity

What style of leadership do you think Charge Nurse A and Sister C used?

Charge Nurse A appeared to be rather participative or democratic, while Sister C
used a laissez-faire style.

Lewin's categories have been used extensively since 1939. Wider categorisation of
leadership styles is diverse and may include:

*   Coercive: using many sanctions and few rewards; gives directives rather than
    directions; useful for simple, straightforward tasks
*   Authoritative: has clear vision and provides long-term direction; is prepared to
    justify and take responsibility for the direction; useful where there is a clear aim
    and people are buying into it

- Affiliative: aims to avoid conflict and develop harmony; avoids confrontation; useful for getting to know people and how things are done around the organisation
- Democratic: encourages participation and seeks consensus; aims to seek commitment through ownership; sometimes useful when the leader is not clear about the most appropriate direction
- Pacesetting: focuses on task accomplishment to an elevated level of excellence; tends to take the lead; useful in managing change
- Coaching: encourages the development of others; identifies strengths and weaknesses; useful for the long-term development of people and the organization (see Chapter 11) (National Professional Qualification for Headship (NPQH), 2005).

It is perceived that the most effective leadership style is that exhibited by democratic leaders. However, it should be remembered that one style will not be adopted for all occasions but that a mixture of styles will be required, depending on the situation.

LEADERSHIP AND FOLLOWERSHIP STYLES

Having noted that there are a variety of clinical leadership styles, it would be useful to analyse one's own ability not only as a leader but also as a follower. Daft (2017: 360–83) suggests that leaders who demonstrate an awareness of their rationality as well as their emotion-driven impulses learn to trust their instincts and realise that these feelings can provide useful information about difficult leadership decisions. So, to be successful, leaders must also look inwards to their hopes and dreams. Part of preparedness for leadership might be to test what sort of style you prefer as a leader by taking a Leadership and Followership Test of the type described by Frew (1977).

This test helps you understand how and why both you and your colleagues react within a situation. As a potential leader, this information can help you to develop and become more effective. This test and the Myers-Briggs® tool will be addressed and explored further in Chapter 5 to demonstrate the benefits of 'knowing' oneself and others.

ASSESSING YOUR ABILITIES/SKILLS

As well as using the Leadership and Followership Style Test set out on the Online Resources website there are other ways of identifying your own abilities. Northouse (2016: 44) notes the difference that *traits* are what you *are*, but *skills* are what you can or have achieved and reflect 'the ability to use one's knowledge and competencies to accomplish a set of goals or objectives'. The three-skill approach relates broadly to technical, human and conceptual skills (Katz, 1955: 34). Further developments of the skills approach are ongoing but newer models become more complex. The NMC (2018a) consulted and defined seven new platforms that an honours graduate of nursing will need to meet to be considered capable, safe and effective. At the point of registration, the new seven platforms are:

1. Being an accountable professional
2. Promoting health and preventing ill health
3. Assessing needs and planning care
4. Providing and evaluating care
5. Leading and managing nursing care and working in teams
6. Improving safety and quality of care
7. Coordinating care.

There are new proficiencies for registered Nursing Associates based on six platforms (NMC, 2018f).

1. Being an accountable professional
2. Promoting health and preventing ill health
3. Provide and monitor care
4. Working in teams
5. Improving safety and quality of care
6. Contributing to integrated care.

The Standards for of Comptence for Registered Midwives (NMC, 2009; 2014) is still current. All other health professions have standards from within the HCPC and the GMC to ensure best practice and safety within the professions always.

Activity (for student and registered nurses)

Outline how you might develop a checklist of the seven platforms for your professional portfolio.

A SWOT analysis is a technique attributed to Ansoff (1987) but originated from the work of Albert Humphrey in the 1960s. It has long been thought of as an admirable way of identifying both individual and organisational Strengths, Weaknesses, Opportunities and Threats (SWOT) (see Table 2.2). Tappen et al. (2004) indicate that, on an individual level, borrowing the SWOT tool from the corporate world can guide you through your own internal strengths and weaknesses, providing an analysis of external opportunities and threats that might help you in your job search or career planning. SWOT analysis is always a useful exercise to undertake and even keep within your professional portfolio. It can be used when applying for a new position or course as it clearly highlights your attributes and how they can be matched against the criteria for the position or course entry. It can also be a basis for the additional information requested when you have to indicate this to appraisers during your annual Development and Performance Review (DPR). Together with identifying internal individual strengths and weaknesses, an external situational analysis can identify how threats might be changed to opportunities in order to enhance individual and organisational performance.

On a wider institutional/organisational level this tool can also be used to focus on where weaknesses might be addressed to increase the efficiency and economy of an organisation. As we hear of some NHS Trusts getting into financial, staffing and environmental difficulties, the thought given to SWOT analysis may assist in changing practices in significant areas. Johnson and Garvin (2017) note the importance of SWOT assessment within health care business planning for advanced health care practitioners.

Table 2.2   SWOT analysis

Strengths	Weaknesses
Skills	Age
Qualifications	Gender
Life experiences	Skills; Experience
Professional experiences	Time keeping
Punctual	Planning/organisation
Hardworking	Narrow/broad focus
'Fit' with the job description	
Opportunities	**Threats**
To be able to rectify:	'Fit' with the job description
Insufficient appropriate skills	Training
Insufficient appropriate experience	Career development
Insufficient appropriate knowledge	New courses
	New experience

PROBLEM-SOLVING STYLES: THE MYERS-BRIGGS TYPE INDICATOR® (MBTI®)

Another point for consideration when leaders are being appointed relates to problem-solving styles. For many, the Myers-Briggs Type Indicator® (1995) is one tool for identifying ways in which individuals differ in gathering and evaluating information for problem solving and making decisions. (Myers-Briggs Type Indicator®, Myer-Briggs®, MBTI® and the MBTI logo® are all trademarks or registered trademarks of the Myer-Briggs Type Indicator Trust in the United States and other countries.)

Four dimensions are considered within the tool, each of which has two polar aspects (see Tables 2.3–2.6).

1. **Introvert (I) – Extrovert (E)** This dimension focuses on where people gain inter-personal strength and mental energy. Extroverts gain energy from being around and interacting with others, whereas introverts gain energy by focusing on personal thoughts and feelings.

Table 2.3 Extrovert/introvert dimensions

	Positive Impact	Negative Impact
Extrovert	Spreads energy, enthusiasm	Loudmouth does not include other people
Introvert	Thoughtful, gives space to others	Nothing worth saying? Uneasy networker

2. **Sensing (S) – Intuition (N)** This identifies how a person absorbs information. Those with a sensing preference gather and absorb information through the five senses, whereas intuitive people rely on less direct perceptions. Intuitivists, for example, focus more on patterns, relationships and hunches than on direct perception of facts and details.

Table 2.4 Sensing/intuition dimensions

	Positive Impact	Negative Impact
Sensing	Practical, concrete, detailed	Dull, unimaginative
Intuition	Creative, imaginative	Flighty, impractical, unrealistic

3. **Thinking (T) – Feeling (F)** This dimension relates to how much consideration a person gives to emotions in making a decision. Feeling types tend to rely more on their values and sense of what is right and wrong, and they consider how a specific decision will affect others' feelings. Thinking types tend to rely more on logic and are very objective in the decision-making process.

Table 2.5 Thinking/feeling dimensions

	Positive Impact	Negative Impact
Thinking	Logical, rational, intellectual	Cold and heartless
Feeling	Empathetic, understanding	Soft-headed, fuzzy thinker, bleeding heart

4. **Judging (J) – Perceiving (P)** This dimension concerns an individual's attitudes toward ambiguity and how quickly a person can decide. People with a judging preference like certainty and closure. They enjoy having goals and deadlines and tend to make decisions quickly based on available data. Perceiving people, conversely, enjoy ambiguity, dislike deadlines and may change their minds several times before making a final decision. Perceiving types like to gather a large amount of data information before making a decision.

Table 2.6 Judging/perceiving dimensions

	Positive Impact	Negative Impact
Judging	High work ethic, focused and reliable	Compulsive neat freak, uptight, rigid, rule bound
Perceiving	Work–life balance, enjoys work	Lazy, messy, aimless and unreliable

Clearly from these four dimensions 16 unique personality types can be identified. Owen (2009: 4) suggests that there is no 'leader type' but there are tentative suggestions that leaders are equally divided between extrovert and introvert types. Leaders – in the main – are intuitive, feeling and judging (i.e. ENFJ or INFJ).

Activity

1. Try the example personality test provided on the book's website to see what sort of personality you or your colleagues might exhibit.
2. You may want to compare the results with the Jung and Myers-Briggs typology test found on the internet site www.humanmetrics.com/cgi-win/jtypes2.asp.
3. Consider what these results tell you about how you are perceived.
4. Do you think your personality type is correct?

Lesley remembers completing a personality assessment and thinking how accurate the assessment was (she was ISTJ), even though she hadn't given the questions much thought. Within clinical practice she found that knowledge of her personality type gave her a greater insight into how she interacted with both patients and colleagues. It made her more aware of how other people worked so that when they were asked to complete a job they went about it in their own way and not necessarily the way she would have done. 'I was probably using my 'emotional intelligence' before it became a leadership construct' she said. Greater discussion related to EI (Goleman, 1995) takes place in Chapter 11.

More recently she undertook the Jung/Myers-Briggs test which provided an SJTI result. Jill on the other hand has an ENFJ Myers-Briggs (MBTI®) test result.

Interestingly, in terms of writing this book, one author sees themself as a linear thinker and the other thinks in circles, arrows and flamboyant diagrams; we see that each style is valued and feel we complement each other's strengths and weaknesses by being able to see and work from different creative perspectives. Effective teams need a variety of personality types; otherwise conflict, complacency and apathy might occur.

REFLECTIVE PRACTITIONER

Since the Francis (2013) Inquiry into failures in the NHS, professional registration for health and social care professionals have been reviewed in the context of professional regulation. Nurses are now required to undertake a peer-reviewed 'revalidation process' every three years for online registration (NMC, 2017a). Revalidation involves a prescriptive focus on the NMC Code (2018b) which focuses on four themes: prioritise people; practise effectively; preserve safety; and promote professionalism and trust. Revalidation also requires the following:

- Documentation of practice hours over three years (450 hours practice for every Nurse or Midwife)
- Evidence of continuing professional development of 35 days with 20 days in participatory learning
- Five written reflective accounts
- Five pieces of practice-related feedback (patients/service users, colleagues or management)
- A reflective discussion with another NMC registrant
- A health and character confirmation
- A professional indemnity declaration.

HCPC registrants need to register every two years (see HCPC, 2017b) and declare that:

- they have either continued to practise the profession since last registration, or not practised the profession since last registration but have met the HCPC's return to practice requirements
- they have continued to meet the HCPC's standards of proficiency for the safe and effective practice of individual profession including the HCPC's (2016) *Standards of Conduct, Performance and Ethics*
- since the last registration there has been no change relating to their good character (this includes any conviction or caution, if any, that they are required to disclose), or any change to health that may affect an ability to practise safely and effectively
- they continue to meet the HCPC's (2017a) *Standards of Continuing Professional Development*.

The GMC (2017) identifies that medical doctors require a licence to practise and usually must revalidate every five years, with a focus on appraisal across four domains set out in the updated standards of practice document *Good Medical Practice* (GMC, 2014):

- Knowledge, skills and performance
- Safety and quality
- Communication, partnership and teamwork
- Maintaining trust.

In all professions, there is an expectation of reflection on practice (GMC, 2013; NMC, 2017a; HCPC, 2017b, 2017c). To do this effectively reflective practice should encompass a systematic approach using a model of reflection.

There are many models of reflection identified within the literature; however, the one selected must be understandable, useable, effective and fit for the intended purpose. Schön (1987) differentiated between reflection-in-action and reflection-on-action; in later literature he also talks of reflection-before-action. Each of these indicates when reflection should take place, that is, before, in or on action. It is thought that reflection-before-action is likely when the practitioner has met a specific situation before and draws on memories and records to influence the way in which the current situation is handled. In-action, on the other hand, is normally limited as the need to act quickly in complex situations is paramount; by comparison on-action takes place once the incident has been dealt with and assists the practitioner to gain insights and make amendments as necessary.

The simplest of reflective cyclical models linked to experiential learning has been proposed by Driscoll (2007) based on ideas by Borton (1970) which identified three simple *questions that can be related to health care practice* (see Figure 2.1).

1. What?
2. So what?
3. Now what?

Activity

Can you use Driscoll's model and explore a recent and significant health care episode or event in which you were involved? Write notes on each of the 'boxed' stages.

Another reflective model often used in health care is one that is described by Gibbs (1988) (Figure 2.2) wherein a series of similar but possibly more academic questions are posed; Johns's (1995) model (Figure 2.3) builds on the questions posed by Gibbs but adds other dimensions, e.g. Influencing Factors and Learning.

Whatever model is used, by answering the questions in order one can work through an experience, learn by it and review it later. Reflection is an excellent

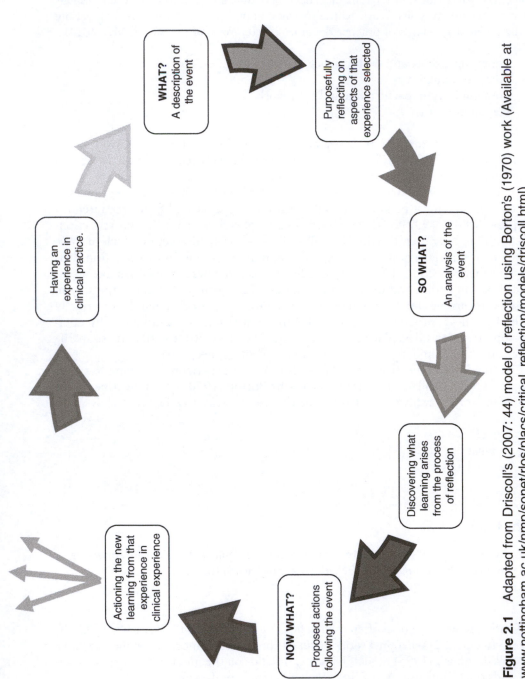

Figure 2.1 Adapted from Driscoll's (2007: 44) model of reflection using Borton's (1970) work (Available at www.nottingham.ac.uk/nmp/sonet/rlos/placs/critical_reflection/models/driscoll.html)

Source: Driscoll, J. (2007)

process by which to learn and this is most certainly the case for the newly emerging leader. To become effective, it is useful to analyse any situation critically, taking care to discover the parts that can be improved upon. Taylor (2010), when talking of the value of reflection, notes that there are three main kinds of reflection:

1. Technical (based on scientific method and rationale)
2. Practical (leads to the interpretation, description and explanation of human interaction)
3. Emancipatory (leads to transformative action).

These are categorised according to the kind of knowledge they involve, and the work interests they represent. Each type is important in developing the effective practitioner within the clinical area.

Activity

- Think about what reflection means to you.
- To what extent does your definition agree with that of the authors mentioned here or in other books you have read?
- Keep a record of your thoughts to refer to as you progress in your career.

I normally use a mixture of Gibbs's and Johns's models of reflection to consider the direction of my career, identifying what I want to change and what I am doing well. It is a way of moving forward. It does, however, feel a bit cumbersome at times, but once you are used to using a model of reflection – and reflecting on action – it goes a long way to improving practice.

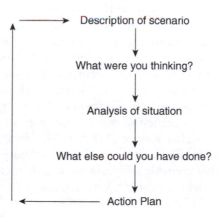

Figure 2.2 Feedback loop as a model of reflection

Source: adapted from Gibbs, G. (1988) *Learning by Doing: A Guide to Teaching and Learning Methods*. Further Education Unit: Oxford Polytechnic

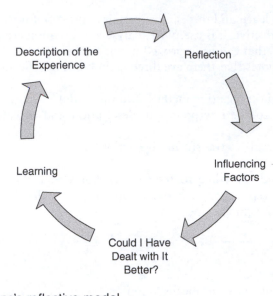

Figure 2.3   Johns's reflective model

Source: republished with permission of John Wiley and Sons

PRACTICE MASTERY: EVIDENCE–BASED PRACTICE

There is a need for evidence-based practice within nursing, midwifery and health-care generally (Pearson et al., 1997; Shorten and Wallace, 1997; Steffaleno and Carlson, 2010; NMC, 2018b: 6). This could be considered as saying that healthcare practice should be based on effective research rather than rituals, traditions and whims. It is this evidence-based movement that is testing the validity of long-standing procedures, seeking to replace them with newer, research-based ones.

Being able to master your own specific professional practice may come after many years in a clinical area. On occasion time can be lost when you put yourself in the hands of others to direct your professional development. Often when people look back, they realise that they could have reached career fulfilment much earlier, if they had relied on their own determination. 'Self-mastery' is about empowering *yourself* to reach your own goals and dreams. This is related to the seminal work of the Harvard professor of business and nurse researcher Kanter (1983, 1991, 1993), which is still held as important in our world of healthcare practice. Kanter's theory of structural power in organisations suggested that knowing and realising an individual's full potential, redis-covering new ways and insights towards taking actions, will enable personal goals to be achieved. Laschinger (2010) used the work of Kanter to link the empowerment of the health professional to the empowerment of the patient for better health outcomes. Bennis et al. (1994) identified that we all have a large amount of untapped potential which can be used within a work situation to achieve personal growth and mastery.

Self-mastery is about being driven by vision and also being able to act as a focaliser, facilitator and synergiser, as well as a co-creator, learner and shaper.

In terms of professional practice, mastery is about continuously focusing on trying to improve your own skills and knowledge. What do you want to learn today? What skills do you want to gain this week, this month, this year? What achievements have you planned for the next five years? Being a 'master' in your particular practice means there is no chance to stay still. Along with new skills, the ability to critically understand how these skills benefit patients and clients, and how they can be improved, is all part of searching and mastering the evidence base underpinning practice.

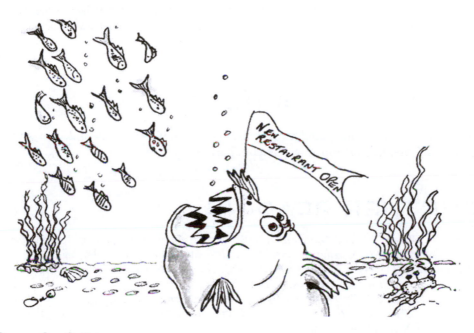

Source: Sue Saillet

The shark is advertising himself as a new restaurant but is he a restaurant or a diner? He may be able to achieve a goal of more food, but self-mastery within the smaller fish community could avert this danger.

Summary of Key Points

This chapter has briefly looked at various aspects of leadership in order to meet the identified learning outcomes. These were:

- **Recognise the importance of clinical leaders in health care** We all learn from observation of our role models.

(Continued)

(Continued)

- **Reflect on personal experiences of leaders in clinical practice** We will learn things that we will not wish to repeat in our practice setting, and at the same time there will be elements that we would wish to carry forward.
- **Develop self-awareness** This development of self-awareness through the use of tools such as SWOT analysis and the leadership–followership tools can only serve to enhance the care we offer as well as our career prospects.
- **Develop practice mastery through evidence-based practice** In all professions it is important to ensure that the care offered is current and based on reliable evidence. It is only in this way that we can develop mastery of our individual professions.

ONLINE RESOURCES

For online resources, including SAGE journal articles, weblinks and videos, visit the book's website: https://study.sagepub.com/barr4e.

FURTHER READING

Jasper, M., Rosser, M. and Mooney, G. (2013) *Professional Development, Reflection and Decision-Making in Nursing and Healthcare* (2nd edn). Chichester: Wiley-Blackwell.

Manion, J. (2011) *From Management to Leadership: Strategies for Transforming Health* (3rd edn). San Francisco, CA: Jossey-Bass.

Silberman, M. (2007) *The Handbook of Experiential Learning.* San Francisco, CA: Wiley.

Taylor, B. (2010) *Reflective Practice for Health Care Professionals: A Practical Guide* (3rd edn). Maidenhead: Open University Press.

3 CULTURE, DIVERSITY AND VALUES

Chapter Contents

Learning Outcomes

By the end of this chapter you will have had the opportunity to:

- Examine the concept of culture
- Discuss the importance of cultural diversity influencing health and healthcare
- Discuss leadership in the context of cultural diversity
- Examine the theoretical models of transcultural care
- Critically reflect on personal transcultural care and leading the culturally diverse

INTRODUCTION

To be an effective leader within the delivery of health care, it is vital that leaders recognise the importance of individuality, and how it relates to the delivery of health care to patients, clients and service users. Health care professionals (and their leaders) bring a richness of individuality into the relationships they have with their patients. Whether we are more reserved or extrovert than others can help us recognise how these traits can be used as leadership strengths. The value of individuality, however, cannot be isolated from the roles and responsibilities required within an organisation such as the health service. This chapter will attempt to relate the notion of cultural diversity and values to the present climate of public accountability for health care teams and the responsibilities for caring for patients.

CONCEPT OF CULTURE

Culture is an important aspect of diversity within the health service yet what do we mean by culture? Sardar and Van Loon (1997: 4–5) highlighted an early definition by the anthropologist Edward Burnett Tylor (1832–1917):

> Culture is that complex whole which includes knowledge, belief, art, morals, law, customs and other capabilities and habits acquired by man as a member of society. (Tylor, 1997 [1871]:1)

More recently, Salzman (2018: 13) explores a wide range of perspectives with respect to the meaning of the concept 'culture', and concludes with a generic version that it is a 'roadmap to living'. This may or may not be helpful as a reflection of the complexity of the term, and the Center for Disease Control in the USA offers a more workable definition:

> *Culture is the blended patterns of human behavior that include 'language, thoughts, communications, actions, customs, beliefs, values, and institutions of racial, ethnic, religious, or social groups'.* (www.cdc.gov/nchhstp/socialdeterminants/definitions.html)

Sometimes students will equate culture with religion or foreigners and forget the various levels of culture even within one ethnic or religious group. Healthcare professionals need to try and understand the importance of their own cultural heritage in the first instance. Helman (2007: 3) emphasises the context of culture and its importance in 'how people live their lives, their beliefs, behaviour, perceptions, emotions, language, religion, rituals, family structure, diet, dress, body image, concepts of space and time, and attitudes to illness, pain and other forms of misfortune'. These issues have implications not only for leaders of individuals in teams but also for all the patients that are part of their care. The relationship between the patient, the health practitioner and the care provided is underpinned by the complex notion of culture.

The richness of diversity across many cultural issues is thus related to the need for sensitive and individualised and patient-centred care. Mendes (2015: 459) signals that to provide truly compassionate person-centred care it is important to be aware of patients' cultural, religious beliefs and traditional customs, and more importantly their feelings when they are decision making regarding care and treatment, regardless of the professional's own personal feelings.

In a global world, health care leaders must be aware of the teams they lead and the importance of the diversity of the workforce. A leading leadership talent acquisition company, 'ThisWay Global' (2017), identified the seven biggest diversity issues in the workplace as being:

1. Acceptance and respect
2. Accommodation of beliefs
3. Ethnic and cultural differences
4. Gender equality
5. Physical and mental disabilities
6. Generation gaps
7. Language and communication.

The 'worldview' of different societal groups helps individuals in defining themselves to form values related to their lives and the world they live in. This gives a sense of the identity, belonging and self-worth required to be mutually supportive and survive in society (Kagawa-Singer and Chung, 1994; Leininger, 1997). Kelly-Heidenthal (2004) identified a model reflecting the ways people differ (Table 3.1).

Table 3.1 Characteristics of culture

- Culture is both learned and taught
- Culture is shared
- Culture is social in nature
- Culture is dynamic and adaptive

Culture and health are linked as a functional aspect in society and relate to the influence of the values, beliefs and practices of promoting one's own health and illness prevention. Culture thus gives a reason for the causation, detection and treatment/care of the ill and the well and determines social roles, expectations and relationships (Helman, 2007). Cultural behaviour can be recognised in our society through the various transparent dress codes, eating habits, music tastes or attendance at different social gatherings outside work, such as the theatre, the mosque, the tennis or golf club, nightclub or even the hen/stag weekend. On the one hand, some of these exhibited behaviours can give an individual a sense of belonging; on the other hand, they may be a superficial cultural identity that could lead to discrimination from outside groups.

Activity

- Identify and jot down issues that are unfair and hence discriminatory in these two case studies.
- Provide an alternative response that would help to promote anti-discriminatory practice in care delivery.
- You may wish to use these questions for discussion with colleagues.

Case Study: Paul

Paul is a 30-year-old man who is HIV positive. He lives with his partner at 23 Lee Street. Paul is dying from an AIDS-related illness. A community nurse has been asked to visit to provide support. Upon arrival at the flat, the nurse discovers Paul's partner is dressed up as a female, with lipstick and make-up. A group of gay friends are there, wearing gay pride T-shirts, chanting songs, making speeches and playing music.

The nurse orders them to be quiet while she carries out an assessment. She becomes cross when they don't stop and asks them to have some respect for Paul while she tries to talk to him. Eventually she can proceed and finish her paperwork.

On her return to the health centre, she comments to her colleagues on what she describes as 'the nonsense' going on at 23 Lee Street, stating that 'these people have such weird behaviour'.

Case Study: Mrs Polaski

Mrs Polaski is a 77-year-old lady who lives in her own three-bedroom, semi-detached house. All her relatives live outside the area and she can only see them when they come to visit on special occasions. Mrs Polaski's neighbour regularly visits to 'keep an eye' on her, doing her shopping and collecting her pension and helping her out generally.

Following a recent fall, she was admitted to hospital. In planning for her discharge, the assessment team advised Mrs Polaski that she should really decide to move into a residential home, where she would be safer. The patient responded by saying that she intended to stay at home as her neighbour was happy to look in and help her out. The nurse advised Mrs Polaski that it was unfair to expect a neighbour to take on all that responsibility. Mrs Polaski then refused to discuss it further, but the assessment team recorded that they recommended the patient needed residential care.

DISCUSSION

You may have thought that in both cases scant regard was given to either Paul's or Mrs Polaski's right to live in the way they wished. Both people were regarded as different. While the nurse visiting Paul may have been quite correct in asking for – not ordering – some quiet, it was wrong of her to pass comments about 'the nonsense' when she got back to the health centre. Of course, one could say that it is human nature to discuss the 'unusual' with one's colleagues. It is important to recognise, though, that the way Paul's friends dress is irrelevant to the care offered. Similarly, while Mrs Polaski was made aware of the potential problems of her staying at home, and this could be documented, her personal views on her choices should also be aired, discussed and documented. It is easy to think that cultures are made up of people who are all the same and that they never change characteristics. However, it is important to see the diversity of deeper values even between people who have a common identity. The values and beliefs held by student nurses, the local Muslim community, members of an Elton John fan club, or members of a city football club may be quite different.

Whatever your views on the current Brexit situation have you stopped to listen to the various viewpoints as to the way forward and the potential implications of new legislation? These are very emotive issues and can highlight not only people's values but also their difficulties with other groups in society. Generational, class and gender differences will underpin the diversity of values. Religious and ethnic group beliefs and values will all change over time. For instance, ideas concerning international issues, such as the ideologies in some of the global war zones or various new reproductive technologies such as gene therapy, can vary considerably even in one cultural section of society. It is therefore useful to engage actively in looking for similarities between diverse cultures to combat the lack of understanding of others' beliefs and values.

DIVERSITY OF VALUES IN HEALTH CARE

It was during the late 1980s that diversity research began to appear and influence management literature. Normally health care is delivered by a team of people engaged in a variety of professions. The make-up and ability of these teams to function well together depends on a good working relationship. It poses the question of how similar and how different the team members should be. It could be argued that where there are more similarities than differences the team may function effectively but not be proactive; however, the wider diversity perspectives may in time offer a broader knowledge base, potentially leading to greater innovation. Borrill et al. (2000) found that the greater the number of professional groups represented in the team, the higher the level of innovation in patient care. Jackson (1996) describes two differing diversities as being either task related (organisational position or specialised technical knowledge) or relations oriented (age, gender, social status and personality), whilst Mathieu et al. (2008) elaborate and offer three definitions of diversity as being functional, personality and demographic diversity.

Recognising diversity creates a tolerance for the richness of values in our society, but on the negative side can lead to the development of stereotypical ideas of people who don't belong to our specific subgroup. It is important to recognise the main cultural groups, where adverse reactions occur in relationships at work and particularly in the health service. The main cultural groups affected as suggested by social research are: ethnicity, religion, age and gender.

ETHNIC DIVERSITY

Ethnic diversity allows people to get to know one another and share cultural aspects, and enhances tolerance between groups. It can reduce the chances of developing prejudice, racism and phobias. Ethnicity has been defined in many ways, but is often equated with race or colour and is even confused with religion on a day-to-day basis. *Race* refers to the grouping of people based on biological similarities, such as genetic features (including skin colour), whereas *ethnicity* is seen as a generic term for how a group perceives its own identity (Kelly-Heidenthal, 2004). *Ethnocentrism* is the term for a belief that one's own culture is better than that of other groups, without considering the values of other groups, and is thus discriminatory. These issues raise concerns in our society as to how we can move cultural integration forward.

Multiculturalism may be related to the diversity in a society, but not in the 'melting pot' approach where minority groups take on the dominant culture but can still maintain their distinctive collective identities and practices (Song, 2017). In the UK there are areas where it is difficult to define what is meant by minority groups, with almost equal proportions of indigenous to ethnic minority populations. This could be perceived to lead to a harmonious culture with tolerance of differences and the continuing integration of the diverse cultures. However, it has been argued that culture is not represented just by ethnicity and other groups may be marginalised even within the same ethnic group such as women, disabled or gay people. These issues obviously then pose challenges for politicians and policy makers as well as health service staff when addressing such inequalities.

Some people describe a feeling of 'twoness' where they live in two worlds: one life at home and the other at work, in education or outside the home. They sometimes find themselves striving to adopt cultural behaviours and attitudes that will help them be successful in a multicultural country, while at the same time maintaining ties to their racial and ethnic community and culture. This leads to the development of sociocultural skills and attitudes as they integrate both the dominant culture and their own (Daft, 2017: 27).

The fish in the cartoon believe that they are different to each other, but they are still fish and so fundamentally the same animal. Similarly, we are all unique but fundamentally all human.

The Race Relations Act 1965 has now been subsumed into the Equality Act 2010, and this has implications of culture awareness for leadership in the health

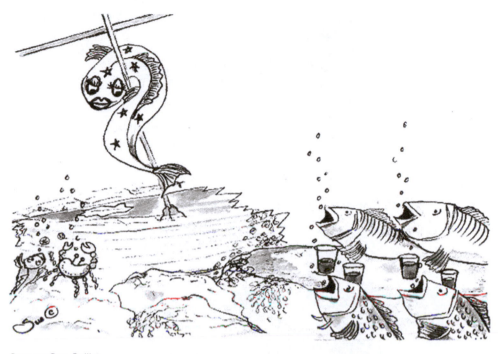

Source: Sue Saillet

service to avoid institutionalised racism. The glass ceiling is the invisible barrier, in ethnocentric organisations, that separates minority groups – such as black ethnic minorities (BME), women, older staff and people with disabilities – from progressing in their career; if members of such groups do achieve better positions their pay now needs to now reflect equality of value.

In 2016 the Annual Population Survey (NHS Employers, 2018) showed that 17% of all the medical and dental NHS workforce are from a non-white background. This continues to highlight the need for further investigation because of the steep reduction of non-white registrars becoming consultants. It also indicates that the medical route (and indeed the nursing route) does offer some opportunities for BME staff to obtain clinical director and subsequently board-level positions as medical and nursing directors. The report provides further data reflecting the underrepresentation of BME staff in NHS middle management (16%) but also indicates a glass ceiling between middle and senior NHS management. The total percentage of staff ratio differs little from the lower bands. One is led to question why, when so many of the students following nurse training today are from an ethnic minority group, many do not appear to be currently working within the NHS post qualification.

See Figures 3.1–3.3 to elucidate the above data.

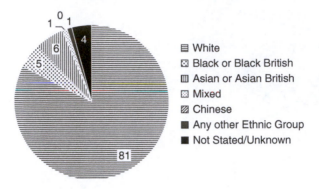

Figure 3.1   % All Medical and Dental Staff in NHS 2016

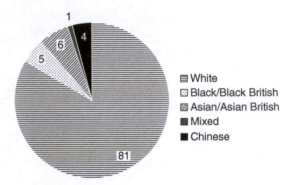

Figure 3.2   % Breakdown Nursing Bands 1–4

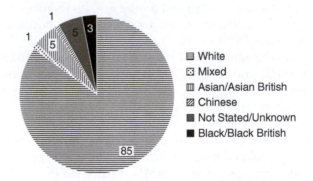

Figure 3.3   % Nursing Band 8a–9

RELIGIOUS DIVERSITY

Caring for patients with diverse religious beliefs is often paid 'lip service', and even though some awareness regarding sprituality needs is accepted, there is a general lack of understanding of a variety of traditions that belong to certain 'faith beliefs'. How any one patient or family member understands their own spirituality or religion in the context of health care may be very variable: a patient may note they are 'Church of England' but was last in a church on their christening; a Jewish, Catholic or Muslim patient may be much stricter about their traditions than another patient from the same religion; a health care professional may share the same religion as a patient, but this does not mean that they share the exact same beliefs (Griffith, 2009).

Mendes (2015) explores how religion may impact on health care choices where a patient of a Sikh faith may refuse to have their hair cut for positioning electrodes for an electrocardiogram because uncut hair is an important religious symbol in Sikhism. Another example may be a Muslim patient receiving end of life care who may request to lie facing Mecca. There are often ethical debates about Jehovah's Witnesses refusing blood transfusions and Griffith (2014) noted how this may be very difficult for health professionals when death may be the consequence. The important aspect for care is to respect patient autonomy and self-determination and that the wishes, beliefs and values of each patient should be determined.

It is also worth noting that the religious diversity of staff may also impact on health care delivery and should be respected within the contract of employment and as part of the 'Equal Opportunities' legislation.

Activity

Check out the following web pages and jot down one item of new knowledge for you regarding Buddhism, Catholicism, Hinduism, Jehovah's Witnesses, Judaism and Islam that can affect your care delivery.

* www.uphs.upenn.edu/pastoral/resed/diversity_points.html
* https://nursing.ubc.ca/sites/nursing.ubc.ca/files/documents/ReligiousAspects ofNursingCareEEdition.pdf

---

I found these sites very interesting; despite being in health care for many years, I always feel I can still learn and be challenged in knowledge to serve a multicultural society. One new issue for me has been that certain medications using animals may be problematic for some Buddhists who may be strictly vegetarian. MRI scans can be very adversely affected by metal objects such as a rosary which some patients who are Catholic may wish to keep near them. Hindu patients requiring intravenous therapy may well be challenged as the right hand is kept for clean tasks such as eating while the left hand is kept for unclean tasks such as toileting. Organ donation and transplantation are allowed and within the beliefs of Jehovah's Witnesses. Patients who are Jewish have relatively quick burials and there may be a request for amputated limbs to be available for burial. Muslim patients may typically prefer 'running water' and thus a shower may be preferred for hygiene needs. They also tend to refuse analgesia as pain may be 'spiritually enriching'. Did anything else surprise you? Maybe you do not know when Ramadan occurs and need to become aware in oder to adapt care for your patients who are Muslim. These dates change yearly.

AGE DIVERSITY

The characteristics between different age groupings have been under research for many years and in particular for business marketing sectors. Marquis and Huston (2017: 450) argued that different generations exhibit different value systems from each other which influence health care (see also Martin, 2003; McNeese-Smith and Crook, 2003) (Table 3.2). There is a view that the older generations of health workers are very respectful of authority, supportive of hierarchy and disciplined (the Silent Generation; Veteran/War Generation; Traditionalists). A younger generation (Baby Boomers) have similar traditional work values and ethics but are more materialistic and willing to work long hours ('live to work'). They have been taught to think more as creative individuals and fit well with independent and flexible roles. Generation X, in contrast, define success differently. They tend to lack an interest in one lifetime career in one place, and value flexible contracts and 12-hour shifts, which give them more scope for other activities during the rest of the week ('work to live'). Generation Y is seen as the first group that is globally aware, seeking roles that will push their limits. They are self-confident, optimistic, team dependent, techno-savvy and socially conscious (Nexters or Internet Gen). Generation Z is seen to be more tolerant than Generation Y of racial, sexual and generational diversity, and less likely to subscribe to traditional gender roles. McCrindle (2018) identified Generation Alpha, noting that even as children they are the most materially endowed and technologically literate generation.

Table 3.2   Different generation value systems (Carter, 2016; McCrindle, 2018)

Year of Birth	Generation
Before 1945	Silent Generation/Veteran Generation/Traditionalists
1946–1964	Baby Boomers
1965–1976	Generation X; Gen X
1977–1995	Generation Y, Millennials
1996–2010	Generation Z/iGen/Centennials
2010–2025	Generation Alpha (still children but brought up on ipads and tablets)

You may observe from your clinical practice that all these generations, apart from Alpha, can work effectively together if they respect where others are coming from and what their individual expectations of team working are. Of course, there may be conflict at times, but this is all part of team working. Stanley (2010) conducted a literature review of the four generational categories in the nursing workforce and highlighted the differing needs and attitudes that these groups bring to the workforce. This resulted in implications for recruiting and retaining staff from these different generations, particularly in the context of nursing shortages. The research also highlighted the emergence of Generation Z which appears to have some key features, i.e. their lifestyle integrates easily with media technology and digital communication, and they were born into the postmodern and globalisation era.

GENDER DIVERSITY

It has been identified that 77% of NHS staff are women and 23% are men; however, of all the NHS staff only 5% of female staff are doctors or dentists and 22% of male staff are doctors or dentists (Table 3.3) (NHS Employers, 2018).

Table 3.3   Gender balance in the NHS (NHS Employers, 2018)

	Doctors or Dentists	Other Occupations in the NHS
Men (23% NHS total)	22% of the total 23%	78% of total for men
Women (77% NHS total)	5% of the total 77%	95% of total for women

From the visualisations below, you can see how the split in the NHS workforce of 23% men and 54% women maps onto the percentage of the NHS workforce that are senior managers (see Figure 3.4).

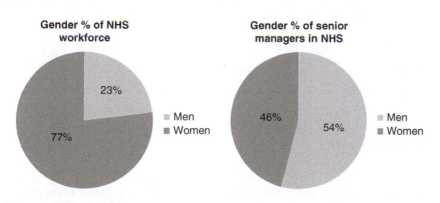

Figure 3.4   Gender split in the NHS workforce

There are thus proportionally fewer women in senior management posts (46%) despite the larger female workforce percentage.

The King's Fund (2013) questioned whether men and women lead differently and reported on a survey which commonly highlighted that women were seen to have a more collaborative, inclusive and empathetic and/or understanding style than men, and noted these aligned with the open and honest culture advocated in the 2013 Francis Report. However, under-representation at a senior level was reported to be partially due to barriers such as challenging masculine cultures and boys' networks, juggling childcare roles, and issues of confidence exacerbated by ethnicity and age factors.

In line with this, Espenshade and Radford (2009) found that although women are more likely to do better overall educationally, men are more likely to gain the highest degrees. They noted that women's confidence in their own academic abilities erodes faster than men's over their time at university, and that they are more hesitant about speaking up in class. The language of men and women also differs, and the notion that women have less self-belief than men may help to explain why men are more likely to take the lead. Grohar-Murray et al. (2010) concur that men and women communicate differently in groups. Women tend to be more passive in groups, and as new leaders or managers are more hesitant in speaking to groups. Ford's (2006) research using an in-depth narrative approach found four themes emerging which reflected a continued masculine model of leadership through the need for:

- macho-management
- post-heroic leadership
- influences from outside
- career paths.

NHS managerial culture may thus still be controlled by a transactional leadership style (Markham, 2005). The emerging need for talent management in the context of coaching (see Chapter 11) and mentoring is now developing within the scope of leadership courses to influence and address gender inequities.

Activity

- How do you feel when having to speak to small groups of peers?
- How do you feel when having to speak to large groups of peers?
- How do you feel when having to speak in groups of people you do not know very well?

I was quite worried about having to talk to group peers because I had always felt that I had nothing of interest to say; they would all know far more than I did about any given subject. Once I got over my initial lack of confidence and found I could contribute to discussions, raise issues and make a reasonable attempt at getting my point of view or experiences over to others, I felt more at ease with this activity. Like all things, it's difficult getting over that initial barrier. It is, however, much easier to speak to a group of people you do not know as you have fewer preconceived ideas of their expectations of you, or your view of them.

Although men and women work alongside each other in the NHS, they are socialised quite differently (Grohar-Murray and DiCroce, 2002). It has been suggested that:

> Women tend to use communication in a personal manner to maintain or establish relationships, share ideas and learn about others and go about it in a quieter and more tentative manner whereas men, on the other hand, tend to use communication in an instrumental way to reach their goals. They also appear to be rather more direct and forceful. (Wood, 2012)

Recognition of these differences in leadership matters because communication styles are an essential element of getting messages through to people, as well as of understanding the needs of people in a team. Chapter 7 will further develop the notion of diversity of communication styles. Managing and leading health care teams involves an underpinning philosophy of the importance of individuals and developing teams who can manage diversity in their everyday work. It is useful to ask teams to develop their awareness of some of the models of transcultural care, and to try and work towards a fully integrated transcultural operational delivery in the health service.

Newly recruited staff may have challenges as they start to be integrated into their professional role. Some might identify with their own traditional culture initially and find difficulty in absorbing the professional expectations, e.g. some staff may be expected to deliver intimate care to the opposite sex giving rise to dissonance and anxiety. Cultural lag may be an issue for leadership; this is the notion related to a changing cultural context driven by technology which may give rise to social problems and team conflict as staff work to keep up with the speed of technological and cultural changes, e.g. the emergence of fertility treatments, organ donation, and potentially some legislation related to end of life care.

ABILITY DIVERSITY

Since 2010 the the Disability Discrimination Act (DDA) 1995, extended in 2005, has been replaced by the Equality Act 2010 which continues to protect the interests of disabled people and makes it unlawful to discriminate against people of differing abilities.

Increasingly, in the delivery of health care, we are meeting with individuals who have unseen disabilities, e.g. dyslexia, dyspraxia, dyscalculia, asthma, deafness … Reasonable adjustments must be made to enable these people to function in the workplace and within their chosen profession. I remember a student who was quite severely dyslexic: he had a laptop that had a programme suited to his needs and he used this, both as a student and a qualified nurse, to record patient assessments; clearly these were all downloaded on completion of his shift to maintain confidentiality.

Prior to 1999 it was impossible for a person with hearing loss to train to become a registered nurse, but following the equality acts these students were accepted into training and were offered help, e.g. interpreters for British Sign Language, note takers in lectures and electronic stethoscopes to listen for manual blood pressure recording, to enable them to study effectively (University of Salford, 2009). NHS eemployers must also make effective working adjustments to ensure the safety of the employee and of course their patients. One nurse talks of being involved with a cardiac arrest procedure (Weaver, 2013):

I offered to do CPR and asked one of the anaesthetists if he could lift his hand each time I had to stop and start, which he did, therefore allowing me to fully participate in a life-saving event.

She needed the hand signal because, for Ms Manning, fast-paced moments like these are silent ones. Profoundly deaf, she relies on observation and training to keep up with the unpredictable nature of her profession. This worked well, and the patient survived; it just takes teamwork and an understanding of each other's needs (emotional intelligence plays a part here) to make the whole experience work.

MODELS OF TRANSCULTURAL CARE

Leininger (1997) offers a model underpinned by the notion that one's cultural background affects the reactions generated by any given situation. The value of a culturally diverse workforce is that patients and clients perceive that health service delivery involves a transculturally sensitive openness. First, the importance of *care as a concept*, within all cultures, should be recognised. However, what is defined as *caring* can be different in diverse cultures. Second, each culture identifies what it considers to be adequate and necessary care. Transcultural care requires an acute awareness of each culture's:

- lifestyle patterns
- values
- beliefs and norms
- symbols and rituals
- verbal and non-verbal communication
- caring behaviours
- shared meanings
- rituals of health, wellness and illness.

Andrews (2017) noted the importance of culturally congruent care in the context of terrorist attacks. This fits with the concept of 'transcultural care'. She defined culturally congruent care as a focus on what unites us as human beings when cultures are in conflict, and concurred with Leininger and McFarland (2006) who recognised that care is central to nursing, and caring is essential for health, well-being, healing, growth, survival, and for facing illness or death.

For example, a few weeks ago when I was looking after an older Asian man with prostate cancer. His son and daughter-in-law asked whether there was any possibility of him being moved to a single room. They were concerned about their mother, who was sleeping in a chair by their father's bed, with limited privacy in the three-bedded men's ward. Some of the staff felt the request was unreasonable and wondered why the mother did not go home to bed as the father 'had been admitted for symptom control not for terminal care'.

Activity

Jot down what you think about the issues of this ethical dilemma.

It is difficult getting single rooms for all families. However, the caring behaviours within this family needed to be understood. The gentleman expected his wife to look after him and be with him at night, even while he was in a hospice. They had been married for thirty-four years. Their caring, sharing, togetherness and closeness behaviours were ingrained within this family unit. Neither spoke good English and both preferred that their children bring them a familiar diet from home. This left them feeling isolated from most of the other families. The mother found sleeping difficult with other men in the room. The outcome was that a single room was eventually found for them until an early discharge plan was organised.

Giger and Davidhizar's (2004) transcultural care model consists of five central concepts underpinning care:

- Transcultural nursing and provision of culturally diverse nursing care
- Culturally competent care
- Cultural uniqueness of individuals
- Culturally sensitive environments
- Culturally specific illness and wellness behaviours.

When undertaking a culturally competent assessment of patients, professionals should recognise the following attributes of every cultural group:

- Communication
- Personal space/touch and closeness
- Social organisation
- Time
- Environmental control
- Biological variations.

Bennett's (1986) model highlighted a staged development of diversity awareness leading to more competent care in health care practice. It must be recognised that new health care students will maybe develop similarly. These stages are:

- Denial (incompetent)
- Defence
- Minimising differences
- Acceptance
- Adaption
- Integration (competent).

Diversity of values and beliefs is to be welcomed in health care teams, but how does this fit with what the public expect from health care staff as a whole? Patients and clients expect some consistency of action and advice from health care professionals. Excellent patient communication skills are essential. There is now a plethora of academic, professional standards and benchmarks associated with each professional health care group. These professional qualifications, codes of conduct and policy drivers invariably influence and shape specific roles in health care.

LEADING A CULTURALLY DIVERSE TEAM

A health care team featuring cultural diversity in terms of ethnicity, religion, age, ability and sexual orientation will be one that reflects the breadth of patient diversity, resulting in a beneficial, culturally mirrored partnership of staff and patients. To work effectively as a team, leaders could reflect on the following recommendations:

- When problem solving, be sure to examine the diversity of the workgroup so you can gather diverse perspectives for the solutions to be more widely accepted.
- Understand how team members respond to conflict and their expectations
- Work towards understanding the benefits of diversity and appreciate all contributions.
- Avoid assumptions that cultural groups act and respond in the same way.
- Avoid labelling.
- Value everyone's differences and recognise similarities; seek out different experiences from the majority.
- Pay close attention to both verbal and non-verbal communication for cultural cues.

- Ask for clarification to avoid assumptions.
- Assist those in minority groups to be successful; include them in informal networking within the team culture.

The challenge for the NHS is the concerning shortfall of doctors and nurses, affected by recent immigration policies, and NHS England has the strategic responsibility for managing this (National Audit Office, 2016; NHS Improvement (2016). Recruitment and retention are therefore linked to a need for a healthy and diverse workforce. The Nuffield Trust (2018) noted that the NHS in England does not have enough staff, with more nurses and midwives leaving than entering the workforce. This is compounded by this workforce group having an ageing demography. Even though the medical workforce has grown, and the number of hospital consultants has increased, there are several specialities where there are staffing difficulties such as paediatrics, psychiatry and general practice. It is also noted that there is also around a 10% paramedic vacancy rate and the Nuffield Trust (2018) has reported that the workforce and financial issues are at a critical stage; with social care understaffing and Brexit looming, there will be challenges for recruiting from the European Union.

Based on this, managers and leaders will need to consider recruitment and retention very carefully for the future. Chugh and Brief (2008: 318–24) suggest that by ensuring recruitment policy promotes diversity and remains unbiased, companies that practise diversity and inclusion in the workplace outperform other non-diverse companies by 15%. These factors are important for individual and human development. Leaders and teams therefore need always to be aware of the diversity of values in working relationships and should seek to be sensitive and responsive to that diversity (Marquis and Huston, 2017: 427–9). Morgan and Vardy (2009: 472) questioned why minority groups encounter more difficulty in securing employment even though they may share the same competencies as majority groups, and noted the sociolinguistic differences between employers and minority job candidates. Health care leaders will need to explore creative and sustainable approaches to attracting, recruiting and retaining a culturally diverse workforce for the quality services of health care in the future.

Recognising the structure of the workplace and the strengths of the team is vital, as not only does this improve the corporate image and attract ethical investors, it is also a much better use of human resources. This notion of equity comes, as does much of the management and leadership theory, from North America where there is a vast amount of published material related to diversity and equality. The values, beliefs and material objects surrounding each person are said to constitute their culture, so when any young person comes to train for work in the health service that move may engender a culture shock as they must become accustomed to a new set of 'norms' – this is known as 'cultural entry gate'. As the new student becomes experienced they will pass their experiences on to the next generation – known as 'cultural transmission'.

Summary of Key Points

This chapter has examined the issues related to diversity, values and professional care in order to meet the identified learning outcomes. These were:

- **Examine the breadth of the concept of culture** This was examined in relation to the uniqueness of individuals and the norms, values and beliefs of various cultures.
- **Discuss the importance of cultural diversity, influencing health and health care** This was also explored within the context of the health service.
- **Discuss leadership in the context of cultural diversity** Leading culturally diverse teams was examined in the context of diversity and recommendations were made.
- **Examine the theoretical models of transcultural care** These were discussed in order to manage anti-discriminatory and anti-oppressive behaviour in the health service.
- **Critically reflect on personal transcultural care** This was examined and related to leading a culturally diverse team.

ONLINE RESOURCES

For online resources, including SAGE journal articles, weblinks and videos, visit the book's website: https://study.sagepub.com/barr4e.

FURTHER READING

Harvey, C. and Allard, M.J. (2011) *Understanding and Managing Diversity* (5th edn). Harlow: Prentice Hall.

4 THEORIES OF LEADERSHIP

Chapter Contents

Learning Outcomes

By the end of this chapter you will have had the opportunity to:

- Identify the evolution of leadership theories
- Compare and contrast the various leadership theories
- Critically discuss the application of these theories in relation to healthcare

INTRODUCTION

This chapter highlights the evolution of some of the work of the main leadership writers and the context in which their ideas surfaced. Despite the discipline of leadership being comparatively young and relatively unchallenged, the main theories noted here still have influence and hold ground today within health care. Attempts will be made to link the theories to the practice setting. It must be recognised that the most effective leaders adjust their style and approach to the prevailing situation. This means that the suggestions made here are just that, suggestions, and not a recipe for immediate success.

EVOLVING THEORIES OF LEADERSHIP

The concept of leadership can mean different things to different people depending on their various perspectives. Old theories still have relevance!! There has been a range of ways identified to classify leadership theories (Rafferty, 1993; Mullins, 2016; Daft, 2015, 2017; Northouse, 2016) but it may be useful to look at leadership in the following forms:

- As a collection of personal characteristics or traits
- As a function within an organisation
- As an effect on group behaviour
- As an influence on forming an organisational culture.

Most of the ideas contained in the above theories can be seen as evolutionary. The emerging research data are seen to contribute to the greater knowledge base in the area of leadership. It could be argued that some of the ideas are not always based on good quality evidence – particularly the older research where we would now consider the research biases to be transparent. Hewison and Stanton (2003) examined the development of management theory in order to compare it to emerging nursing theory and identify the implications for health care. They concluded that health care management was based on the 'fads and fashions' of the prevailing theory at the time and questioned whether many ideas were scientifically valid. The complex development of management/leadership theories has been influenced by the prevailing psychological or sociological theories of the day. More specifically, the school of behaviourism within the psychology discipline and the school of functionalism within the discipline of social science underpin some of the leadership theories. Therefore, most of these ideas and theories relate to both social science and psychology as relevant perspectives.

The basis of psychology is the study of how individual people attempt to make sense, through cognitive processes, of their social world, of how their social contexts affect their social behaviours, and of how individuals share their representation of the social world with others (Cardwell et al., 1996). Social science relates to the study

Activity

Write a few notes on the following:

- Have you learnt about psychology previously?
- What is the basis of this discipline?
- Have you learnt about social science previously?
- What is the basis of this discipline?

of how social groups in society behave. There is an overlap of the two disciplines, but the former focuses more on individuality and the latter on group processes. In this chapter, four simple perspectives of how leadership is classed have been mapped against the various disciplines and ideas (Table 4.1).

Table 4.1 Comparative classifications of developing leadership theories (Van Seters and Field, 1990; Crainer, 1996; Sadler, 2003)

Leadership Classification	Development of Leadership Theories
Leadership as a collection of personal characteristics or traits	Personality era
Leadership as a function within an organisation	Influence era
	Situational era
Leadership as an effect on group behaviour	Behavioural era
	Contingency era
	Transactional era
	Role development
Leadership as an influence on forming an organisational culture	Organisational cultural era
	Transformational era
	New leadership era
	Systems leadership era

LEADERSHIP AS A COLLECTION OF PERSONAL CHARACTERISTICS OR TRAITS

Trait or 'Great Man' theory was popularised around the 1900s and focused on the idea of some universal traits of leaders. 'Great Man' theory is based on the belief that leaders possess exceptional qualities. It has been argued that trait theory was born out of the philosophy of Aristotle (384–322 BC) who believed that some are *born to lead* and others are *born to be led*, thus linking back to the notion of leadership and followership (see Chapter 2). It also raises the assumption that some people have specific leadership qualities and others do not. This assumption could be seen as a way to identify potential leaders for the future.

Activity

Q:

- What do you think about effective leaders?
- What characteristics do you think they need?
- Are they different now from those that were needed in the last century?
- Write down any other leadership characteristics that you think are important from what you have experienced or have heard about.

A:

You may have a list that includes the following:

- Someone who knows what's got to be done
- Someone who gets things done
- Good communicator
- Admirable
- Good persuader
- Good at bringing about change.

You may have found this difficult as the way some people lead others varies by time and place; sometimes it is hard to identify characteristics that they all share. This may be because in different contexts leaders require different attributes. You are not alone in such difficulties. The literature is still confusing and there is much debate about the value of trait theory in the world of work today. Leadership traits seem to become more noticeable in retrospect, alongside recognition of a significant achievement. Bennis (1999) highlighted that past research showed that there were seven attributes essential to leadership:

- Technical competence in one's own field
- Conceptual, abstract or strategic thinking
- Track record
- People skills
- Taste to cultivate talent
- Judgement
- Character.

Marquis and Huston (2017: 40) identified certain characteristics of leaders in terms of their intelligence, personality and abilities (Table 4.2).

Table 4.2 Characteristics of leaders

Intellect	Adaptability	Capabilities
Knowledge	Inspiration	Able to Enlist Cooperation
Judgement	Cooperativeness	Interpersonal Skills
Resoluteness	Alertness	Mediation
Oral Fluency	Self-Confidence	Prestige
Emotional Intelligence	Personal Integrity	Social Participation
Independence	Emotional Balance and Control	Charisma
Likeable	Non-Conformity	Collaborative Priority Setting
Skilled Communicator	Critical Thinking	Discretion

Source: adapted from Marquis, B.L. and Huston, C.J. (2017) *Leadership Roles and Management Functions in Nursing: Theory and Application* (9th international edn). Philadelphia, PA: Lippincott.

However, in the mid-1940s trait theory was challenged as the research was found to be inconclusive and contradictory, especially as the relationship between leaders and the context of the situation were seen as more important. Trait theory has also been criticised because it does not seem to take account of organisational culture, and may even negate the part that social class, gender and race inequalities play in maintaining the status quo in leadership positions. Indeed, Bennis and Nanus (2004) identified the following myths about leadership:

1. Leadership is a rare skill
2. Leaders are born not made
3. Leaders are charismatic
4. Leadership exists only at the top of an organisation
5. The leader controls, directs, prods, manipulates
6. The leader's sole job is to increase shareholder value.

Senge (1990), Gardner (1990) and recent NHS leadership policy agree that leadership qualities and skills can be developed and are not inherited. This then leads us to ask a number of questions pertinent to the style you might adopt in your quest to become an effective leader.

Activity

- Do you believe you have inherited leadership qualities?
- Do you believe you have developed your present leadership qualities from experience?
- Do you believe you could develop further leadership skills?

The answers you reached in this Activity will depend on your individual views of what leadership is about and the results you got from the leadership/followership test you completed in Chapter 2. In terms of developing present leadership qualities, for instance, you may have included such influences as observing and emulating senior colleagues in the way they have dealt with specific situations. Similarly, reading about leadership theory may help you to develop; you might feel that you learn more through leadership workshops and exercises, i.e. 'learning whilst doing'.

You could perhaps subscribe to the 'Great Man' theory first suggested by Carlyle in 1841, who said that 'the history of the world is but the biography of great men and that great leaders emerge to deal with specific situations'. However, this theory has largely gone out of fashion today in favour of other theories which discuss the development of leaders through study and experience. As such, the nature/nurture debate is still ongoing. More recently leadership has been linked to the intelligence debate; studies that correlate family IQ suggest that reasoning and spatial ability are more linked to the nature argument. The emergence of the 'Flynn' effect (Flynn, 2009) has also been noted. This theory highlights that IQ has been seen to be increasing in all countries over time, predominately due to environmental effects; this and the Bell Curve notion of intelligence (Lynn, 2008) make IQ a complex area in research. Lynn's work relates to the social stratification of global race to IQ and thus genetic predisposition. This is hugely controversial but has implications for leadership selection involving trait theory. There is evidence that trait theory is also still valued. In trying to set desirable attributes and competencies for job positions in the health service, you will see that essential and desirable criteria for the roles are based on trait assumptions.

These position/role attributes give rise to questions such as, 'Are leaders born or made?' and 'Is leadership an art or a science?' The work of Boerma et al. (2017) in debating the issue of whether leaders are born or made examined research on genetics, twin studies, historical evidence, and even examined stickleback fish to conclude there was a combination of nature and nuture but with a 30% genetic link. Whatever you think, in the first instance, if you are being interviewed for a clinical leadership post, you can argue both ways. If you believe leaders are born you could argue for inherited trait theory based on your leadership experience. However, if you think leaders are made you could discuss developmental training which could enhance deficits in the attributes you have for the post.

Activity

Write 50 words to reflect on how trait theory influences practice in health care today.

You may have considered the fact that potential leaders go 'on courses' to teach them how to lead, but how many of them actually come back and deliver what they have been taught? According to Marquis and Huston (2006) this may be because they are not the sort of person who likes to make decisions and direct people, indicating that they may not have the trait required to be an effective leader. However, Marquis and Huston (2017: 39) have more recently argued that the skills for leadership and management are critical to the long-term viability of health care organisations and thus the traits for both are valued.

I well remember a colleague who was promoted to a post that had 'leader' in its title. However, she would have been unable to lead the rats out of Hamelin – even with the help of the Pied Piper! She simply didn't know how to lead effectively.

When you are in the clinical area, look to see which person you would be most likely to ask for advice. This may not be the person with 'leader' in their title but someone who is seen to be approachable, knowledgeable and willing to impart that knowledge – the traits, according to Bennis (1999), of a good leader.

LEADERSHIP AS A FUNCTION WITHIN AN ORGANISATION

The theories connected with this category relate to social functionalism. These theories relate to how social organisation is maintained and how it functions. The nature of social structures, their integration, harmony and evolutionary stability towards the organisation as a whole underpin these theories (Weitz et al., 2011). Ideas within this category centre on the nature and consequences of these structures and how leadership as a structure supports the function of the organisation to carry out its work with attention given to:

- sources of power and influence over others
- how various roles relate to the functions in an organisation to meet its needs.

The role leaders play, in relation to any organisation, highlights the emphasis not on *what they have* but on *what they actually do*, who they *influence* and how this *relates to the function* a particular leader plays in an organisation. In examining what leaders actually do, Fayol (1925) first identified the main management functions seen as essential at the time as Planning, Organising, Coordination and Control, while Gulick (1937) expanded the scope of these functions to include:

- Planning
- Organising
- Staffing
- Directing

- Coordination
- Reporting and
- Budgeting.

(These functions are denoted by the acronym **POSDCORB**.)

These were, however, set in the context of scientific management and administration, rather than relating to the specific concept of leadership, and were underpinned by the assumption that the 'manager knows best'. Daft (2017: 13–14) confirms that the five functions to managing effectively are still planning, organising, staffing, directing and controlling. The functional approach relates the overlapping ideas of appointed leaders and naturally emerging leaders in an attempt to argue that there are some similarities in the two roles as well as some differences. Again, this will highlight the nature/nurture debate while being aware of the needs of staff in their developing roles. Kotter (2008) suggests that organisations should 'grow' their own leaders to function effectively within that organisation, i.e. current employees should be encouraged to develop their leadership skills in order to advance their careers within that particular organisation or Trust.

Activity

Debate the notion of 'growing' your own leaders vs appointing 'new' blood to enhance organisational and procedural change.

In terms of connecting the functions of the organisation to the people, Adair (2010: 24) uses the idea of 'action-centred leadership' where the group leader, in order to be seen as effective, needs the ability to meet three functions:

- To achieve the required task(s)
- To maintain the team
- To meet the needs of individual team members.

Activity

How could this model of leadership apply in clinical practice?

Clinical practice fits with this simple model. When exploring patient care, the *task needs* are related to specific aspects of care being undertaken at the time and the resources required to undertake those tasks; *individual needs* relates to ensuring staff understand what is expected of them and have an understanding of the purpose of their task, but it is also to do with ensuring that individual needs are addressed. If these elements and group cohesiveness are achieved, then the integrity of *team maintenance* to meet *team needs* should follow. His three-sphere model highlights the overlapping areas of functions that the leader must be aware of in order to achieve the desired outcomes (Figure 4.1).

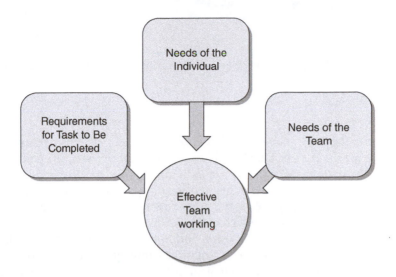

Figure 4.1   Functional needs to be fulfilled for effective team working

TASK NEEDS

An organisation must undertake various activities in order to fulfil its objectives. In health care, there are a number of tasks that are undertaken by various levels of staff. These tasks often involve an overlap of input from members of the multidisciplinary team. The tasks, the required resources and the organisation of the skills mix all contribute to the overall task being completed. For instance, a diabetic patient may require blood glucose monitoring. At first sight this may look easy as it appears simply to involve time, the patient and a health care professional to take the blood, but on further analysis it can be seen to be a much more complex process. More specifically, the task may be analysed as set out in Table 4.3.

Table 4.3   Task needs

The individual task	Monitor the blood glucose of patients
The allocation of resources to achieve that task	Calibrated blood glucose monitoring equipment
	Haematology laboratory facilities/technology
	Time
The organisation of the skills mix in order to ensure the quality of performance	Trained health care professionals to judge the level of monitoring required
	Trained health care professionals who can take and test the blood samples
	Trained health care professionals who can interpret and take action – including advising the patients, referral to other professionals as necessary, and documenting the relevant issues

Activity

Do you think that the task described can be easily learnt by an individual within a team?

In health care, the 'task' not only relates to the delivery of effective and efficient physical care for the patient but should also be about addressing the emotional care required by the patient. All patients are individuals; they have very different needs physically, socially and mentally. Individual staff have to know how to deal with all these aspects of care as they are carrying out the tasks for, or with, patients. Teams also vary; some teams are more effective than others and leaders need to understand how each person works within the team, and how their skills and strengths can be best utilised – this relates to the use of Emotional Intelligence (see Chapter 11).

Leading out on this complexity is challenging. Leaders in health care have to think about the type of work and jobs that have to be done for the health service to address the needs of patients. For example, there are certain tasks that have to be planned and organised in a surgical unit.

Activity

Can you think of any examples of ward tasks required for patient benefit, for instance, around midday?

In relation to the Activity, there are patients who will be hungry and thirsty after returning from their surgery and will want to be offered something to eat and drink. Others may have only just returned from surgery and airway management is required. They or their relatives will expect to see their doctors to discover whether there are any results from the surgery or diagnostic tests, and medical rounds/consultations have to be organised. There may be patients who will need to be prepared for afternoon theatre or other procedures such as X-ray or MRI scans. New patients may be arriving into the area and will need to be 'admitted' and some will be waiting for discharge from hospital. These various patients' needs will have to be addressed in order of priority. In the community there are similar tasks that have to be done, such as the administration of referrals, telephone contacts, visits to book, patient/client visits to make and clinics to run as well as management meetings to attend. Filling the car with petrol is also a task that has to be fitted in!

Part of effective communication may be stating what appears (to you) to be obvious. Here one fish is telling the other that they can hear the sea. Given that the sea would be the natural habitat of the fish involved it is obvious that they would hear

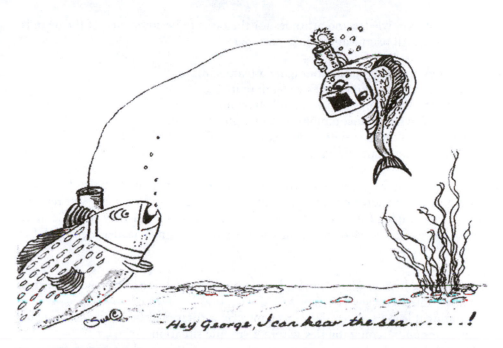

Source: Sue Saillet

sea sounds. Managing and leading teams will require leaders to think about *how* the following activities will be achieved:

- Setting and achieving goals and objectives to get the required work done
- Communicating goals and objectives to the rest of the team
- Defining the tasks to meet the objectives
- Planning the work
- Bargaining for and mobilising resources, for example, beds, linen, people
- Delegating the work, organising responsibilities and supporting the team
- Monitoring performance and quality management
- Reviewing progress.

Leading from the front in order to ensure all eight elements are addressed is an accepted part of effective leadership, whichever style is adopted.

THE NEEDS OF THE TEAM

When we consider the *team*, we must consider training needs, communication systems and team development in order for the multiprofessional teams to function. Teams require leaders and followers (Chapter 2) who may not always be the same people, as various roles change and take shape. The people in a team should have the right skills, knowledge and attitudes for the tasks to be completed, if the team is to be a success. All team leaders must consider:

- Team development and encouraging a team spirit
- Encouraging a working cohesive team unit
- Setting standards and professional behaviour
- Setting up systems of communication within the team
- Learning and training within the team
- Delegating and team growth.

These features may be addressed formally within a team meeting as part of the recognised agenda or addressed within an informal situation – say a night out ten-pin bowling, encouraging team growth, team spirit and cohesion. It may be difficult at times to address the needs of the team where there is no single leader identified, for example:

- **Job sharing leaders** When one leader has one way of doing things and the other holds a different view
- **Rotational leaders** Where leaders change on a rotational basis or with specific functions and accountabilities within a specific situation
- **Distant leaders** Where the team members are working throughout the geographical community and only have limited face-to-face contact. (Barr and Dowding, 2016: 59).

Differing philosophies and styles may affect how the team functions, but through open discussion a central path and philosophy can be devised to satisfy all concerned.

THE NEEDS OF INDIVIDUALS

This area focuses on a leader giving attention to personal needs or individual problems while giving praise and status to those concerned. Again, professional development and training has to be recognised in order to raise the quality of care delivery. Individuals will have personal as well as professional needs. They will come to work for a variety of reasons besides financial gain. They will want to be valued and developed within the working team. Leaders may well need to think about the following:

- Appraising and listening to the needs of individuals
- Attending to personal issues
- Giving praise and status to individuals
- Reconciling conflicts between team needs and individual needs
- Training and developing individuals
- Clinical supervision and reflective practices.

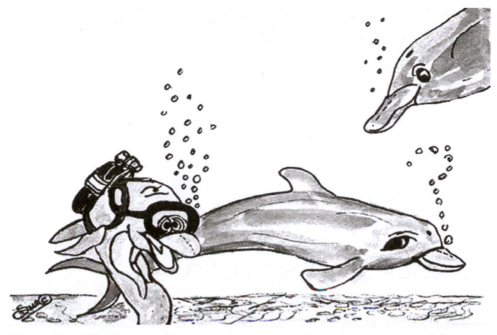

Source: Sue Saillet

Within the strategy addressing personal needs there will always be an individual that needs additional reassurance. The smaller dolphin has yet to realise that they can breathe on their own and does not require scuba equipment.

Working within the three spheres of Adair's model (Figure 4.1) is challenging for any leading individual. The ideal is, of course, to occupy the position in the centre where all three areas are integrated, needs are adequately met and the team or group is satisfied. Adair (2006) suggested the seven qualities of a strategic leader as being:

- Direction (purpose and aim of the business)
- Strategic thinking (bridging the gap between now and the future)
- Making it happen (details)
- Relating the whole to the parts
- Establishing allies and partners outside the business
- Releasing corporate energy
- Developing leadership in others.

The implications of this focus within the complexity of the Health Service are related to the need to build the capability and capacity within the leadership of the NHS. The Institute for Innovation and Improvement (DH, 2007) recognises this will bring huge benefits for patients, carers and staff as well as increased quality and value. The latest developments – of GP consortia commissioning and the impact of the Health and Social Care Act 2012 overall – have stimulated mounting debate for many stakeholders in the shaping of the future of the NHS.

LEADERSHIP AS AN EFFECT ON GROUP BEHAVIOURS

This category overlaps with 'Leadership as a Function' but has a greater focus on the behavioural aspects of people relationships. The Human Relations Management era greatly influenced the humanistic view of leadership and the importance of people over productivity. The theories that emerged within this category focused initially on how leaders behaved towards their team; but later the importance of the effects of team behaviour *on leadership* was realised. The various *leadership style* and *motivational* theories, which concern how to get the best out of people to get the work done, are seen as wide ranging. The motivational theories of people such as Herzberg (1966), Ouchi (1981), Maslow (1987) or McGregor (1987) 'fit' within this section but will be discussed in greater depth in Chapter 7.

LEADERSHIP STYLES

The way an individual leads, within an organisation or a team, has been seen in terms of their style of behaviour and relates to the underpinning behavioural theories. Lewin (1951) and White and Lippitt (2006) identified various types of leader behaviour that signalled different styles. One way of looking at leadership style is in connection to the *power* that a managerial leader exerts over any subordinates in a team and these were situated on a continuum (Figure 4.2).

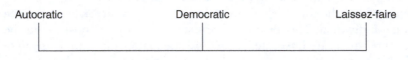

Figure 4.2 Leadership behaviours

- **The autocratic or authoritarian style** The leader exercises ultimate power in decision making and controls the rewards and punishments for the subordinates in conforming to their decisions.
- **The democratic and participative style** The leader encourages all members of the team to interact and to contribute to the decision-making process.
- **The laissez-faire style** The leader *conscientiously* makes the decision to pass the focus of power on to the subordinate members in a genuine laissez-faire style. This is distinct from abdication or 'non-leadership' when the 'leader' refuses to make any decisions.

A person's leadership style has a great deal of influence on the work environment. For many years it was believed that leaders employed a consistently dominant style. It was also felt that autocracy and laissez-faire styles were less acceptable than democratic leadership. Later on it was felt that there was a continuum of styles between autocratic and laissez-faire behaviours and those leaders moved dynamically between styles in response to new situations. Go back to Chapter 2 and look at the results of your leadership/followership quiz to see where you might 'fit' in Table 4.4. The table highlights how this categorising of styles is influenced by situations and is, therefore, more complex than was first suggested.

Table 4.4   Comparative elements of leading styles

Comparative Criteria	Autocracy Style	Democracy Style	Laissez-faire Style
Situations where valued	Where predictable group action is required to reduce group frustration and develop group security Useful in crisis situations	Where groups are together for long times and cooperation and coordination are necessary	Where problems are poorly defined and all views can be considered to find solutions
Possible negative outcomes	Creativity, self-motivation and autonomy are reduced	Time-consuming and frustrating when decisions need to be made in a short time Less efficient than autocracy	Group apathy, disinterest leading to frustration
Possible positive outcomes	Well-defined group actions reducing frustration and producing security	Promotes autonomy and growth in individual workers Communication flows up and down	Group cohesion when trying to deal with ambiguity
Cultural issues	'You' and 'I' signal the different status Coercion is used to motivate Decision making does not involve others	'We' is emphasised Rewards are used to motivate Decision making involves others	The group is emphasised Motivation by support when requested Decision making is spread within the group

The notion of a continuum model from laissez-faire to autocratic leadership has also been challenged. The work of Tannenbaum and Schmidt (1958) highlighted that the continuum model is too simplistic, that a mixture of autocracy and democracy is needed, and elements such as leadership skills, the situation, and the abilities of the group are required for effective leadership.

The ideas of Hersey and Blanchard (1977), Blake and Mouton (1985), Blake and McCanse (1991) and Yukl et al. (2002) are also reflected in this section, concerning the multiple dimensions involved in leadership behaviour.

EMERGENCE OF CONTINGENCY THEORIES

Theories that identified the impact of the situation on the behaviour of a leader highlighted that leadership styles of individuals *could* be changed. From this a range of contingency theories emerged in order to explain the variety of contexts which influenced leadership (Fiedler, 1967; Vroom and Yetton, 1973; Vroom and Jago, 1988). In essence one can think of these theories as being quite fluid and manoeuvrable – an 'if/then' sort of relationship between a number of variables – so that *if* a certain situation arose *then* it would be dealt with in the most appropriate manner. Within the clinical situation we work a good deal within the confines of such theory; we rarely know what is going to happen next, so we have to adapt to each situation as it occurs.

FIEDLER MODEL

The work of Fiedler (1967) concluded that no one particular style of leadership met the needs of every situation so developing the contingency model of leadership. Fiedler came from a background in psychology and used the assumption that personality is relatively stable but that *situations* changed the effectiveness of the leadership style. The relationship between the leader and the group was affected by the leader's own ability, the task to be met and the positional power of the leader. Fiedler's interpretation of his research was that there were leaders who were good in terms of developing interpersonal relationships with the team. Conversely, there were leaders who derived most satisfaction from knowing that a specific task had been completed, rather than considering the implication of relationships within that achievement. However, as a piece of scientific research this has been challenged over the years. Fiedler's work has been subject to much criticism but it is worth recognising the contribution it has made both to gauging leader effectiveness and stimulating further research.

THE VROOM–JAGO CONTINGENCY MODEL (1988)

This model focused on the degrees of people relationships of the leader and their impact on decision making (see Figure 4.3). The starting point is the idea that a solution is needed to solve a problem and the amount of involvement of others depends on the leadership influence. The model is made up of three main parts:

- Leader participation styles
- Diagnostic questions
- A set of decision-making rules.

The seven diagnostic questions that accompany this model relate to the following:

1. The importance of the decision for the organisation
2. The commitment of the group to implement the solution
3. The level of leadership expertise in the decision
4. Likelihood of group commitment to the decision
5. The group's support for the organisational goals
6. The group's expertise
7. Competence of the group to team problem solving.

This model is complex but interesting in its view of the relationship between the group, the organisation and the leadership. It has since been integrated into a computer-based model to add more complexity. Despite being less than perfect, it is a useful model for managers learning to make timely, high-quality decisions (Daft, 2017: 81–8).

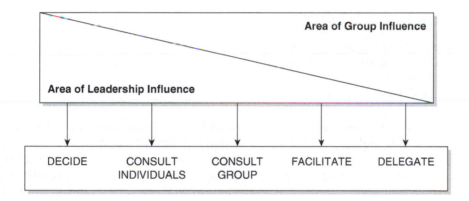

Figure 4.3 Vroom-Jago Contingency Model

LEADERSHIP AS AN INFLUENCE ON FORMING AN ORGANISATIONAL CULTURE

Having examined the last three forms of leadership theory (see p. 58), the latest era concerns the different cultures set within the organisation in which the leadership operates. Transactional culture and transformational culture have been differentiated as being part of organisational life. The *transactional era* stems from the work of Bass, who stimulated new management thought around transactional leadership between the 1960s and 1980s. This was a time when there was more employment stability in the UK and transactional leadership was based on the notion of a *contract process* between the leader and the group. Bass (1985) noted that transactional leadership concerned:

- rewards and incentives to influence motivation
- the ability of the leader to monitor and correct subordinates in order to work effectively
- an explicit promise of tangible benefits for followers
- an ideological appeal.

The bureaucracy of the National Health Service benefited from the contractual or transactional leadership style in the stable environment at the time. The growth in policies, procedures and employment law started around then. It was also felt that leaders and groups found mutual satisfaction within these transactional relationships by 'knowing where they stood'.

Marquis and Huston (2017: 50) identified the characteristics of a transactional leader as someone who:

- focuses on management tasks
- is committed
- uses trade-offs to meet goals
- does not identify shared values
- examines causes
- uses contingency rewards.

Transactional leadership has been criticised in less stable environments where creativity is needed to deal with today's more complex business worlds.

However, a culture of 'following the rules' has been noted to be effective, especially where planning, organising and budget management are essential – as in Britain's NHS. When traditional industry in Britain was changing in the 1980s and 1990s there was a shift away from a culture formed through transactional leadership. We began to lose our manufacturing base for employment and the information revolution started to take hold on a global basis. Traditional ways of working, where employees had a job for life and were rewarded for their loyalty to the employer, were starting to dissipate. More creative problem solving was required to look for new markets, new products and services and 'fit' within the emerging global economy. This environment also affected the health services, within the public services, and quasi management modelling, based on the private sector, occurred. *Transformational leadership* theories started to surface, in contrast to transactional leadership theories. Transformational theories of leadership are based on the idea that leaders are people who *motivate* others to perform by encouraging them to see a vision and change their perception of reality. Such leaders are seen as committed individuals with long-term vision and a need to empower others, and who are interested in the consequences. They use:

- charisma
- individualised consideration

- intellectual stimulation to produce greater effort, effectiveness and satisfaction in followers
- inspiration through symbols. (Bass and Avolio, 1990)

Burns (2010) identified that the transforming process is one in which leaders and followers raise each other to higher levels of morals and motivation. So values such as liberty, peace, equality and humanitarianism are often emphasised rather than values based on individual benefits. However, it has been noted that transformational leaders can have the potential for accruing a good deal of control and power, which can lead to the exploitation of large numbers of followers. Great leaders can be seen as very positive; however, there may be transformational leaders who are portrayed in a negative light (Table 4.5).

Table 4.5 Positive and negative transformational leaders

Positive	Negative
Pope John Paul II	Adolf Hitler (WW2 leader)
Mohandas Gandhi	Saddam Hussein (Iraqian leader)
Martin Luther King	Bashar al-Assad (Syrian leader)
John F. Kennedy	
Nelson Mandela	

Other criticisms of transformational leaders may be that they tend to focus on the bigger issues of life and because of their high visibility are unwilling to spend time facilitating the implementation. Thus, to followers, it may seem that leaders are autocratic and success is about the detail of getting things done. The old adage, 'the devil is in the detail', might be appropriate here.

Activity

- Have you ever been inspired and motivated by someone else's charisma in practice?
- Jot down three reasons why you think they made such an impact on you.
- How do you think these ideas relate to trait theory?

An anaesthetist I worked with was amazing with children; he was so calm that the parents left knowing that their child was in good hands, irrespective of how ill they were. I'm not sure why he made such an impact on me but I think it was that calm, quiet way he went about his work. I believe the fact that he was so positive in his outlook, and encouraging to junior colleagues, made him approachable when one didn't quite understand an element of care.

ANTI-LEADERSHIP ERA

It is interesting that some management theory from the 1970s recognised the important relationship between leaders and their team workers and, although the focus of the time was on leadership styles, the relevance of the team situation was underplayed. Hersey and Blanchard (1977) highlighted that the characteristics of the team ethic *influenced* their leadership behaviour. The readiness of the work team to take on board the required organisational tasks was reflected in the way their managers/leaders approached them (Table 4.6).

Table 4.6 Team readiness and leadership approaches

Team Readiness	Leadership Approach
Low	TELLING
Moderate	SELLING
High	PARTICIPATING
Very high	DELEGATING

This is an interesting perspective for healthcare work teams. More recently there has been a developing perspective of anti-leadership theory moving towards the importance of teams of 'followers'. Servant leadership theories are more recent and may combine views from any of the other theories above.

Greenleaf (1977), as a director of the communication company AT&T, first raised the idea of servant leadership. He noted that successful managers led in a different way and put 'serving others' as a priority. He noted they had certain qualities:

- Listened deeply to others to try to understand
- Kept an open mind without judging
- Dealt well with ambiguity and complexity
- Shared critical challenges with all and asked for input to solutions
- Shared clear goals and gave direction
- Served, helped and taught first
- Chose words carefully to avoid damage
- Used insight and intuition
- Had a sense of the whole and relationships/connections with that.

Howatson-Jones (2004) highlights that understanding the followers' perspective in servant leadership offers a valid way to promote health care effectiveness. The style involves mature mutual trust, collegiality and empowerment of multidisciplinary or multi-agency professionals. Greenleaf (1998) noted that, contrary to traditional leadership, the two leadership stages involved in servant leadership are reversed:

1. Serving the needs of followers to empower them to reach their potential
2. Aspiring and maturing into leading.

There seems to be more acceptance of servant leadership in the health industry (Lucas, 1999; Mullaly, 2001) because of the complexity of professional relationships. However, it has been debated whether vision and direction get lost in this type of leadership; as the direction of the NHS is well set within the total goals and governance of quality patient care, this may not be a valid argument here (Snow, 2001).

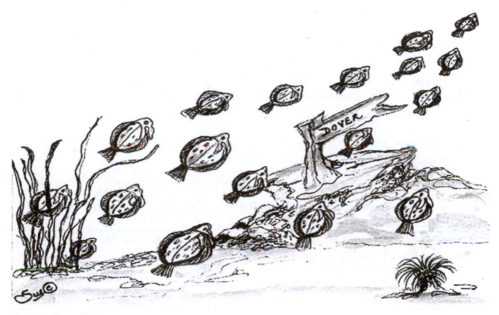

Source: Sue Saillet

McAlpine (2000), however, challenged the idea of serving in a moral and ethical style and drew an analogy between Machiavelli (1469–1527) and organisational achievement. In highlighting the role of leaders and followers, the principles that are not good indicators for success are that:

- leaders require the souls of their followers; given that some theories state that leaders require the souls of their followers, the illustration shows a shoal of Dover Soles heading for their destination
- leaders should never fail to express gratitude and appreciation; followers need flattery as recognition of their success
- leadership loyalty, fairness, trustworthiness in prosperity and adversity are key to success
- true leaders have a sense of history and awareness of the present position
- leaders must never blame or penalise followers for their own misjudgement
- leaders should resist exchanging old friends for new.

Jealousy, competition, skulduggery and treachery keep the power and leadership in place; an interesting idea in politics but when patient care is the centre of the business these principles could also work against the quality of service provision. How these ideas may influence an organisational culture will need to be evaluated and an interesting contemporary health service question is this: who has the right to lead out on clinical excellence and patient safety, who is competing for this power and how can managers and clinicians work together to be accountable to the public purse?

The relationship of leaders with their teams or followers is also an interesting phenomenon. Kelley (1992) identified five types of followers:

- Alienated: deep and independent thinkers who do not willingly commit to leaders
- Passive: do as they are told but do not think critically and are not active followers
- Conformist: participative but do not challenge
- Pragmatic: middling in their independence, engagement and general contribution
- Exemplary: excel in all tasks, strongly engage with the team, and provide intelligent yet sensitive support and challenge to the leader.

Activity

Reflect on this 'followership' typology and your own role relationship with a health service leader. Jot down which of these 'followership' styles reflect your perceived behaviour and how this related to your 'leader's style.

Reflect on a past leadership role you might have had and note whether you think you had any of these types in your team.

I can reflect on a past role I had and saw all of these types present within the team I was leading. This had implications for taking projects forward in that various communication strategies were required to enable members of staff to fulfil their role expectations, particularly the 'passive' and 'alienated'. Sometimes strategies required the exemplary and pragmatic members of staff to be harnessed to provide more peer-group support and drive to enable the effective functioning of the team. Daft (2017:15) promotes this idea of aligning followers to reach the team goals.

Leadership has thus emerged in the context of changing cultures and dynamics, which is especially important within different health care environments, even within the NHS. Schein (1985) felt that leadership needs to be seen in context and the culture of that context is important: 'Leadership is entwined with culture formation'. The type of leadership required in health care is therefore one that fits with the culture of the organisation in which that health care is delivered. Schein (1992: 237) defined organisational culture as:

The pattern of basic assumptions that a given group has invented, discovered or developed in learning to cope with its problems of external adaptation and internal integration and therefore taught to new members as the correct way to perceive, think and feel in relation to those problems.

These levels of culture (Table 4.7) can be seen within the organisation of a hospital or community placement and also within university life itself.

Table 4.7 Levels of culture (www.valuebasedmanagement.net/methods_schein_three_levels_culture.html)

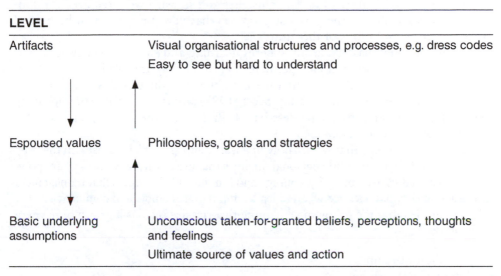

LEVEL	
Artifacts	Visual organisational structures and processes, e.g. dress codes
	Easy to see but hard to understand
Espoused values	Philosophies, goals and strategies
Basic underlying assumptions	Unconscious taken-for-granted beliefs, perceptions, thoughts and feelings
	Ultimate source of values and action

Induction at the start of a new course, meeting up with lecturers, mentors and other students on the course as well as people who have nearly finished their courses, integrates us into what is expected in terms of our behaviour within the university. During our induction into new clinical placements we note the way other professionals behave and react to patients/clients and their relatives. This idea will be explored further in Chapter 7.

NEW LEADERSHIP

New roles and expectations are driving health care professionals into a more prominent position. Non-medical prescribing, nurse–consultant led clinics, integrated community teams, hospital and community matrons and nurses managing doctors are signs of this challenge for clinicians. Kanter (1991) identifies some specific skills for new leadership:

- Self-mastery
- Strategic visioning
- Continual learning
- Creator of partnerships
- Team facilitator.

Multi-agency teams will be a feature of the future and they too will require appropriate leadership. Mintzberg (1998: 588) highlights vision, shared ideals, creation of organisational pride, developing environments for energies and innovation as essential attributes of leadership. He also identifies that a unique and essential leadership function is to build an organisation's culture and shape its evolution. He goes on to suggest the leadership roles of designer, teacher and steward were required for contributing to leadership in the past but proposes that new meanings will be needed for 'learning' organisations of the future.

Through personal mastery, group synergy, learning and sustainable development, a new leadership theory will emerge. Bennis et al. (1994) and Malby (1994) support this view and identify that the time is right for leading in this way within a framework of increased accountability. Scott (1998) points to the value of improving relationships between settings, process-based skills and professional judgement for the future of clinical leadership.

Daft (2017: 15) noted that we are now in a leadership era which focuses on the need for leaders to show more subtle personal qualities that are not transparent but are powerful, such as enthusiasm, integrity, courage and humility. He identifies that management encourages emotional distance whereas leadership requires emotional connectivity.

It is identified that the following emerging theories are seen as a group of new era leadership:

- Servant leadership
- Interactive leadership
- Moral leadership
- E-leadership
- Level 5 leadership
- System leadership.

These ideas have connected themes within leadership theories. E-leadership concerns the situation found in many industries, where communication is often not on a face-to-face basis and with increasing amounts of e-communication there are thus further challenges for leaders. Building trust, maintaining open lines of communication and being open to subtle cues of concern are crucial in what are seen as virtual working environments. Level 5 leadership emerged from a five-year study by Collins (2001), where a model of five hierarchical states to top leadership was proposed. Not everybody can climb to be a level 5 leader, but in line with many of the new leadership theories the ultimate leader is not seen as someone who is egotistical and overly ambitious, rather as someone who works ethically and humbly and gives credit to others.

Kouzes and Posner (2007) focused on leadership as a human relationship and noted the five exemplary practices of leadership:

- Model the way
- Inspire a shared vision
- Challenge the process
- Enable others to act
- Encourage the heart.

Level 5: Level 5 Executive
Builds enduring greatness through a paradoxical blend of personal humility and professional will.

Level 4: Effective Leader
Catalyzes commitment to and vigorous pursuit of a clear and compelling vision, stimulating higher performance standards.

Level 3: Competent Manager
Organizes people and resources toward the effective and efficient pursuit of predetermined objectives.

Level 2: Contributing Team Member
Contributes individual capabilities to the achievement of group objectives and works effectively with others in a group setting.

Level 1: Highly Capable Individual
Makes productive contributions through talent, knowledge, skills and good work habits.

Figure 4.4   The level 5 hierarchy model

Source: Good to Great by Jim Collins © 2001. Used by permission of Curtis Brown, Ltd. All rights reserved.

Daft (2017: 11) indicates that the *humble* leader is now more likely to succeed than the *charismatic hero* leader of yesterday. Leadership today involves complex change challenges requiring learning environments, sharing vision and shaping cultural values which are important in the complexity of organisational life. Weberg (2012) proposes the value of 'Complexity (adaptive) Leadership' to provide a newly coined framework of continual process that focuses on collaboration, complex systems and innovation mindsets with the promise to improve costs and quality in healthcare. It has its roots in chaos theory and situational and servant leadership as well as the shared leadership approach of Mintzberg. Leadership professor Jim Clawson noted that a leader is not about status but about a perspective (2013:1). In his opinion, leadership has three elements:

1. Seeing what needs to be done
2. Understanding all the underlying forces at play in the situation
3. Having the courage to initiate action to make things better. (Clawson, 2013: 3)

This fits in well with Radcliffe (2012: 29) who developed his recent model to stress that successful leadership is not about leadership personality or characteristics, or even whether leaders are born or made, but shaped on what *needs to be done* through three ingredients that focus on the:

- Future
- Engagement
- Delivery.

He noted this FED recipe signified effective leadership:

> Powerful and effective leaders are guided by the future they want. And more than this, the leader is stronger when that future is powerfully connected to what he/she cares about. If you need others then you need to engage with them and encourage and support them to deliver. (Radcliffe, 2012:19)

AUTHENTIC LEADERSHIP

Authentic leadership is a relatively new model idea of leadership. Northouse (2016: 195–223) infers that the focus is where there is a genuiness and moral link between leaders and followers and concerns intrapersonal perspectives or processes. It is felt that authentic leadership develops over time and influenced by personal life events. George (2003) identifies five characteristics of authentic leaders:

- Sense of purpose and passion
- A set of moral values and behaviours
- A belief in relationships and connectedness
- Sense of self-discipline and consistency
- Compassion and 'heart'.

Authentic leaders are seen as important in helping colleagues find significance and association at work so that they can deal with the novel, chaotic and vigorously altering work surroundings and are essential in organisations today. On the other hand, there needs to be more research into the validity of this model as it is still so new and focuses on positive higher order characteristics which would be difficult to measure (Northouse, 2016: 208). Mubarak and Noor (2018) used research to explore the relationship that exists between authentic leadership and employee creativity in project-based organisations. They found that employee creativity is significantly associated with authentic leadership, work engagement and psychological empowerment. They also revealed that extra engaged employees at work were more creative and had a sense of empowerment affected by the relationship between authentic leadership and employee creativity. Creativity is needed in the health service, but a compromise needs to be made with having too much creative change.

SYSTEMS LEADERSHIP

The King's Fund (2011) identified that the NHS needed to move away from models of heroic leadership of institutions by individuals towards one where leaders engage with systems of care and engaging staff in delivering results. The complexity, turbulence and changing boundaries in the NHS mean that leadership needs to be 'shared, distributed and adaptive' (The King's Fund, 2011: 22). It needs to have the patient at the core of any activity. The requirement for a better integration of primary, community and secondary health care has long been seen as challenging in continuity of care and work across the systems in these sectors. Systems leadership concerns collaborative working across a number of organisational structures to bring about effective improvement. Collective leadership involves taking responsibility for the success of systems in the healthcare organisations involved, with a focus on learning and improving the quality of care delivered to patients and service users (The King's Fund, 2015). Macdonald et al. (2016: 12) note, however, that systems leadership is also about a social process, so it is more about relationships than power. Manley and Titchen (2017) utilised emancipatory action research with nurses, midwives, health visitors and allied health practitioners who were working at a higher level of practice, and recommended that policy makers, governments and commissioners recognise the role of facilitation skills for clinical systems leadership to achieve quality, productivity and effective person-centred services.

As for the best leaders, the people do not notice their existence. The next best, the people honour and praise. The next, the people fear, and the next the people hate. When the best leader's work is done, the people say, 'we did it ourselves!'. (Lao-Tsu, 604–531 BC, cited in Robertson, 1997: 278)

Summary of Key Points

This chapter has briefly looked at various aspects of leadership theory in order to meet the identified learning outcomes. These were:

- **Identify the evolution of leadership theories** There is a direct link to psychology and social sciences in the adopted styles of the leader; however, it is generally felt that – depending on the situation – the role of leadership may change.
- **Compare and contrast the various leadership theories** Trait theory originated prior to the turn of the twentieth century and around the time of the second Industrial Revolution. It was felt that leaders exhibited distinct qualities or traits in order for them to function effectively. Conversely, what leaders do in terms of Action Centred Leadership to meet the needs of an organisation was discussed. However, it is necessary to be aware of the effects different leadership styles have on the overall behaviour of the group in order for that group to become effective.
- **Critically discuss the application of these theories in relation to health care** A wide range of leadership theories has developed over time and these theories have contributed to the drive to make the health service more effective and efficient. However, it has been debated whether these theories have always been scientifically substantiated. The influence of these theories can be seen through the recruitment, work practices and appraisal processes in organisations, and these have an impact on the performance of the individual or the team.

ONLINE RESOURCES

For online resources, including SAGE journal articles, weblinks and videos, visit the book's website: https://study.sagepub.com/barr4e.

FURTHER READING

Prosser, S. (2002) Servant leadership, *Professional Nurse*, *18* (4): 238.

PART 2

THE
TEAM

5 TEAM LIFE

Chapter Contents

Learning Outcomes

By the end of this chapter you will have had the opportunity to:

- Define what is meant by 'group' and 'team'
- Examine the values of team membership
- Discuss the value of group/team unity
- Discuss the importance of group/team formation
- Debate the classification of work groups
- Investigate the application of team leadership
- Evaluate the notion of effective leadership teams and their impact on the learning environment

INTRODUCTION

Over the last four chapters, you have been considering yourself as an individual preparing for or reflecting on the role of leader, considering the expected behaviours, beliefs and values you may hold. It is now prudent to scrutinise the team from the point of view of group/team formation, team dynamics and how you might expect individuals to react within a given situation. It is important to recognise the dynamics of the team to lead effectively for best patient-care outcomes. To enable us to do this we must examine group formation and dynamics prior to studying the effects these elements have on leadership skills. Following this, we will attempt to offer suggestions as to the best method or style of leadership within given hypothetical health care situations.

GROUP AND TEAM CHARACTERISTICS

Individuals do not often work in isolation; rather they are members of a group. Indeed, you may well be a member of one or more groups related to both work and leisure activities. Groups are an essential feature of any organisation; their power cannot be underestimated and so the ways in which they work together are fascinating phenomena. It is interesting to study children at play to see how they interact with each other. If you watch what is going on in the playground, crèche, or any group of children you will see different behaviours emerging – from leader to subservient member. The effective leader should consider the impact of diversity such as age, gender and ethnicity on group processes and work pressures. These pressures can, in turn, have an enormous influence over the behaviour of group members, e.g. society expects health care workers to dress and act in a particular way. It is useful to think of other areas where expectations in fads and fashions influence the way groups of people dress and act together – where group members must dress in a particular way in order to be accepted into the society. Those who like to have a gym workout and be seen wearing tight, brightly coloured lycra outfits and fluorescent trainers, for golfers maybe trousers and Argyle sweaters,, and for those who want to sneak in at the back of classes baggy joggers and T-shirts. The norm of the 'formal work suit' of the middle/executive class has now been replaced by a more casual mode of dress.

Activity

- What do you think a group is?
- Write a definition.
- How many groups do you belong to?

Thornton (2016: 1) explores how our lives are lived in groups and how the quality of relationships gained impact on personal satisfaction and 'pleasures in life'. Honey (2001: 88) notes that a group is seen as 'a collection of individual people who come together to achieve some purpose'.

Sullivan and Garland (2013: 78) concur with this but differentiate between:

- formal groups – existing within the organisational structure to complete a specific task, e.g. Task and Finish Groups
- informal groups – evolving naturally from social interactions despite organisational structure, e.g. golfing or theatre work societies.

Mullins (2016: 271) offered the suggestion that any number of people who interact with one another are psychologically aware of one another, and those who perceive themselves to be a group are therefore a group. Whatever groups you may have listed, the identified group members should share a common purpose with shared norms, values and beliefs.

It is often fudged but it is important to explore the difference between groups and teams. Ellis and Bach (2015: 24) define *a group* as a number of people sharing something in common, such as an interest, belief or political aim. They also go on to say that:

a team is a number of people organized to function co-operatively as a unit. They exist to get a job done effectively and efficiently.

Thornton (2016: 1) concurs with this difference between groups and teams. She notes that all teams are groups, but all groups are not teams; a team has an explicit shared purpose and task in an organisation.

Honey (2001: 185) distinguishes a group from a team in that the latter evolves from the former and performs at a much higher level of cohesion than a group needs to. Sullivan and Garland (2013: 79) discern that there is a blurred boundary between groups and teams. They note that not all work groups are teams, giving a General Practice (GP) as an example; it may have six General Practitioners (GPs) working alongside each other but they will not necessarily work as a team to care manage their patients. The practice management administration will, however, need to work as a team to arrange appointments, maintain records and ensure referrals are managed appropriately. This could be seen as a 'community of practice' which is a concept where individuals work together with a shared practice goal (see Chapter 6). Whether we concentrate on work or leisure activities, we all have roles to play within a team or a group and we all seem to function better when we work with others rather than working in isolation.

Xyrichis and Ream (2008: 238) undertook a systematic concept analysis and proposed the following definition of team working in health care, which demonstrates the significance of team leadership:

A dynamic process involving two or more health professionals with complementary backgrounds and skills, sharing common health goals and exercising concerted physical and mental effort in assessing, planning, or evaluating patient care. This is accomplished through interdependent collaboration, open communication and shared decision-making. This in turn generates value-added patient, organizational and staff outcomes.

Loyalty within a team or a group is often seen as a requirement. Those who question the actions or decisions of the group may run the risk of being ostracised or subtly made to conform. For instance, within the workplace allied health professionals may work in directorate groups, standard setting groups and workplace audit groups to name a few. There are also the Royal College of Nursing (RCN) Forum groups, supporting different professional groups such as operating theatre, rehabilitation, primary care nursing, emergency care working. If you wish to maintain membership of these groups then you might, at times, feel a need to suppress or restrain your feelings to retain your membership without any loss of face. So, it is clear that group and team formation is an important area to understand when endeavouring to lead; it is this knowledge that will help the effective leader to understand better the ways people behave. If leaders or managers are to avoid the negative aspects of a group, it is vital that they understand the dynamics of work groups and the advantages and limitations of using them to accomplish different types of tasks.

Visit the book's website for a self-assessment of how you work in teams through the companion website. If you answered mainly yes to these statements, your role is seen as having a people focus within the role of dealing with groups and teams. It is important to realise that a work team strongly influences the overall behaviour and performance of individual group members. Belbin (2011: 16) noted that 'teamwork' was a fashionable term having replaced the more usual reference to the group; therefore, every activity conducted by a group is referred to as teamwork.

There were many changes in the way people viewed groups during the twentieth century. However, it appears that for universal purposes the word 'group' is taken to have a general sense, whereas 'team' has a more specific context; thus to 'get the job done', a team needs to be formed. In general, we refer to the 'group' or 'team' according to the focus of attention and the spirit, style and perception of the group/team. Confusion arises due to the duality and interchangeability of the terms and many writers do not differentiate between the two. The dynamics of the group are about the forces within a group that are ever-changing in order to meet specific situations; they are also about the science investigating the action of these forces relating to the strength of the demands of given situations on individual members. They affect not only the way we interact at work but also how we behave when we are in our homes and within our individual communities.

RELEVANCE FOR PERSON-CENTRED CARE

If we now consider the relevance of groups and teams in relation to person-centred care it is clear that, by considering the patient as a person rather than a condition, care can be devised to meet individual needs. Person-centred care aims to be user focused, promote independence and autonomy, provide choice and control, and be based on a collaborative team philosophy. It considers service users' needs and views and builds relationships with family members. Considering services from a user's point of view is an excellent way of helping the professionals involved to take a step back and see their services from a new perspective. This becomes a powerful motivator and driver for change and can help to increase clinical engagement in the project. When staff hear how patients experience their services, the need for improvement is immediately apparent and the case for change becomes compelling.

The Health Foundation (2015) suggests person and family-centred care involves a framework built around four principles:

- Affording people dignity, compassion and respect
- Offering coordinated care, support or treatment
- Offering personalised care, support or treatment
- Supporting people to recognise and develop their own strengths and abilities to enable them to live an independent and fulfilling life.

It is the Care Quality Commission (CQC) that has a specific role within the Health and Social Care Act (2012), the Care Act (2014), and the Health and Social Care (Health and Safety) Act (2015). The CQC has a responsibility to monitor, inspect and regulate health and care services to make sure they meet fundamental standards of quality and safety and to publish findings including performance ratings to help people choose care. Their fundamental standards relate to the following:

- Person-centred care
- Dignity and respect
- Consent
- Safety
- Safeguarding from abuse
- Food and drink
- Premises and equipment
- Complaints
- Good governance
- Staffing
- Fit and proper staff
- Duty of candour
- Display of ratings.

The CQC inspections will determine whether the organisation is safe, effective, caring, responsive and well led. (Chapter 13 will explore quality issues further.)

It is noted that *The Five Years Forward View* (NHS England, 2014), which set out the future agenda to improve the NHS, does not transparently indicate the value of patient-centred care. It was developed by the partner organisations that deliver and oversee health and care services including the Care Quality Commission, Public

Health England and NHS Improvement. *Next Steps on the Five Year Forward View* (NHS England, 2017), which then found the need to focus on urgent care, GP, cancer, mental health, elder care and an 'NHS 10-point Efficiency Plan', is also service improvement and public health focused, and thus related to system effectiveness and efficiency. The balance for a patient centred service and a public centred service is one of challenge. However, the National Information Board (NIB) published its framework for action, *Personalised Health and Care 2020* in 2014 to set out a framework for better use of data and show how technology can improve health as well as transform the quality and reduce the cost of health and care services. It is hoped that patients and citizens will have more control over their health and well-being, that carers will be empowered, that the administrative burden for care professionals will be reduced, and that there will be support for the development of new medicines and treatments.

We make many assumptions that we, as clinicians in whatever speciality, know what it is like for patients and carers, but taking the step of actively finding out and involving them is critical, not only when designing or changing a service, but also when we devise our own professional plan of care for the current need episode.

It is necessary to validate and prioritise problems with patients, clients and their families to meet with their individual values and life goals. In 2012 the National Institute for Health and Care Excellence (NICE) produced clinical guidance on *Patient Experience in Adult NHS Services: Improving the Experience of Care for People Using Adult NHS Services* which clearly promotes an individualised and person-centred approach to all care (NICE, 2012). The use of standard care plans should be adapted on an individual basis and ensure that patients with communication difficulties are not compromised. Hibbert and Peters (2003) highlight the complexity and quantity of information given to patients and that the skill of the professional is in how to present and target that information for patients so that it is actually used in their decision making.

Activity

How do you think the use of standard care plans might assist or inhibit personalised care planning and taking the patients' individual needs into consideration?

You might have thought about the constraints of using a model of assessment as inhibiting choice, but by the same token it could enhance the situation because you will have the basic building blocks on which to discuss how changes in lifestyle, treatment or therapy can help move the person towards their optimum health and activity. An example of personalised care might be thinking of the patient with diabetes who is at increased risk of circulatory problems, so it is vital that the subject of diet, cessation of smoking and taking effective exercise needs to be raised. The rise of integrated care specialists goes some way to deal with the problem of helping the patient adapt to their new lifestyle, perhaps by attending combined clinics where diabetes and cardiovascular specialists are present to share expertise, or there may be sessions where guest speakers talk about their experiences in coping positively with the situation. Diabetes care has evolved and will continue to do so over the years. The introduction of new technical advances and changes in working practices has provided health care professionals with excellent opportunities to deliver best practice, thereby improving patient outcomes.

VALUE OF GROUP/TEAM MEMBERSHIP

Activity

Why do you think working in a group is so popular?

What benefits does it offer to individuals?

There are both positive and negative aspects to the use of work groups or teams. On the positive side you might have thought about the feedback, support and praise you get from others as you attempt to complete a task. There is also the togetherness and friendships formed which may give you a feeling of self-worth. Look at the success of websites like Facebook, where people can reach out to members of groups they have lost contact with in order to see how they are getting on. On the negative side, group membership may apply peer pressure on an individual to perform at a certain level. Similarly, an individual may find the behaviours of the group unacceptable, but due to the power within the group may find it difficult to rail against the 'norm' which is a form of 'groupthink' (Janis, 1982). (This concept will be discussed further in Chapter 8.)

Thornton (2016: 1) notes the power of groups which if harnessed can lead to creativity, collaboration and adaption. Specific benefits from teamwork may also relate to:

- achieving goals more quickly and efficiently than individuals working alone
- supporting each other to improve skills
- becoming more confident and developing interpersonal skills
- taking more risks
- becoming more flexible
- showing commitment to the task and each other
- sharing information, knowledge and feelings
- becoming more self-motivated
- enjoying the work by being with other people
- being easier to lead.

Activity

Do you agree with this or does team working seem to take too much time?

The work of West (2012: 14), highlighting research work, established a relationship between staff working in teams and patient mortality. The leadership team processes and innovation in clinical contexts can be seen to have practical and theoretical implications. Mukamel et al. (2009) suggested that a higher quality of care was linked to better team-work in nursing homes. Dackert's (2010) quantitative research in Sweden examined the positive importance of team climate and innovation in nursing the elderly.

It is interesting to read how management theory and research relates to the benefits of teamwork. The classical approach to management and organisational behaviour tends to ignore the importance of groups/teams. Indeed Taylor (1947), commonly thought to be the 'father' of scientific management, described the concept of the 'rabble hypothesis' wherein he made the assumption that people should carry out their work as solitary individuals, unaffected by others and with no interaction. He may also have thought that allowing people time to mix would only lead to trouble and rebellion! This assumption was challenged by the Hawthorne experiments at the Western Electric Company in America (1927–1932). These experiments were designed to demonstrate a positive correlation between the amount of light in the workplace and worker productivity. One of the experiments took a group of 14 men working in a bank wiring room. It was noticed that the men formed their own sub-groups and that, despite financial incentives, the group had decided that 6,000 units per day was a fair level of output. The group felt that if they started to produce more than the 6,000 units then it would ultimately become the 'norm'. Although 6,000 units was well below the level the group was capable of producing, group pressure not to 'over work' was stronger than the financial incentive, so the actual output was kept to the perceived 'reasonable' limit.

The four general conclusions drawn from the Hawthorne studies were that:

- **The aptitudes of individuals are imperfect predictors of job performance** Although they give some indication of the physical and mental potential of the individual, the amount produced is strongly influenced by social factors.
- **Informal organisation affects productivity** The Hawthorne researchers discovered a group life among the workers, and also showed that the relations supervisors develop with workers tend to influence the manner in which the workers carry out directives.
- **Work-group norms affect productivity** The Hawthorne researchers were not the first to recognise that work groups tend to arrive at norms of what is 'a fair day's work'; however, they provided the best systematic description and interpretation of this phenomenon.
- **The workplace is a social system** The Hawthorne researchers came to view the workplace as a social system made up of interdependent parts.

The notion of the Hawthorne effect arose from these experiments. The effect can be defined as 'an increase in worker productivity produced by the psychological stimulus of being singled out and made to feel important', hence team or group members experienced a boost to their self-esteem when their work was being valued (www.nwlink.com/~donclark/hrd/history/hawthorne.html). For decades, the Hawthorne studies provided the rationale for human relations within the organisation. Then two researchers (Franke and Kaul, 1978) used a new procedure called *time-series analyses*. Using the original variables, and including the Great Depression and the instance of a managerial discipline in which two insubordinate and mediocre workers were replaced by two different productive workers – with one who took the role of straw boss – they discovered that production was most affected by the replacement of the two workers due to their greater productivity and the effect of the disciplinary action on the other workers. Early social scientists readily embraced the original Hawthorne interpretation since it was looking for theories of work motivation that were more humane and democratic.

Activity

How do the groups you identify with meet your social needs and enhance your social identity?

Do they stifle your individuality and freedom?

It can be argued that better ideas emerge when a few people work on a problem separately and come together later than when they work face-to-face in a group. This is possibly because group situations can inhibit the generation of ideas from less vocal members. Which begs the question: why form work groups or teams? Groups will often take greater risks (possibly because the responsibility is shared and is therefore less threatening) and make fewer errors because there may be more rescuers, i.e. members who see potential problems and set out to rectify these before they become problems. In a group there is also greater total knowledge and information. By discussing the situation, a more thorough review is accomplished, and a proposal strengthened. Most importantly, problems require decisions that depend on the participation and support of a few individuals. By forming groups, more members will accept a decision based on the group solving a problem than when one person solves it alone. Furthermore, communications relating to the decision can be speedy in the group process; communication breakdowns are reduced when the individuals have ownership.

GROUP UNITY

Group unity is an important aspect of work group dynamics. When establishing a new work group, it is important to cultivate a feeling of unity among the group members at an early stage. Unities in a group develop slowly as members open up and learn about each other. In the beginning, members are not sure whether they will be accepted and may hold back until they feel more secure. If the group has an unfriendly atmosphere or there is a chance of rejection, unity may not develop at all. As a leader, you can help the group become more unified by providing a safe environment for all. Today, for the most part, groups are usually composed of people possessing some basic idea upon which they are all agreed and which they are trying to express through the medium of their clashing personalities and frequently in obedience to someone in a leadership role. Groups also come together in order to exploit and use methods which are regarded as essential to attaining the prevailing definition of 'successes'. Whatever degree of unity is achieved in such groups is often based on expediency or good manners. Ambition, conflict, hurt feelings and bruised egos can still be the 'normal' in-group experience. Several factors have been identified which affect the cohesiveness of a group.

Size As the size of a group increases, its cohesiveness tends to decrease.

Achievement of goals The attainment of goals increases cohesiveness, especially if the group establishes the goals.

Status of the group Generally, the higher a group ranks in the hierarchy of an organisation, the greater its cohesiveness. A group can achieve status for many reasons, including:

- Achieving a higher level of performance or attaining other measures of success within the organisation
- Achieving recognition because individuals within the group display a high level of skill
- Conducting work that is dangerous or more challenging than other tasks
- Recognition that members of the group are considered for promotion more often or more quickly than those outside of the group. However, it should be noted that a sense of 'eliteness' might cause friction with other groups.

Dependence of members on the work group The greater individual members' dependency upon the group, the stronger will be the bonds of attraction to the group. A group that is able to satisfy a number of an individual's needs will appear attractive to that individual. These needs may include status, recognition, financial rewards, or the ability to do their job more easily.

TYPES OF GROUPS

In every organisation, people are assigned to groups to perform tasks that one person could not accomplish alone. Some work groups, such as departmental teams, are formal parts of the organisation's structure, e.g. operating department teams and ambulance teams, while some are ad hoc groups established to meet a short-term objective. Other groups may be formed where members operate individually but with equal commitment to achieving a set goal, such as integrated teams/ multi-agency teams. An example of this type of group may include nurses, radiographers, physiotherapists, speech and language therapists, and doctors working with patients in a stroke care unit. Still others are informal working arrangements that evolve to meet the various needs of the organisation, e.g. a pastoral church group that visits housebound parishioners.

The formal group is one created to accomplish a defined part of the organisation's collective purpose. It has specific tasks allocated to it for which it is officially responsible. On the other hand, the informal group is a collection of individuals who influence one another's behaviour within the formal group. The informal group normally develops spontaneously and the people within the group talk and joke with one another; they have 'in jokes'; they associate with one another outside of the working environment and may be referred to as 'cliques' or be part of the grapevine system of communication within an organisation.

FORMATION OF GROUPS

A discussion related to the formation of groups must start with an examination of the members of the proposed group. They are a collection of people who will meet for the first time and then go on to form a group. Forsyth (2010) notes the work of Tuckman and Jensen (1977) who suggest that generally groups pass through five clearly defined stages of development that they call Forming, Storming, Norming, Performing and Adjourning (sometimes listed as Mourning). They admit that not all groups go through all the stages; some find that they are stuck in the middle and remain inefficient and ineffective. With others, passage through the stages may be slow, but that passage appears to be necessary and inescapable. These stages are explained further below.

FORMING

This is the orientation phase where individuals have not yet gelled. Each person is busy finding out about the others' attitudes and backgrounds; from this, ground rules (i.e. codes of behaviour) for the group are established. Members often like to establish their personal identities and a leader is chosen. Task-wise they seek clarity/ instruction about what they are being asked to do, what the issues are, and whether everyone in the group understands the task.

HOW TO ADDRESS THE FORMING STAGE

Help team members get to know one another using name badges or by introducing each other to the group. Make sure the purpose and task are clearly defined and share management expectations of the group. Give the team time to get comfortable with one another but move the team along as well.

STORMING

This is a conflict stage in the group's/team's life and can be quite an uncomfortable period. Members bargain with each other and try to sort out their position within the group; occasionally hostility may result as differences in goals emerge. The key element for the leader here is to manage and resolve the conflict. The fish image below is made up with many smaller fish working as a cohesive group to overcome the threat of something much larger.

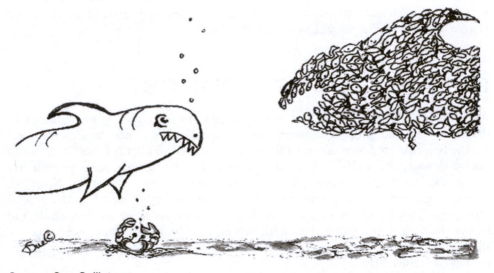

Source: Sue Saillet

HOW TO ADDRESS THE STORMING STAGE

Do not ignore the storming stage. Acknowledge it with the team as a natural developmental step. Facilitators should acknowledge the conflicts and address them. This is a good time to review ground rules and revisit the purpose and related administrative matters of the team.

NORMING

In this cohesion stage, members of the group/team develop closer relationships with each other; overall working roles like norms of behaviour and role allocation are established, and group cohesion becomes obvious.

HOW TO ADDRESS THE NORMING STAGE

At this stage, the team has established process fairly well. The task will take on new significance, as the team will want to accomplish its purpose. Facilitators should keep this in mind and remind the team of the task. In addition, facilitators should be more diligent in adhering to the road map, providing time for feedback or closure.

PERFORMING

Here the group/team has developed an effective structure and is concerned with getting on with the job. Interestingly, not all groups reach this stage, with many becoming 'bogged down' in an earlier and less productive stage. Within the performing stage members are equally happy to work alone, in subgroups or as a single unit.

HOW TO ADDRESS THE PERFORMING STAGE

Teams at the performing level are generally self-regulating. Road maps, processes, decision making, and other matters of team management will be handled independently by the team.

ADJOURNING/MOURNING

In this final stage, the group may disband or shift its dynamics, as its work is complete. The final stage (adjourning) is a more recent addition because it is thought to be a natural performing conclusion as the purpose of the team has been achieved. Tuckman and Jensen (1977) go on to suggest that groups may oscillate between the stages and pass through some stages several times without ever becoming effective.

Activity

Consider the teams you are a member of and think of the following:

- What stage are you at in the formation of your team?
- If you believe you are at the performing stage, did it take you a long time to get there?
- Has there been a change in membership of the team?
- If so, has it affected the performance level of the team?

Humphries (1998) discusses the need to identify team roles, recognising that each team member will have two roles: their professional role and their team role. He then lists seven team roles:

- Natural leader
- Activator
- Thinker
- Organiser
- Checker
- Judge
- Supporter.

He suggests that the role undertaken will be related to the personality of the team member but will not be under the control of that person, i.e. you would not be able to select the role you think you might wish to undertake. As each role has some advantages, it is useful to have a mix of the attributes within the team so that as the team leader you would be able to develop the positive features and reduce the negatives. In an ideal world, a team would have one member from each category together with several supporters. Belbin (2000) lists eight similar roles but gives slightly different descriptions of each role, the overall intent being for the leader to recognise and utilise these roles effectively. It might be useful to go to Belbin's website (www.belbin.com) in order to compare and contrast the team roles described. Barr and Dowding (2012) reflect on the member roles identified by Belbin (2015) and conclude that whilst one is a Coordinator/Energiser/ Evaluator/Recorder mix the other is an Information Seeker/Opinion Seeker/ Elaborator mix. They work well together and complement each other's skills. Griffith and Dunham (2015: 24) (Table 5.1) further identified three types of team roles for tasks, relationships and individuals.

Table 5.1 Team roles and functions

Task roles	Function
• Information seeker	• asks for facts, opinions, clarification and ideas from team
• Information giver	• contributes facts, opinions and new ideas to the team
• Discussion facilitator	• assists the discussion by engaging the team
• Task manager	• keeps the team on task and gives a practical focus
• Sceptic	• challenges ideas and explores solutions
• Recorder	• note taker who records group decisions
Relationship roles	
• Encourager	• endorses, confirms and supports others
• Harmoniser	• team conflict manager
• Process observer	• Makes commentary on the progress of the group
• Advocate	• Helps quieter members speak up

Individual roles

• Resister	• negatively opposes team ideas
• Dominator	• dominates and intimidates others in team
• Avoider	• attempts to do as little as possible
• Attention seeker	• seeks attention to meet personal needs

Source: adapted from Griffith and Dunham (2015)

Activity

Look at the table above and see if you can identify any of these roles as ones that you or others play in a regular meeting you attend.

Come back to this activity when you have read Chapter 9 and think about how different roles relate to conflict and conflict management.

It could be that the negative behaviour listed on the right-hand side is not meaningfully destructive but simply indicates that the individual has found no other arena in which to convey their work dissatisfactions; leaders need to confront these dissatisfactions in a one-to-one supportive meeting. These individuals may be seen as helpful in raising creative expressions of the value systems of the team, but it must be noted that an individual may feel excluded from the team unless the leader manages this positively. Their behaviour will continue to impact negatively on the team's ability to reach its goals unless the individual feels valued as a member and has their concerns taken seriously.

HOW TO HANDLE THE 'NOT ALWAYS HELPFUL' ROLES

There are several ways team members may appear to be unhelpful ranging from outright hostility towards the change to quiet but grudging acceptance. To recognise and address these issues it is vital that the team leader is aware of the non-verbal as well as the verbal manifestations of the members' concerns by understanding the roles described by Belbin. Strategies for dealing with these 'not always helpful' roles can include the following:

- **Set clear time limits for making decisions and remind people often of the time** Jokers are less likely to intrude or delay if they are regularly informed of the time and process.
- **Clarify expectations** Get a team 'buy-in' upfront for the work to be done. Agree by consensus that everyone will accept responsibility for any extra work. If the 'Busier Than Thou' person begins to complain, remind that person of their agreement.

In general, individuals disrupt meetings for myriad reasons. Skilled facilitators will acknowledge the fears or anxieties behind the behaviour and then move on.

Activity

Have you worked with people in the clinical area who fit into the categories mentioned?

I well remember a colleague who clearly functioned within the 'dominator' role. I seemed to spend a great deal of time reassuring new members of staff that it was 'just her way' of achieving objectives and that her attention to detail when delegating work was not personal – she did it to everyone irrespective of their role or position within the hierarchy. Once they had realised that it was not personal, members of staff were able to function effectively and not take her comments to heart. In this situation I was seen as the 'harmoniser'; the new staff became effective 'followers' until they took on their preferred roles.

Whilst, in the main, diversity within a team may lead to creativity, it can also contribute to a healthy level of conflict. The effective leader must remember that there can be negative effects of teamwork. Sullivan and Garland (2010: 180–1) highlight the negative aspects of 'groupthink' (Janis, 1982) which is a phenomenon occurring in highly cohesive, isolated groups in which group members start to think alike. In turn, this can interfere with critical thinking and may lead to inappropriate decision making.

You may have found that it took you longer to reach the performance level in one group than it did in another; indeed, you may never have reached high performance in one of your groups and found that you remained at the storming stage for most of the time until the group was disbanded. The problem may have stemmed from the lack of effective leadership, where the leader may have been unaware of the roles of some of the group members. Dynamic leaders will inspire followers towards participative management by how they work and communicate in groups. Effective leaders will need to keep group members on course, draw out the shy, politely cut off the talkative, and protect the weak. At all times leaders must be aware of the team but also remember that they should not be 'hung up' on the roles yet recognise that all those roles are valuable. The long-term consequence of this is 'labelling' a person, which may lead to the 'halo' or 'hero' effect (Hartley, 1997).

CLASSIFICATION OF WORK GROUPS

Mullins (2016: 269–349) noted the classification of work groups as being either formal or informal. These groups may coalesce to accomplish a specific task or arise naturally in order to meet the needs of a particular group of people working within the organisation. Understanding the functions of these groups is important in becoming an effective leader.

FORMAL GROUPS

These include a variety of groups and teams whose roles can be clearly defined. In the main, they are permanent groupings of personnel specified in the organisational chart. Within the NHS these groupings could be speciality based, e.g. operating theatres, ambulance trust, ward based, community and NHS Trusts that are concerned with the commissioning of care in the community setting. Subordinates report directly to a designated supervisor and the relationships among personnel have some formal basis. This might take the form of duty rotas where there is a rota chart that relates to who is working with whom on what days, in order to ensure all care is given to the patients/clients within a specific area. Other formal groups may be termed 'task groups' and are formed by a number of personnel assigned to work together to complete a project. There are different levels of task group. Task groups may comprise personnel from two or more departments and are thus cross-departmental. A 'committee' is a special-purpose task group. The purpose of committees is to:

- exchange views and information
- recommend action
- generate ideas
- make decisions.

Here the term 'committee' refers to a group of people whose job is to define the parameters of tasks, while a 'work group' is assigned the job of accomplishing tasks.

Activity

Go back to the purposes of a committee above where the exchange of views and information, recommending action, generating ideas and making decisions are identified.

What views do you have about the effectiveness of the committees you know?

You might wonder about the outcome or output of many committees. One can think of areas where a committee may be necessary in deciding a long-term strategy or business plan, but it sometimes seems out of touch with reality. Indeed, remember that 'a camel is a horse designed by committee' (Issigonis, n.d.). It's an ironic expression that Issigonis was said to have used to illustrate his dislike of working in groups. Often it feels as though nothing ever comes from a committee; we hear of people/managers 'going to meetings' but then go on to ask, 'What has been achieved?'. The routine of meetings for meetings' sake has to be challenged and there are now more references made to task and finish groups in order to prevent stagnation. Task groups in the form of unilateral or multidisciplinary teams may also be charged with reviewing policies and procedures governing clinical practices. Here we may think of a project such as ensuring all procedures are documented and updating any research that informs practice towards better quality patient care.

Advantages to teamwork include broader experience and wider knowledge, and members may be more committed to implementation if they have the opportunity to share in the decision-making process. Disadvantages might include any decisions that come from a group process being open to social pressures, with decisions made for the wrong reasons and weaker members being strongly influenced by stronger ones.

INFORMAL GROUPS

Within a work setting, people may band together informally to accomplish an objective. This objective may be related to the work of the organisation; for example, a group of people such as nurses, physiotherapists, pharmacists, and dieticians may join up to produce a health education poster. Informal groups are likely to develop when the formal organisational structure does not accommodate their joint needs. Another example is where all the paramedics within a shift might get together informally to compare notes, talk about practice, and socialise in the context of clinical support groups. Workers who want to promote a particular interest or point of view also form interest groups within an organisation; these are the most important non-formal groups for the manager to consider.

'Friendship groups' are informal associations of workers developed as an extension of their interaction and communication in the work environment. They are formed for a variety of reasons, including common characteristics (such as age or ethnic background), political sentiment, or common interests. In this book, we will not explore friendship groups in detail. However, managers should be aware that many actions (such as assignment of tasks and the establishment of other types of working groups) influence the interaction and communication patterns among subordinates, causing individuals to affiliate with each other so that interests and friendship groups inevitably emerge. These groups can have both positive and negative consequences for an organisation, and managers should be alert to ways in which these informal friendship groups affect overall performance.

THE EFFECTIVENESS OF TEAM LEADERSHIP

Many researchers have attempted to identify the effectiveness of potential leaders to manage the teams for organisations through the development of psychometric testing and MBTI® (see the book's website) is one such tool. The Hogan Personality

Inventory (HPI) is another tool that is used with senior medical staff. It measures how individuals relate to others when at their best (Hogan and Hogan, 2007). Partipants can check out their leadership potential profile with Hogan's tests (Table 5.2).

Table 5.2 The Hogan Personality Inventory (HPI)

Scale name	Low scorers tend to be	High scorers tend to be
• **Adjustment**	Open to feedback	Calm
	Candid and honest	Steady under pressure
	Moody and self-critical	Resistant to feedback
• **Ambition**	Good team players	Energetic
	Willing to let others lead	Competitive
	Complacent	Restless and forceful
• **Sociability**	Good at working alone	Outgoing
	Quiet	Talkative
	Socially reactive	Attention-seeking
• **Interpersonal Sensitivity**	Direct and frank	Friendly
	Willing to confront others	Warm
	Cold and tough	Conflict averse
• **Prudence**	Flexible	Organized
	Open-minded	Dependable
	Impulsive	Inflexible
• **Inquisitive**	Practical	Imaginative
	Not easily bored	Quick-witted
	Uninventive	Poor implementers

Source: www.hoganassessments.com/assessment/hogan-personality-inventory

Moving on from this we can revisit the application of information from the MBTI® (see Chapter 2). From the results of the indicator and by learning to know yourself – and how you prefer to work – you can construct your 'style compass' (Owen, 2009: 8) (Figure 5.1) in Excel, as we have.

Following this, you can use your judgement of what you know about others to plot their shape over yours (Figure 5.2). Now you will see how alike/different you are and note the degree of overlap. Clearly, it would not be of great benefit for us all to be the same otherwise nothing would be achieved; there needs to be a balance so that decisions can be made, thus making it easier to move forward as a team. The style compass is only a quick way of thinking about any style and can be adapted to highlight interactions among people within a team.

Certainly, while as colleagues, we both appear to be extroverts, I appear to be more judgemental than my colleague is but she has more perception of what is required – hence, we work well together, recognising each other's differences and building on each other's strengths.

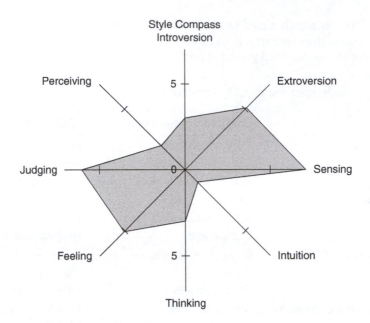

Figure 5.1 Individual style compass

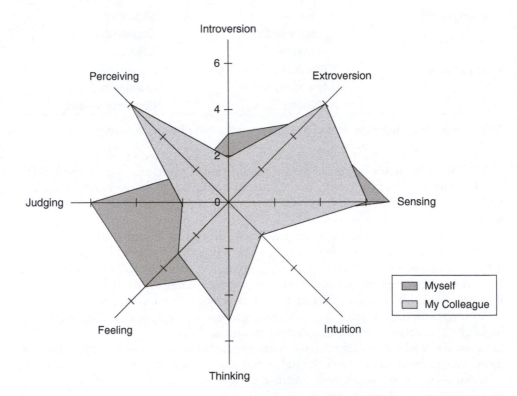

Figure 5.2 An example of a style compass for two people

Activity

Now, you can plot your own style compass and that of a colleague. Having completed the Myers-Briggs MBTI® type test (discussed in Chapter 2) you can plot the initial totals by constructing a graph in a spreadsheet program; this is most useful for visual learners. Highlight where you differ and discuss how these differences may enhance your ability to lead effectively and how you might function in a team.

By understanding yourself you can work more effectively in teams, become a good leader, and demonstrate capabilities of management. Also, where there might be weaknesses there is a possibility that you could, by being more aware, undertake activities that will strengthen these.

GROUP CONFLICT

Effective team development can help to resolve conflict. Initially the group needs to plan what they are going to do, identify goals and decide, if appropriate, on a mission statement (Marriner Tomey, 2008). There are techniques that can be utilised in order to do this, the best known of which is 'nominal group technique'; alternatives include 'consensus', 'majority rule' and 'independent listing', so that items can be considered in order of importance. This is very similar to nominal group technique, which has the following pattern:

- First, the group members are asked to list, on paper, what the group wants to achieve and how they will behave to reach that identified goal.
- Second, each person will read out one item from their list, which will be recorded on paper or a whiteboard for all to see, discuss and agree to.
- Third, discussion will take place to prioritise the items prior to them being typed up for everyone to have a copy.

By having all members of the group agree to the list of objectives and behaviours a feeling of identity is engendered and the group should function well.

LEADERSHIP TEAMS

In general education, the notion of distributed leadership is becoming the 'norm'. It is a notion that has been around for a long time as either delegated or shared leadership. It is essentially about sharing out leadership across the organisation. However, we are aware that while there is a strong belief in the idea, there is not a great deal of evidence about how it works in practice. Therefore, we need to explore the idea in some depth. We know that effective leadership makes a difference, so it follows that the caring professions need effective leaders at all levels.

Leadership teams, it is believed, are one way of giving power to everyone. As the caring professions and the NHS in general become more complex to manage and lead, we need many more leaders than ever before, enabling us to create pools of talent from which we can grow tomorrow's leaders. A key to successful planning and implementation is the development of teams. Table 5.3 provides a description of three types of teams and their relative advantages and disadvantages.

Table 5.3   Three types of team and their relative advantages and disadvantages

Model	Features	Advantages	Disadvantages
Functional	A manager and subordinates for a particular function in organisation (e.g. ward nursing team)	There is a whole team focus on implementing continuous nursing care across a 24-hour period for patients on the ward Skills can be learnt within the team and cost effective to use different grades of staff Hierarchical management to ensure policy/ procedures are followed	There may be difficulties communicating the needs of patients to other specialities (medical, physiotherapy, pharmacy, etc.) on a regular basis Cross-sector communication to community teams may also prove difficult Rigidity of change
Cross-functional	Experts in various specialities or functions working together on specific organisational tasks (e.g. Accident and Emergency staff in a Trust)	Uses the skills and knowledge of a breadth of practitioners (e.g. surgical, nursing, radiology, social work functions) for the care management of complex trauma needs of patients	Complexity of functional cultures where poor communication issues may affect care and thus patient outcome
Self-directed	Self-managed teams work without managers to deliver services to internal or external customers (e.g. alternative health therapy centre)	Problem solving and decision making left in the hands of each consultant, practitioner or therapist	Difficulties when specialist is off work to cover their speciality Difficulty in internal monitoring of quality provided by each specialist

When we talk about sharing leadership, we ought to mean sharing learning-centred leadership. We should create and develop many leaders who influence and improve the quality of learning and teaching. Although distributed leadership is not a difficult idea, when put into practice it can take many different forms. For example, you will find that there are assortments of teams within the health service that have powers in a variety of situations (Table 5.4). It is useful to understand how they work to function effectively.

Table 5.4 Team and administration responsibilities

Management Team	Governance Team Responsibilities	Administration Responsibilities
Vision (planning)	Creates, reviews and approves	Recommends process, develops and plans (decides what) and implements plans (decides how)
Structure (policy)	Creates, reviews and adopts	Recommends and implements
Advocacy (communication)	Represents public interest, seeks public input	Acts in public interest, seeks and provides public information
Accountability (evaluation)	Monitors progress towards goals, evaluates the board standards and personnel in accordance	Implements the evaluation of programmes

Barr and Dowding (2016: 96) highlighted the relative features, advantages and disadvantages of leadership teams that are seen to be necessary to ensure the smooth running of a business or institution such as the NHS. The Executive teams are normally quite small (3–8) and able to make decisions quite quickly, whilst District teams are often mid-sized (15–20) where key representatives are present to ensure their views are considered. However, when teams or committees get bigger than this (Community Teams can be 25–30) there are often so many individual issues to be satisfied that decisions take longer to be made and opportunities may be missed.

When a unit has leadership in teams, the whole institution can evolve towards becoming a learning organisation. Learning organisations can retain staff by their commitment to those staff. It is therefore part of the role of the effective leader to ensure students and staff are supported within their clinical areas, which in turn requires effective mentorship programmes and updating of staff to ensure accurate and professional assessment within that clinical area. The following characteristics may go some way to define the effective learning environment:

- People feel they are doing something that matters – to them personally and to the larger world.
- Every individual in the organisation is somehow stretching, growing or enhancing their capacity to create a learning, caring environment.

- People are more intelligent together than they are apart.
- The organisation continually becomes more aware of its underlying knowledge base in the hearts and minds of employees.
- Visions of the direction of the enterprise emerge at all levels; the responsibility of the administration is to manage the process whereby new emerging visions become shared visions.
- Employees are invited to learn what is going on at every level of the organisation, so they can understand how their actions influence others.
- People feel free to enquire about each other's assumptions and biases.
- People treat each other as colleagues.
- There is a mutual respect and trust in the way they talk to each other, no matter what their position is.

All this is led by the effective leader and done within the framework of the team. Staff retention and team morale will be supported and maintained; together with this, students will feel that there is a place for them within the organisation and as they complete their individual courses they will apply for a permanent post.

Summary of Key Points

This chapter has briefly looked at various aspects of team life in order to meet the identified learning outcomes. These were:

- **Define what is meant by 'group' and 'team'** The various definitions and interchangeability of the two labels were discussed. Ultimately, it seems from the literature, there is ongoing debate related to whether or not there is a need to differentiate between the two.
- **Examine the values of team membership** Teams are valued because they can achieve cohesiveness and effectiveness within our working environments. The Hawthorne Experiment demonstrated the ability to enhance worker productivity through boosting self-esteem due to work being valued.
- **Discuss the value of group/team unity** This is an important aspect of work group dynamics. As a leader, you need a unified team in order for the workplace to become effective.
- **Discuss the importance of group/team formation** It is important to remember that groups and teams form for specific purposes. The stages of formation are important if the effective leader is to encourage the team to meet their final objectives.
- **Debate the classification of work groups** Here we note that there are two main classifications of groups: formal and informal. Each has its own role and responsibility but working effectively relies on all types of groups/teams.

- **Investigate the application of team leadership** Effective team leadership is vital. In order to achieve this, a number of tools have been developed to identify personal strengths and weaknesses to enable team leadership to work effectively.
- **Evaluate the notion of effective leadership teams and their impact on the learning environment** Learning from general education we can see that employee retention is affected by staff perception of involvement with the decision-making process. The knock-on effect of this may be to enhance the learning environment.

ONLINE RESOURCES

For online resources, including SAGE journal articles, weblinks and videos, visit the book's website: https://study.sagepub.com/barr4e.

FURTHER READING

Archibald, R., and Archibald, S. (2015) *Leading and Managing Innovation: What Every Executive Team Must Know about Project, Program, and Portfolio Management, Second Edition (Best Practices and Advances in Program Management.* Boca Raton, FL: Auerbach.

Ellis, P. and Abbott, J. (2011) What new leaders need to understand about their teams, *British Journal of Cardiac Nursing*, 6 (3): 144–6.

Granger, K. (2011) *The Bright Side.* Available from Amazon Kindle Books.

Granger, K. (2012) *The Other Side.* Available from Amazon Kindle Books.

Kay, L. (2010) Leading other midwives: experience of midwife team leaders, *British Journal of Midwifery*, 18 (12): 764–9.

National Institute for Health and Care Excellence (NICE) (2012) *Patient Experience in Adult NHS Services: Improving the Experience of Care for People Using Adult NHS Services.* Available at www.nice.org.uk/Guidance/CG138 (accessed 13 March 2018).

Rashid, C. (2010) Benefits and limitations of nurses taking on aspects of the clinical role of doctors in primary care: integrative literature review, *Journal of Advanced Nursing*, 66 (8): 1658–70.

The Point of Care Foundation (2018) Patient and Family-Centred Care tools overview. Available at www.pointofcarefoundation.org.uk/resource/patient-family-centred-care-toolkit/patient-family-centred-care-tools-overview (accessed 8 March 2018).

6 INTERDISCIPLINARY AND INTER-PROFESSIONAL WORKING

Chapter Contents

Learning Outcomes

By the end of this chapter you will have had the opportunity to:

- Critically discuss the importance of interdisciplinary and interprofessional working in health for effective patient care and safety

- Critically explore the opportunities and challenges of interprofessional working in the contemporary context
- Identify issues of practice communities, tribalism and professional identities, and the importance of interprofessional education

INTRODUCTION

In Chapter 5 we explored the nature of team life and the importance of leadership in relation to team behaviour and management of demanding situations. We also explored the importance of team working in relation to improving patient/client outcomes. This chapter aims to explore another facet of the notion of teams within the context of working across boundaries with people from diverse backgrounds. The importance of effective interdisciplinary and interprofessional team working for quality health care has long been underpinned by research, inquiries and policy (Reeves et al., 2010; HM Government, 2013). Interdisciplinary and interprofessional working does need leadership for success.

Failings in the NHS have become more evident in the last few years, especially concerning the quality of patient care. There is an emphasis on interprofessional team working across several NHS agencies and partnerships. The Kennedy Report into child heart surgery in Bristol in 2001 identified several poor interdisciplinary practices (DH, 2002). Then Francis (2013) in his independent inquiry into care provided by a Midland NHS Foundation Trust noted that 'patients were seen intermittently by various members of the multidisciplinary team but there was little evidence that there was a planned multidisciplinary approach to their care'. Bender et al. (2013: 165) noted the challenge of formal collaborative processes and resulting fragmentation of care that exists throughout the health care system today.

Ineffective interdisciplinary and interprofessional leadership is seen as a cause of concern. With the need for more effective and efficient health services – and with the finances of public health services being under government scrutiny – working with different disciplines and professions will be essential. The Keogh review of care quality in July 2013 also signalled the importance of healthcare leadership and proposed the following improvement issues:

- **Patient Experience** Understanding how the views of patients and related patient experience data are used and acted upon (such as how effectively complaints are dealt with and the 'visibility' of feedback themes reviewed at board level)
- **Safety** Understanding issues around the Trust's safety record and its ability to manage these (such as compliance with safety procedures or Trust policies that enhance trust, training to improve safety performance, the effectiveness of reporting issues of safety compliance or use of equipment that enhances safety)

- **Workforce** Understanding issues around the Trust's workforce and its strategy to deal with issues within the workforce (e.g. staffing ratios, sickness rates, use of agency staff, appraisal rates and current vacancies) as well as listening to the views of staff
- **Clinical and Operational Effectiveness** Understanding issues around the Trust's clinical and operational performance (such as the management of capacity and the quality – or presence – of trust-wide policies, how the Trust addresses clinical and operational performance) and in particular how Trusts use mortality data to analyse and improve quality of care
- **Governance and Leadership** Understanding the Trust's leadership and governance of quality (such as how the board is assured of the performance of the Trust to ensure that it is safe and how it uses information to drive quality improvements).

The National Nursing Research Unit (NNRU) (2013) identified that research shows there is a close correlation between staff experience and patient care. Patients receive better care by staff working in teams that are well led, have clear objectives, and have the time and resources to provide that care. On a wider scale, NHS England is very committed to collaborative activity for more joined-up decision making across the whole of the NHS and provide a collaborate model for commissioning agreements (www.england.nhs.uk/publication/model-collaborative-commissioning-agreement-multiple-contract-option/). Another example related to the 'Coalition for Collaboration Care (C4CC)' which was set up in 2014 to help make person-centred care for people with long-term conditions a reality. The C4CC brings together like-minded organisations, including NHS England, who want to bring about change; they work in co-production with people who have lived experience of long-term conditions. This innovative partnership of more than 45 national organisations across the health, social care, voluntary and community sectors is focusing on changing the relationship between people with long-term health conditions and the professionals supporting them. This allows the expertise of both to be used most effectively to help people manage their condition and maximise their wellbeing (http://coalitionforcollaborativecare.org.uk/aboutus/our-partners/).

Activity

Jot down what you understand by the terms 'interdisciplinary', 'interprofessional' and 'multidisciplinary' working.

There are several similar terms – such as interdisciplinary and interprofessional – which are often used interchangeably.

The term *interdisciplinary*, as an adjective, relates to two or more disciplines collaborating together towards a shared goal. In health care, this may be care activity which involves the various disciplines within one profession. So, one example may be that of the disciplines of a children's nurse and a senior adult nurse working in

Accident and Emergency collaborating on addressing the needs of children requiring emergency care in that hospital. Another example may be a locality district nurse and a general practice nurse collaborating to work on tissue viability treatments offered in the home and at the surgery for consistency. Interdisciplinary communication will also be required when patients cross boundaries from the community into hospital or on discharge from hospital to home. A breadth of international, national and regional interdisciplinary networks and forums have been set up around certain conditions or concerns such as cardiac/coronary care, child health, learning disabilities or mental health.

Interprofessional as a term relates to two or more professionals collaborating towards a shared goal. In health care this could involve nurses, doctors, allied health professions (such as occupational, speech, podiatrists or physiotherapist), therapists and social workers collaborating in working out a management plan to discharge an older person with complex needs following a cerebral haemorrhage.

The term *multidisciplinary* implies that health care providers from different professions work together to provide diagnoses, assessments and treatment, within their scope of practice and areas of competence. However, this term is somewhat less used as it is now felt that it does not demonstrate an interactive relationship but is probably how health care practice usually manifests itself.

The term *collaboration* has also been defined by Goldman and Kahnweiller (2000: 435) as a 'mutually beneficial and well-defined relationship entered by two or more organizations to achieve common goals'. Petri (2010) undertook a concept analysis of *interdisciplinary collaboration* in the context of health care and developed a definition as:

> an interpersonal process characterised by healthcare professionals from multiple disciplines with shared objectives, decision – making, responsibility and power working together to solve patient care problems; the process is best attained through an interprofessional education that promotes an atmosphere of mutual trust and respect, effective and open communication and awareness and acceptance of the roles, skills and responsibilities of the participating disciplines. (2010: 79)

HISTORICAL AND CONTEMPORARY CONTEXT OF INTERPROFESSIONAL WORKING

Historically, different health care professionals have tended to work alongside each other. From the 1500s the development from craft guilds to professions has been documented by Reeves et al. (2010). They note the separate development of professions rather than an integrated development and thus health care tension arose. From a sociological perspective, linked to Freidson's (1970) theory of professional closure, different health and social care workers developed their own 'closed' organisation through professional training and indeed cultural values. The early professionalisation of medicine hence resulted in a hierarchical dominance over these other disciplines.

For this chapter, it is important to note that some areas of multiprofessional and multi-agency care have resulted in having more attention given to them than others and thus have attracted more developed national policy, regional and local policies and procedures. This has resulted in more mature attention being paid to vulnerability, risk assessment and multiprofessional and interagency care management and safeguarding. We need to be mindful of vulnerable children, which has been seen to lead the way in safeguarding, and then vulnerable adults, which may reflect the elderly, as well as those at risk of domestic and institutional abuse from a broad range of categories and the challenge of global human trafficking. The challenges of this range of 'social problems' have placed considerable stress and strain on all healthcare practitioners, multiprofessional and interagency working and health care leadership over the last few years. It must be said that despite these developments, children and vulnerable adults are sadly still hurt and die.

Child vulnerability set the way for working collaboratively. It was only in the mid-1970s that the UK started to collect data on child abuse and set up interdisciplinary child protection management systems. Several child deaths, such as that of 7-year-old Maria Colwell who died in 1973, led to the Fisher review which concluded there was a lack of communication between the agencies that were aware of her vulnerable situation. Eventually child abuse registers were set up in the 1980s; since the late 1980s, health policy has advocated effective interagency collaboration. This is in the context of several serious child deaths where reviews note the breakdown of interprofessional communication influencing effective child protection. The death of 4-year-old Jasmine Beckford in 1984 also triggered changes in child protection services; and as other children continued to be abused and died, the services and the government attempted to address policy and interagency practice. The rise in recognition of this social problem influenced another high-profile case, the 1988 'Cleveland child abuse' scandal, which emerged with what the media felt were overzealous medical and social professions removing over a hundred children from their families, most of whom were found to be wrongly diagnosed as abused. However, this posed issues of tension for interagency protection working to focus on the needs of children and the needs of families.

Ongoing policy documentation influenced the Children Acts of 1989 and 2004. Following the first Laming Inquiry, prompted by the death of Victoria Climbié, further child deaths such as those of Baby P and, in 2013 another child, 4-year-old Daniel Pelka who suffered at the hands of his parents, the lack of poor interagency working together was again identified. More interagency legislation has developed over the last few years:

- Female Genital Mutilation Act 2003 (www.legislation.gov.uk/ukpga/2003/31/pdfs/ukpga_20030031_en.pdf)
- Safeguarding Vulnerable Groups Act 2006 (www.legislation.gov.uk/ukpga/2006/47/pdfs/ukpga_20060047_en.pdf)

- Children and Young Persons Act 2008 (www.legislation.gov.uk/ukpga/2008/23/pdfs/ukpga_20080023_en.pdf; www.legislation.gov.uk/ukpga/2008/23/pdfs/ukpga_20080023_en.pdf)
- Children and Families Act 2014 (www.legislation.gov.uk/ukpga/2014/6/pdfs/ukpga_20140006_en.pdf)
- Children and Social Work Act 2017 (www.legislation.gov.uk/ukpga/2017/16/pdfs/ukpga_20170016_en.pdf)

This reflects the breadth of interagency policy to address the social problem to safeguard children. HM Government (2018) has updated the *Working Together to Safeguard Children* statutory guidance. All relevant professionals should read and follow the guidance, so that they can respond to individual children's needs appropriately. Policies in themselves do not prevent abuse, it is the commitment and best safeguarding practice of all those who work with children that do this.

Activity

Discuss with a colleague the role you both play in safeguarding children.

As a member of the public or as a healthcare professional, it is important to recognise that we all have a role to play in safeguarding children. Vigilance is imperative in society today whether you encounter children in your care or within your home or holiday community.

In terms of the vulnerable adult, adults are now living longer; relatives of those who are more vulnerable are often faced with caring for older and more dependent parents and family members. Historically the extended family or interprofessional community care provision was more accessible and available. Domestic challenges prove to be a social issue as more people look after their relatives in their own homes and the cost of professional care becomes too high. Along with this, the growth of the independent sector in care and nursing homes has meant that often older people without families become more vulnerable in institutional care. The White Paper (DH, 2015) *No Secrets: Guidance on Protecting Vulnerable Adults in Care* sets out a code of practice for the protection of vulnerable adults, with strong recommendations for an interagency framework and policy to manage potential and actual elder abuse. The Care Act 2014 attempted to address the care of vulnerable adults.

This Act explained how commissioners and providers of health and social care services should work together to produce and implement local policies and procedures. They should collaborate with the public, voluntary and private sectors and they should also consult service users, their carers and representative groups. Local authority social services departments should coordinate the development of policies and procedures. The importance of protection of vulnerable adults (POVA) has since been developed to note the 'safeguarding of vulnerable adults (SOVA)'. Policy and legislation has now been underpinned by this 2014 Act.

Activity

Explore this document on government policy and reflect on how this may affect your health care role.

www.gov.uk/government/publications/safeguarding-policy-protecting-vulnerable-adults/sd8-opgs-safeguarding-policy

The Care Act principles appear to fit well with all codes of professional practice:

- Empowerment
- Prevention
- Proportionality
- Protection
- Partnership
- Accountability.

However, often those dealing with vulnerable groups on a day-to-day basis may well feel unempowered themselves and thus not have the knowledge, power and skills to signpost to those who can take action. As an adult example, domestic abuse is possibly an issue not only for older people but also younger people and across men and women. Many people also suffer physical, mental and sexual abuse from their partners, family or carers. Health care professionals tend to deal with the resulting medical or psychological issues and rarely have time to address the deeper safeguarding adult issues.

Hague et al. (1996) undertook a two-year research study into multi-agency work which was supported by the Joseph Rowntree Foundation. They noted the variation in domestic abuse services across the country. There was concern whether the interagency collaborative approach was pioneering work or just a 'smokescreen'. They concluded that there was a need for a national commitment to resourcing interagency work in a structured, coordinated way. There is now more political pressure for health visitors and other health and social care professionals to screen families for domestic violence (Early Intervention Foundation, 2014). They link domestic abuse to what is termed the 'toxic trio' of domestic abuse, mental health issues and substance misuse.

Activity

- Have you considered domestic violence as another possible risk factor when you have cared for a patient with a mental health issue and/or substance abuse?
- Check out whether you are aware of any domestic violence screening assessment tools.
- Has this section raised your awareness of the health issues related to child abuse, elder abuse and domestic violence?

Screening for domestic violence has been developed in America but at the moment the NICE guidelines do not recommend it in this country. On 13 May 2014, the BMJ online identified that there was no evidence to support domestic abuse screening (www.bristol.ac.uk/news/2014/may/domestic-violence-screening.html). You may think these issues are not related to your role but perhaps feel you want to raise awareness of this social problem in your own working team or the wider multidisciplinary team if seen as relevant. Population screening is not advocated but raising awareness of services is important.

Another key emerging public health issue requiring multiprofessional working is that of global human trafficking. This has been identified as the trading of humans for the purpose of forced labour, sexual slavery or commercial sexual exploitation for the trafficker or others, and organ donation. It can involve vulnerable grooming and forced marriage and is linked with organised crime, coercion and exploitation (Aronowitz, 2009; Kampadoo et al., 2016). Ronda-Perez and LaParra (2016) commented that the health sector has a key role to play in this public health and social problem which makes victims invisible immigrants. They note that collaboration by 'actors' in health, social services, law enforcement, justice systems and non-governmental organisations in each global society is necessary to provide child and adult protection. However, Foot (2016) explores the complexity and multifaceted challenges, conflict and human challenges in collaboration in the context of gender, race, poverty and power. Health care leaders have a responsibility for raising awareness of human trafficking in their teams and the 2014 Jay Report which highlighted the recent shocking violations in the Rotherham experience between 1997 and 2013 that were taking place on our own doorstep.

EXPERIENCE OF INTERPROFESSIONAL WORKING

There may be positive or negative perceptions of interprofessional experiences by health care staff. Regan et al. (2016) concluded in their Candian research into perceived interprofessional collaboration that empowerment and authentic leadership promotes professional practice environments and enhanced interprofessional working. What are your perceived experiences? Chapter 2 identified several reflective models including Driscoll's (2007) simple model which is a useful tool for exploring interprofessional working events and their impact. The basis of this reflective model can be seen in Table 6.1.

Table 6.1 Reflection Model

What?	Report the facts and events of an experience objectively
So What?	Analyse the experience
Now What?	Consider the future impact of the experience on you and the wider community

Activity

Using the reflective model in Table 6.2, reflect on a recent interprofessional experience.

The activity shown in Table 6.2 may be useful for realising the complexity of working in an interdisciplinary way while caring for patients and clients and links to improving your health care leadership skills.

Table 6.2 Your reflection

Features	Underpinning Ideas	Your Practice Reflections
What? *What happened?* *Knowledge and comprehension*	**Describe event** Describe the situation: achievements, consequences, responses, feelings and problems	
So What? *Analysis/Evaluation*	Debate, compare and contrast Discuss what has been learnt: learning about self, relationships, models, attitudes, cultures, actions, thoughts, understanding and improvements	
Now What? *Application and synthesis*	Demonstrate, construct, predict Identify what needs to be done in order to improve future outcomes and develop learning What did you learn professionally and what skills do you need to learn about for the future?	
Can you now write three personal action points relating to improving your interprofessional working skills?		1. 2. 3.

CONTEMPORARY HEALTH CARE PRACTICE ACROSS ACUTE AND COMMUNITY SECTORS

The NHS as an organisation is an important and governmentally scrutinised public service element of what is known as the health industry in the UK. However, there are a great many health and social care industries that organisationally impact on the health of the nation – or even on global health.

Generally, the local arrangements for health care in the UK have a three-part structure:

- Primary Care (community care/walk-in centres)
- Secondary Care (acute/hospital care)
- Tertiary Care (residential nursing/care facilities).

Primary care usually involves the services that patients and clients can access directly from their home locality and does not require referral to specialist services. However, there are many views about what exactly it involves, and a specific definition is hard to pin down. It may be a number of services accessed via the local general practice or health centre but 'walk-in' centres or even Accident and Emergency provision are seen as primary care, although they may be located in both acute and community centres. The World Health Organization (WHO) is also now less specific about a definition but notes that the goal of primary healthcare is better health for all. There are five key elements identified to achieving that goal:

- Reducing exclusion and social disparities in health (universal coverage reforms)
- Organising health services around people's needs and expectations (service delivery reforms)
- Integrating health into all sectors (public policy reforms)
- Pursuing collaborative models of policy dialogue (leadership reforms)
- Increasing stakeholder participation.

The WHO Report (WHO, 2008) noted the importance of primary healthcare in global terms, now more than ever, in economically challenged health industries. Secondary care usually requires referral from a primary care service for more specialist services in an outpatient service or more directly via the hospital inpatient system. Interestingly, district nurses were formerly perceived as a primary care service, but in today's context an external referral is usually required and patients cannot always self-refer. Tertiary care usually means a service referred from secondary or even primary care, e.g. a specialised rehabilitation service, a nursing home or a hospice. The notion of quaternary health care is also emerging as a concept of highly specialised or even experimental treatment, but this is not yet clearly defined.

The boundaries between these care services are sometimes very blurred for patients as well as professionals.

Professional groups have in the past either seen themselves as working in community services or within institutionalised acute hospitals or specialist treatment centres. This has sometimes caused challenges for patient care when the patient moves from the community to hospital or when being discharged from hospital to the community services.

There have been several other models that aim to ensure that the patient journey from primary and community care into secondary or tertiary care, or secondary care back to primary care, is well planned and seamless. Services set up as 'inreach' community provision bring staff from community across into hospital services, a residential home or even prison services. Nelson et al. (2009) conducted evaluative research into an innovative inreach nursing and physiotherapy service in a residential home. They noted the challenges of cultural differences between the various services but concluded there was successful up-skilling by the staff in the home. Outreach specialised services are about bringing the hospital specialised services out into the home territory. There are also differences between skills, even within the same discipline. In community nursing there is a tendency for nurses to develop generalist skills covering a wide range of skills around medical conditions, in a comparable way to the practice of general practitioners. In contrast, those nurses who work in the acute sector tend to specialise in certain conditions in line with the medical direction of the clinical area. Generalist skills and specialisms in midwifery, mental health and learning disability are also evident. Interdisciplinary conflict may manifest itself when either a generalist or a specialist professional feels threatened. However, the generalist and specialist model of care offers the best of both worlds for patient journeys even while the challenge may be about the transition from primary to secondary to tertiary care. Also, another challenge for patients may be transition from one acute Trust to another where complex needs demand a variety of specialist referrals.

POLICY, LEADERSHIP AND WORKING TOGETHER

The government's structural framework for the National Health Service continues to stress the importance of interprofessional working for the needs of patients and children. Clinical Commissioning Groups (CCGs) were created following the Health and Social Care Act in 2012. CCGs are clinically led statutory NHS bodies responsible for the planning and commissioning of healthcare services and are:

- composed of membership bodies, with local GP practices as the members
- led by an elected governing body made up of GPs, other clinicians including a nurse and a secondary care consultant, and lay members
- responsible for approximately two-thirds of of the total NHS England budget, or £73.6 billion in 2017/18

- responsible for commissioning health care including mental health services, urgent and emergency care, elective hospital services, and community care
- independent, and accountable to the Secretary of State for Health through NHS England
- responsible for the health of populations ranging from under 100,000 to 900,000, although their average population is about a quarter of a million people.

The NHS Clinical Commissioners (NHSCC) (2015) set out a vision for the future of clinical commissioning, allowing more flexibility on local issues and solutions. Local collaborative partnerships were actively encouraged. The vision focused on the following:

- Delivering a healthier future
- Leading local partnerships
- Shaping healthy cities and economies
- Support from the start
- Excellence in commissioning diabetes care.

NHS England has the responsibility of developing CCGs, ensuring they are fit for purpose, and commissioning highly specialised services. CCGs work closely with NHS England, and as co-commissioners they work with NHS England's regional teams to ensure joined-up care. As local authorities are responsible for public health, CCGs work closely with them through *health and well-being boards*. They work together to achieve the best possible outcomes for the local community by developing a joint needs assessment and strategy for improving public health. There are now 195 CCGs in England (https://www.nhscc.org/ccgs/).

Team working, with various professions involved, requires skills and competencies in interdisciplinary collaborative working. All professional-based pre-registration education identifies multidisciplinary team working skills. Leadership in collaborative practice for patient care is recognised as an advancement competency. The NHS Leadership Academy (2011) highlights the NHS Healthcare Leadership Framework that was introduced in November 2013, as a development from the original seven dimensions of the NHS leadership framework.

The nine dimensions of the Healthcare Leadership Model are:

- Inspiring shared purpose
- Leading with care
- Evaluating information
- Connecting our service
- Sharing the vision
- Engaging the team
- Holding to account
- Developing capability
- Influencing for results.

You will find the framework a useful improvement tool to review your own SWOT analysis.

Activity

Explore how your own SWOT analysis aligns with the NHS Healthcare Leadership Model. Can this model provide any ideas for your own future career planning?

RATIONALE FOR COLLABORATIVE WORKING PRACTICES

It is generally seen as important that we work together across the disciplines and professions in order to address the following:

- Population health needs and demographical changes which reflect complex issues that cannot be addressed by a unilateral approach
- Public protection where health care staff support each other but are also charged with public protection in their codes of conduct and standards of practice
- Consumerism/public confidence
- Governmental targets
- Resource management
- Budget control
- Complexity of work
- Role expansion/extension
- Specialism vs generalist skills.

However, from some patient/public perspectives, the notion of interprofessional working has presented challenges. The public often have a much simpler perspective on the NHS and perceive it as made up of doctors and nurses. Depending on their experience of their care/treatment, however, patients/the public come to realise several other professional groups are involved – though they do not always understand the differing expertise or skills. The patient experience does not always receive consideration by interprofessional services and patients do not always feel at the centre of the activity (Howarth and Haigh, 2007).

In terms of the perspectives of the patient, interprofessional working has therefore provided some challenges. Some older people have found the complexity of various personnel roles, uniforms and badges they have met during a hospital stay somewhat confusing. If they need a home service, they may be confused by the number of professions who ask to assess their needs. A patient once stated that she had just experienced a 'circus' of visits from healthcare professionals which was tramatic, troublesome and extremely tiring – particularly as they often asked the same questions, sometimes within an hour of each other. Often a number of professionals fail to introduce themselves in a hospital and there is no overall record of who has seen the patient, and this further adds to the confusion for patients, their families, and also ward staff.

Activity

Can you identify the discipline/professional groups that could be involved in the scenarios in Table 6.3?

Table 6.3 Interprofessional scenarios

Health Event	Professionals and Support Staff Involved
Having a baby	
Bringing up a child until age 18	
Screening events:	
• Cervical	
• Breast	
• CVD	
• Prostate	
• Bowel	
Mental health episode	
Surgical intervention	
Eye issue	
Foot issue	
Stroke	
Problems with getting pregnant	
Children with a diagnosed learning difficulty or developmental delay	
A challenge where an older person in a family is told they are terminally ill	

EFFECTIVE COLLABORATIVE TEAMS

Activity

What do you think makes a good interdisciplinary or interprofessional team?

You may have had experience of interprofessional team working that provided satisfaction for you on a few personal and professional levels. The factors you may have thought about would relate to any kind of team effectiveness:

- Patient-centred goals
- Openness
- Collaborative decision making
- Clear communication channels
- Good conflict management
- Good leadership.

One aspect of effective interdisciplinary or interprofessional teams is how well the members of each teams collaborate with each other. McCrae (2011) noted that the multidisciplinary context of care has provided challenges for nursing models and thus the nursing-based theory that was taught in the 1970s and 1980s tended to be unilateral in focus. Sommerfeldt (2013: 519) concurred and noted that practice, assumptions, stereotypes, power differentials and miscommunication can complicate the interactions of healthcare professions where there is lack of clarity of knowledge, skills and roles in nursing.

Professional power is a complex concept, especially in its relationship to patient empowerment. Gilbert (1995) suggests that you need to understand power to realise the real meaning of empowerment. Bradbury-Jones et al. (2007) note that power is a contested concept:

- It has a diversity of interpretation.
- Everyone has an opinion of what it means.
- Power has a value (nebulous).
- Power is perception.
- The concept of power is interwoven with empowerment.

Activity

Jot down four ideas linked to the notion of power in health care practice.

You may have thought about the various power issues linked to different professions such as doctor, social worker and pharmacist. You may have thought about the types of knowledge they use or their skills in health and social care. Wilkinson and Miers (1999) highlight the work of Freidson, a medical sociologist who saw the profession as an occupation that had succeeded in controlling its own work and been granted legitimate autonomy, usually through the state. This in itself is a form of hierarchical occupational power in society. Some occupations are considered professions and others semi-professions. Social work and nursing may have been consigned to the category of 'semi-profession' on account of the perceived limitations of their knowledge base, training and autonomy (Etzioni, 1969). Democratic accountability and bureaucratic hierarchies are presumed to imply a degree of lay interference in professional activity which does not correspond with the traditional ideal of professionalism.

Orchard (2010) notes the importance of interprofessional patient-centred collaborative practice. The relative importance of the health care team and the patient/family and their choices, however, are often seen as being in competing spheres. Patients may 'move' into the sick role and don't realise or even desire a role in major decisions about their care within the context of the interprofessional team. The patient needs to be helped to retain control over their own care within the context of having access to the knowledge and skills of the interprofessional team. For instance, patients often feel confused when facing complex symptoms relating to the involvement of more than one medical specialty and dealing with various hospital and GP appointments. Bergman (2014) highlights that the health care world has a good deal of conflict among caregivers, patients and their families. He notes that medicine's scientific, psychological, and language complexities, high stakes, fragmentation of care, multiplicity of players, time constraints, institutional politics, cultural differences, competing philosophies and economic dimensions can hinder patient/family understanding. For those requiring acute secondary care, hospital life in itself also compounds the situation.

Public involvement in shaping health care is fraught with difficulties in engaging with ill patients or the multi-interest factors, but as the health service moves away from a paternalistic culture, public involvement is now a key principle for policy, research, delivery and medical education (Coulter, 2011). Pollard et al. (2010: 186) identify that policy has helped in the shifting of power, though they note the ongoing challenges of the role of 'lead professional' and that of information sharing. Snape et al. (2014) identify the various values involved with public engagement and question whether this agenda addresses the power imbalance. Laverack (2005) argues, however, that in professional practice someone can only possess a certain amount of power if another person loses an equivalent amount of the same. Do you think this is true?

Foucault (1995) noted in his work on the deconstruction of power that:

- it is 'exercised rather than possessed'
- it is not a thing, it cannot be relinquished
- it is embedded in everyday practice and interaction.

In exercising power this can be seen in:

- control
- politics
- wealth
- hierarchy
- a reaffirmation of the social order.

Cooke (2006) noted that those 'without power' are marginalised. Disempowerment, then, can reaffirm one's own identity with others in the same issues, leading to a solidarity movement embracing loyalty and conformity for those within the marginalised group. The issues of power present within each professional group are an interdisciplinary challenge as well as an interprofessional one. Some groups of nurses feel less powerful and marginalised than other groups of nurses. Similarly, this is true for allied health professionals, social workers and doctors. Urisman et al. (2018) researched the introduction of interdisciplinary ward round process in a surgical intensive care environment in San Francisco in the USA, using a mixed qualitative and quantitative approach. They concluded that this model of ward round improved collaboration and had a positive impact on the quality of patient care delivery.

OTHER CHALLENGES TO EFFECTIVE INTERPROFESSIONAL WORKING

The issues of power obviously pose a challenge in working with different teams but there are specific issues relating to interprofessional working.

Activity

What do you think are the main barriers to good interprofessional team working?

You may have thought of the following challenges or barriers:

- Differing professional philosophies, priorities, funding and status rewards
- Differing professional education and training
- Different professional uncertainties
- Gender/class differences
- Staff vacancies
- Agendas – personal
- Structural barriers within health care.

Stereotyping how we perceive different professions and even disciplines can hinder how well we communicate with each other. If we perceive the doctor as the top of the hierarchy, then upward communication may be more of a challenge. Nurses may either be seen as angels, battleaxes, handmaidens or sex objects. Doctors are an admired group in society but often perceived as male. Physiotherapists are linked with fitness and activity. Social workers have been described as wearing sandals and tank tops and health visitors linked with twinsets and pearls. Of course, these are all inaccuracies but it's a way of identifying the pigeon-holing and stereotyping of the range of professions. Rushmer (2005) in her research identified blurred boundaries between professional groups. She noted that informally staff are encouraged to blur the boundaries, in order to reduce protectionist and rigid demarcations which adversely affect service provision. Pollard et al. (2010) highlight the difference between the 'old' models of professionalism, stressing autonomy and specialist expertise which may inhibit health care transformation, and 'new' models of professionalism that emphasise the importance of teamwork and reflective practice. Tang et al. (2018) explored the collaborative experiences of eleven junior physicians and eight nurses in Singapore via themed analysis of interviews. Although a small sample, it was concluded that heavy clinical workloads, organisational constraints and differing power relationships affected interprofessional collaboration, and managers should encourage ward round participation and active contribution in the decision-making process of patient care. It appears that interdisciplinary and interprofessional working is an idea that requires commitment and experience to accomplish positive outcomes.

It is therefore seen to be necessary for professionals to be more flexible in their approach to working with other professional groups. They question what blurring of the boundaries may actually involve and whether it offers a way forward in resolving the difficulties experienced by differing health professionals in working together. Some of the challenges here concern what is termed 'professional tribalism', which is discussed in the following section.

COMMUNITIES OF PRACTICE, TRIBALISM, POWER AND PROFESSIONAL IDENTITIES

Lave and Wenger (1991, in Walmsley et al., 1997) argue that many professional groups behave in similar ways to tribes and suggest the notion of communities of practice:

Communities of practice are formed by people who engage in a process of collective learning in a shared domain of human endeavour: a tribe learning to survive, a band of artists seeking new forms of expression, a group of engineers working on similar problems, a clique of pupils defining their identity in the school, a network of surgeons exploring novel techniques, a gathering of first-time managers helping each other cope. In a nutshell: Communities of practice are groups of people who share a concern or a passion for something they do and learn how to do it better as they interact regularly. (http://wenger-trayner.com/introduction-to-communities-of-practice/)

Walmsley et al. (1997) suggest that individuals belonging to the same professional group exhibit many attitudes in common, especially at the ideological level. Individuals working in common circumstances, in similar positions, hold certain views in common, and this has implications for professional boundaries.

Activity

Can you suggest a variety of attitudes concerning care delivery in your present practice?

As a paediatric link health visitor in an outpatient clinic, I was mainly concerned with child development progress, nutrition and growth as well as home support via the health visiting service across the city. The liaison social worker was mainly concerned with supporting parents – with benefit and charity advice as well as social work and housing support in their district – but also focused on child protection social work liaison across the city. The paediatrician had requested the liaison roles in the clinic but her main role concerned the medical condition of each child and their medical treatment. Interestingly, as a team, this was seen as a holistic approach to care. The downside was that these morning clinics often overran into the afternoon as the needs of each child/family were considered from our triple perspectives.

Child protection issues remain a political challenge to interprofessional working and often in the media limelight, reflecting the dilemmas of safeguarding vulnerable children and supporting parents. Errors of judgement have been seen in too many cases over the years, but as the health and social care context of our society becomes more complex – with the mobility of families, complex family structures and the diversity of health and social care services – it is envisaged that safeguarding children will now pose a major future societal challenge. However, it must also be recognised that although children are a vulnerable group, there are many other vulnerable groups such as older people, those with learning disabilities or severe mental health difficulties, victims of domestic violence, and more recently the slavery of women involved in human trafficking. It is a sad indictment that safeguarding vulnerable adults has not garnered the same political emphasis. Many older people, the mentally ill or those with a learning disability are abused by families, carers and even staff in the caring services. These are often seen as the forgotten groups, overlooked by the political strategists.

Activity

Do you agree that poor interprofessional working in adult care has not been addressed with the same importance as childcare?

Why is this?

You probably work with a wide range of patients and clients, but you will obviously see individuals and families who appear more vulnerable than others. Adults often find difficulty getting health and social care support, particularly if they have some mental or learning disability challenges. There are limited safeguarding laws to protect these groups, and often the individuals involved do not have the capacity to understand fully the risks to them. It is, therefore, important that interprofessional care encompasses a more interprofessional learning model for the future.

LEARNING AND WORKING TOGETHER

Education plays an important part in collaborative working skills and knowledge. Interprofessional education (also known as IPE) refers to students from two or more professions learning together during all or part of their professional programme, with the objective of cultivating collaborative practice (CAIPE, 1997) for providing client- and/or patient-centred care. Laurenson and Brockelhurst (2011), using a tri-angulated method of research into interprofessional care in long-term conditions, concluded that educational providers and professional awarding bodies need to enshrine interprofessionalism within curricula and qualification accreditation, thereby intrinsically instilling collaboration into care provision. As noted, professional pre-registration UK courses now include interprofessional education as part of their curricula based on positive outcomes. Barr (2002) conducted a systematic review of the literature concerning interprofessional education (IPE) in health care, and from the literature noted that successful IPE needed to demonstrate/include the following:

- Service users at the centre of the programme
- The promotion of collaboration
- A reconciliation of competing objectives
- A reinforcment of collaborative competence
- A clear rationale for IPE both in learning and practice
- The incorporation of interprofessional values
- Common and comparative learning
- A range of interactive learning methods being utilised
- That it could be used towards self-assessment and qualifications
- Evaluation programmes
- The dissemination of findings.

Activity

- What are your experiences of IPE?
- Can you say whether they have been positive or negative?
- Did they fit with the recommendations of Barr (2002)?

Horsburgh et al. (2001) undertook research with a multiprofessional group of health care students in New Zealand and found that most students reported positive attitudes towards shared learning. The benefits of shared learning, including the acquisition of team-working skills, were seen to be beneficial to patient care and likely to enhance professional working relationships. However, professional groups differed: nursing and pharmacy students indicated more strongly that an outcome of learning together would be more effective team working; medical students were the least sure of their professional role and considered that they required the acquisition of more knowledge and skills than nursing or pharmacy students. The research concluded that developing effective team working skills is an appropriate focus for first-year health professional students. The timing of learning about the roles of different professionals may yet need to be resolved though. More recently, Bar et al. (2018) examined the attitudes of health care professional students in Israel towards interprofessional collaboration using a descriptive cross-sectional design, and concluded that perceptions of the role of other health care professions improved relationships and patient health care, and could be enhanced by interprofessional education and practice-based learning.

CONFIDENTIALITY AND ETHICAL ISSUES

One of the challenges for interprofessional working relates to the ethical issue of patient confidentiality. The Nursing and Midwifery Council (2018b: 5) identify confidentiality as a fundamental part of professional practice that protects human rights. This is identified in Article 8 (Right to respect for private and family life) of the European Convention of Human Rights which states:

- Everyone has the right to respect for his private and family life, his home and his correspondence.
- There shall be no interference by a public authority with the exercise of this right except such as is in accordance with the law and is necessary in a democratic society in the interests of national security, public safety or the economic well-being of the country, for the prevention of disorder or crime, for the protection of health or morals, or for the protection of the rights and freedoms of others.

They also note that it is not acceptable for nurses and midwives to:

- discuss matters related to the people in their care outside the clinical setting
- discuss a case with colleagues in public where they may be overheard and leave records unattended where they may be read by unauthorised persons.

Discussing the care of patients across the boundaries of a single care delivery setting is less clear. Sharing of information between medical teams in the NHS and social work teams in the Local Authority has been a long-term challenge. The important ethical consideration is about patient choice and consent when information sharing would benefit patient outcomes. Safeguarding children is a specific area where the rights of the child are more important than those of the adults involved.

INTERPROFESSIONAL WORKING AND GLOBAL HEALTH

On an international level, the importance of interprofessional collaboration has been more recently highlighted in trying to deal with global health inequalities. As the economic downturn across the world impacts on the health industry, the need for more effective use of the skills and knowledge across the professions globally will be even more imperative.

The World Health Organization (WHO) convened a WHO Study Group on Interprofessional Education and Collaborative Practice in 2007 to review the inequality issues, tackle the challenges within a global health workforce and maximise human resourcing. A framework for world health interprofessional education and collaborative practice was produced in March 2010: *Framework for Action on Interprofessional Education and Collaborative Practice* (WHO, 2010). It highlights the status of interprofessional collaboration around the world, identifies the mechanisms that shape successful collaborative teamwork, and outlines a series of action items that policy makers can apply within their local health system. It also provides strategies and ideas that can help health policy makers implement the elements of interprofessional education and collaborative practice that will be most beneficial in their own jurisdiction.

Summary of Key Points

This chapter has briefly looked at various aspects of team life to meet the identified learning outcomes. These were:

- **The importance of interdisciplinary and interprofessional working in health for effective patient care and safety** This was seen in the context of inquiries into poor health care standards but more positively in terms of working to improve patient care outcomes nationally and globally.
- **Critically explore the opportunities and challenges of interprofessional working in the contemporary context** The issues of policy attempting to address the

(Continued)

> (Continued)
>
> economic recession, stereotyping and the diversity of cultural differences between professional groups were explored. The opportunities for leadership and effective team working were highlighted.
> - **Identify issues of practice communities, tribalism, professional identities and the importance of interprofessional education** These issues were explored to raise awareness and support the need for improved interprofessional education.

ONLINE RESOURCES

For online resources, including SAGE journal articles, weblinks and videos, visit the book's website: https://study.sagepub.com/barr4e.

FURTHER READING

Day, J. and Wiggens, L. (2006) *Expanding Nursing and Health Care Practice: Interprofessional Working*. London: Nelson Thornes.

Freeth, D., Hammick, M., Koppel, I. and Barr, H. (2002) *A Critical Review of Evaluations of Interprofessional Education*. York: The Higher Education Academy.

Her Majesty's Inspectorate of Constabulary (HMIC) (2014) *Everyone's Business: Improving the Police Response to Domestic Abuse* – Domestic Abuse Inspection. Available at www.rotherham.gov.uk/downloads/file/1407/independent_inquiry_cse_in_rotherham (accessed 17 May 2018).

NHS England (2014) C4CC. Available at https://www.england.nhs.uk/ourwork/patient-participation/patient-centred/c4cc (accessed 29 January 2019).

National Society for the Protection of Cruelty to Children (NSPCC) (2018) *Child Protection System in England*. Available at https://learning.nspcc.org.uk/child-protection-system/england (accessed 29 January 2019).

7 COMMUNICATION AND LEADERSHIP

Chapter Contents

Learning Outcomes

By the end of this chapter you will have had the opportunity to:

- Describe various forms of communication networks and their effects in clinical practice
- Discuss the importance of effective communication and the 6Cs in the context of 'Leading change, adding value'
- Consider the benefits of therapeutic communication, active listening and Neuro-Linguistic Programming
- Explore communication, leadership and motivational theory and its place in the clinical area

INTRODUCTION

Leadership involves communication as a vital necessity at a number of levels in order to provide safe effective care. Within any organisation there are formal and informal communication pathways. An example of formal communication may be shift-handover reports or the ward round. However, within all departments there will also be the informal communication pathways as the day or night progresses with new admissions, discharges or changes in patient statuses. There are quite distinct communication pathway cultures between day and night staff where day staff get ready to take on board the business of mealtimes, drug rounds, multidisciplinary input and a range of diagnostic tests, procedures and surgical agendas. There is thus a huge amount of information that needs to be shared for safe patient care. The reduced night staff take over patient care where on the wards the focus is patient monitoring, drug rounds and rest, as well as other allocated administrative duties. Similarly there is less business at weekends and thus communication is different from that on weekdays. Changes in policies, training, consultation, appraisal meetings and 24/7 staff changes add to more complexity. Leadership must be aware of the differing formal and informal communication networks within their areas of control. This chapter sets out to discuss the breadth of communication forms and effective communication, as well as theraupeutic care and communication for staff motivation.

FORMS OF COMMUNICATION

Communication is a two-way process, complete only when the message is received (Weightman, 2004). It is important that the effective leader can adapt their communication style to each situation depending on the needs of the audience. That is not to say this is always a conscious decision. Communication styles, like leadership styles, are often intuitive, but they ultimately affect the overall performance of the organisation. It is useful, therefore, to understand how communication can be made more effective to reduce the risks of misunderstanding and unplanned confusion.

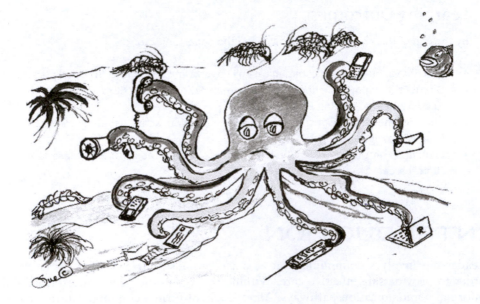

A model, as a representation of reality, may help to describe the communication process and consecutive stages through which someone or something must pass to achieve a specified aim (Weightman, 1999: Figure 7.1). The model also acts as a checklist to ensure each stage has been negotiated successfully, i.e. preparation for communication; delivery of the message; receipt of the message; analysis of how effectively you deliver the message and take corrective measures where necessary. However, exponents of models recognise that, as with many theories, the effective communicator is often unaware of using a model as they are doing 'what comes naturally' to them.

	PROCESS	CHECK POINTS
Encoding	Formulating the message. Selecting the right words or symbols. Understanding the person.	Clarify your objectives; is the message clear to the other person? What will be the emotional impact of the message?
Transmitting	Selecting the right method. Sending the message. Giving non-verbal signals.	Make sure there are no more than approximately seven ideas to transmit. Are verbal and non-verbal signals consistent? Is the language suitable?
Environment	Coping with distractions. Dealing with distortions.	Avoid noise and interruptions. Is the seating right?
Receiving	Understanding the message. Active listening.	What phrases, facts and inferences am I looking for? How can I test my understanding of the message?
Decoding	Making sense of the message. Understanding the other person.	What do they mean? What is the hidden agenda? How will I handle it?
Feedback	Encoding the response. Starting the message.	Nod, smile and agree to continue. Look interested, stop eye contact to stop.

Figure 7.1 The basic communications model

Problems may occur at any point of the model, so it is worth sitting down and working out where the potential problems might originate so that they can be addressed. This is applicable within all individual or group interactions. The overall purpose of communication is to ensure that messages are received and understood to make life easier, both in working and in home environments. Of course, the system goes pear-shaped at times and communication is not as effective as it could be, but if we understand what is happening then we can do something about it.

Another example of a communication model is one described by Shannon and Weaver (1954) and depicted in Figure 7.2. Whatever way the cycle is depicted, there is a purpose and direction for messages to travel for effective communication to take place. It assumes the communicator wishes to influence the receiver and therefore sees communication as a persuasive process. However you think of them, models are a simplified description of a complex entity that allows you to understand the process and so make it work for you.

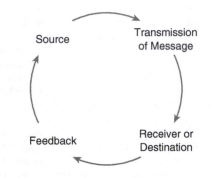

Source   Transmission
              of Message

Feedback   Receiver or
              Destination

Figure 7.2 Communication feedback loop
Source: adapted from Shannon and Weaver, 1954

Health care organisations tend to use a top-down model to communicate issues within the workforce and where directives are passed down, i.e. downward communication (Figure 7.3). However, bottom-up or upward communication (Figure 7.4) is encouraged within the realms of humanistic management techniques whereby the workforce is encouraged to share ideas with their managers and be involved in decision-making processes. Both types have their place within an organisation, but the effective leader *must* recognise which will be the most effective within any given situation.

The main methods of communicating any message are through verbal, non-verbal, written and visualisation mechanisms. Verbal communication occurs via face-to-face situations, by telephone or other electronic means such as television media, Skype or Facetime. Non-verbal communication involves gestures, body language, and even the way we dress or present ourselves. Written communication concerns emails, memoranda, reports, journal articles, health care records, newspapers, and material posted and accessed on the internet or other media. Visualisations include pictures, photographs, maps, diagrams, graphs and logos.

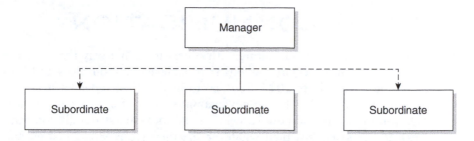

Figure 7.3 Downward communication

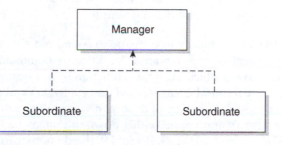

Figure 7.4 Upward communication

Activity

- Consider the stages of communication and attempt to formulate a message for a patient within your sphere of practice.
- Ask whether the patient can move their right arm up and down.
- Apply this same messaging task to a patient who is deaf, then for one who is blind, then for one who does not speak English.

You might have discussed the need for written material, Braille or an interpreter; you may also have thought of the type of environment you were in to see if it helped or hindered conversation/communication. I am sure we have all tried to carry on a conversation in a nightclub or where there is a loud TV, where it is difficult to hear yourself think let alone understand what is being said. Following anaesthesia there may be distortions in understanding due to the drugs. It is important to check that the receiver understands the matter being communicated by considering their response or by asking further relevant questions following the transmission of a message.

EFFECTIVE COMMUNICATION

Effective leadership means communicating with others in such a way that they are influenced and motivated to perform actions that achieve common goals and lead towards desired outcomes (Daft, 2017: 260), so to be an effective leader it is vital to be a good communicator. This chapter will examine various forms of communication to enable you to understand how knowledge and ideas are shared. If you can't get your message across clearly, then whatever the message is won't matter, and nothing will happen. Maxwell (1999: 23) stated:

> Educators take something simple and make it complicated. Communicators take something complicated and make it simple.

This alludes to the fact that things can be made to sound more complicated than they really are by poor or ineffective communication. Effective communication can thus be seen to influence the ways in which a team will function by motivating through planning and effective delegation. It must be remembered that leadership and communication are always affected by the overall structure of the organisation. Where there are many layers of line management, information passed either down or up may become distorted.

The NMC (2018b: 7 and 2018f: 3.4) require the demonstration of competency to provide good communication, including verbal, non-verbal and written communication, as a requirement for registration to practise as a clinician. However, despite the acknowledged importance of communication, there is no consensus definition of 'effective communication' in general health care (Chang et al., 2018). The importance of effective communication in health care has long been recognised, and there is extensive literature on this in general health care. Doyle et al. (2013) reviewed patient experiences and impact on clinical safety and effectiveness of outcomes. They noted clear information, empathic two-way communication and respect for patients' beliefs and concerns could lead to patients being more informed and involved in decision making, and create an environment where patients were more willing to disclose information. Evidence was also strong in the case of effective communication and adherence to recommended medical treatment. Ames et al. (2017) reviewed the role of effective communication in decision making in the context of childhood immunisations. All pre-registration health care programmes include communication in their curricula that reflects the importance of quality patient care.

Furthermore, Hargie (2017) suggests that for health care professionals effective communication leads to success in both personal and professional contexts. Hargie and Tourish (2009: xv) also say 'a highly educated, articulate and assertive workforce no longer wishes to be consulted and listened to – Generation Y demand and expect that this will be the case. One result of this is that the workforce wants communication like modern food – instant and always available when they need it', but beware of the 'rumour clubs,' the 'gossip mongers' and the 'coffee machine' conversations and information – what is transmitted may have been somewhat embellished!

Activity

- Think back over the last 24 hours.
- Make a note of how much time was spent in communication with someone else.
- What form did that communication take?
- What purpose did the communication serve?

You might have identified any of the vast number of communication forms that can be used, e.g. speaking/verbal (v), writing (w) and non-verbal (nv). Some of these are formal (f), some informal (if), and some mixed (m), e.g. department meetings (m), team briefings (m), saying hello (if), coffee break conversations (if), shift change-overs (m), memos (f/w), eye contact in the corridor (if/nv) … and so the list goes on. Effective communication should ensure that messages are received and understood by relevant parties, especially in health care environments – whether in an institution, an ambulance or a patient's home. Clarity is vital and particularly in this digital age where messages, texts or emails can be constructed quickly, sent quickly, and if they are not proofread effectively may give incorrect information or a poor impression, thereby hindering communication.

Health care managers often try various strategies to enhance team communications to get a balance between effective top-down and bottom-up communication. Team meetings, 'away days', and WebEx-conferencing may help to encourage and achieve better organisational communication or even across organisations, and may be helpful for large or small groups. Barr and Dowding (2016: 127) suggested a few reasons why you as a leader may communicate with others:

- To ensure that everyone gets the same message (Regulation)
- To change someone's behaviour (Innovation)
- To sort out a problem and raise motivation (Integration)
- To give factual information that people need to proceed efficiently with their work (Information).

LEADING CHANGE, ADDING VALUE AND THE 6CS

Communication is held as a crucial factor for quality patient care and Cummings's (2012) development of the 6Cs highlighted the importance of this as one of the six:

1. Care
2. Compassion
3. Comptetence
4. Communication
5. Courage
6. Commitment.

These values were one of the great legacies created through 'Compassion in Practice', a three-year strategy that concluded in March 2016. NHS England (2016) however suggested that the 6Cs are now embedded into everything nursing, midwifery and care staff do. They also noted the need to bring the same focus to measuring the outcomes, experiences and use of resources involved in health care. NHS England (2016) highlighted that the updated *Leading Change, Adding Value* (see Figure 7.5) framework for nursing, midwifery and care staff was also important and can be used by everyone in health care. It is aligned with the *Five Years Forward View* (NHS England, 2014) and embeds the 6Cs into the adding value model.

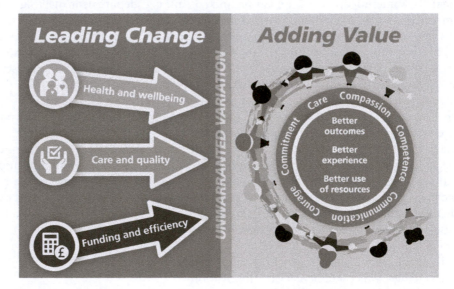

Figure 7.5   NHS England's (2016) 'Leading Change, Adding Value' and 6Cs model

Source: Reproduced with permission under the terms of the Open Government Licence.

To remind you of the 6Cs we can consider these as:

1. **Care** is our core business and that of our organisations and the care we deliver helps the individual person and improves the health of the whole community. Caring defines us and our work. People receiving care expect it to be right for them consistently throughout every stage of their life.

2. **Compassion** is how care is given through relationships based on empathy, respect and dignity; it can also be described as intelligent kindness and is central to how people perceive their care.
3. **Competence** means all those in caring roles must have the ability to understand an individual's health and social needs, and the expertise, clinical and technical knowledge to deliver effective care and treatments based on research and evidence.
4. **Communication** is central to successful caring relationships and effective team working. Listening is as important as what we say and do, and essential for 'no decision about me without me'. Communication is the key to a good workplace with benefits for those in our care and staff alike.
5. **Courage** enables us to do the right thing for the people we care for, to speak up when we have concerns, and have the personal strength and vision to innovate and embrace new ways of working.
6. **Commitment** to our patients and populations is a cornerstone of what we do. We need to build on our commitment to improve the care and experience of our patients, to take action to make this vision and strategy a reality for all, and meet the health and social care challenges ahead.

Activity

How have you considered the 6Cs in your last week of practice?

Discuss these with your peers/colleagues.

THERAPEUTIC COMMUNICATION

The communication skill base of therapeutic communication techniques has developed in the context of treatment, behaviour change and health promotion. Solution-focused therapy and cognitive behaviour therapy (CBT) are relatively well known. Other examples, which are less well known, are motivational and promotional interviewing techniques. Motivational interviewing (MI) originated from the early work of Miller and Rollnick where they defined it as a client-centred, directed method for enhancing intrinsic motivation to change by exploring and resolving ambivalence (Miller and Rollnick, 2002). The five key principles are:

1. Expressing empathy by use of reflective listening
2. Exploring the discrepancy between client goals and current problem behaviour
3. Avoiding arguments by assuming the client is responsible for the decision to change

4.   Avoiding resistance and confrontation
5.   Supporting self-efficacy and optimism for change.

Active listening is a way of listening and responding to another person which improves mutual understanding. Klagsbrun (2011) suggests the importance of active listening in the therapeutic context; professional active listening helps patients clarify their inner thoughts and concerns. She explores the situation of patients, many of whom often feel isolated and invisible in a hospital setting; it is the skill of active listening which can help the patient rebuild their sense of self.

In more general terms, when people talk to each other, they don't listen attentively. They are often distracted, half listening, half thinking about something else. When people are engaged in a conflict, they are often busy formulating a response to what is being said. They assume that they have heard what their opponent is saying many times before, so rather than paying attention they focus on how they can respond to win the argument. You can see this time and again when watching game shows that require a speedy answer – contestants often do not need to hear the whole question to come up with the correct answer, but equally if they buzz too soon they can get it wrong, so in order to become more active in the process the listener must take a structured approach to listening and responding that focuses the attention on the speaker.

In a professional situation the listener must take care to attend to the speaker fully and then maybe repeat, in the listener's own words, what they think the speaker has said. The listener does not have to agree with the speaker; they must simply state what they think the speaker said. This enables the speaker to find out whether the listener really understood. If the listener did not, the speaker can explain some more. Elements that tell the speaker that you are listening can be seen in eye contact, posture and gesture.

We can all tell if someone is listening to us. How many times have you been involved in a conversation and the listener is looking all around the room rather than at you, or they are sitting with their arms folded and leaning away from you? One gets the feeling that they are just not interested in what you have to say, and this can make you angry enough that the point of the conversation is lost.

ACTIVE LISTENING

Active listening has several benefits. Firstly, it forces people to listen attentively to others; secondly, it avoids misunderstandings, as people must confirm that they do really understand what another person has said; and thirdly, it tends to open people up, to get them to say more. When people are in conflict they often contradict each other, denying the opponent's description of a situation. This tends to make people defensive, and they will either lash out or withdraw and say nothing more. However, if they feel that their opponent is really attuned to their concerns and wants to listen, they are likely to explain in detail what they feel and why. If both parties in a conflict do this, the chances of being able to develop a solution to their mutual problem become much greater.

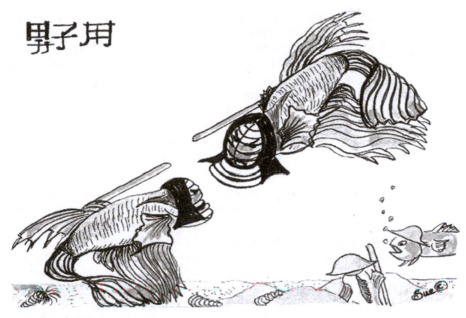

男子用

Source: Sue Saillet

The skills associated with active listening are normally denoted by the mnemonic SOLER, proposed by Egan (2013), which stands for:

Squarely face the person

Open your posture

Lean towards the sender

Eye contact maintained

Relax while attending.

Active listening is used in many ways by healthcare professionals, e.g. counselling, advocacy, restating/interpreting what other professionals have said to the patient to aid understanding and ensure that person knows what their treatment options are. There are several tactics that can be employed in order to effectively listen and understand the other person's point of view.

Paraphrasing is a useful tool. By restating a message, but often with fewer words, the listener is encouraged to interpret the speaker's words in terms of feelings. So, instead of just repeating what happened, the active listener might add 'I gather that you felt angry or frustrated or confused when ... [a particular event happened]'. Then the speaker can go beyond confirming that the listener understood what happened by indicating that they also understood the speaker's psychological response to it. This tests your understanding of what you heard and communicates that you are trying to understand what is being said. If you're successful, paraphrasing indicates that you are following the speaker's verbal explorations and that you're beginning to understand the basic message.

Clarifying helps you to understand exactly what is being said. It brings vague material into sharper focus so that the unclear or wrong listener interpretation is disentangled, more information is given, the speaker sees other points of view, and it identifies what was said, e.g. 'I'm confused, let me try to repeat what I think you were trying to say', or 'You've said so much, let me see if I've got it all.'

Perception checking again helps you to understand by giving and receiving feedback and checking out your assumptions, e.g. 'Let me see if I've got it straight. You said that you love your children and that they are very important to you. At the same time, you can't stand being with them. Is that what you are saying?'

Summarising is about pulling together, organising and integrating the major aspects of your dialogue, paying attention to various themes and emotional overtones, putting key ideas and feelings into broad statements but *not* adding new ideas. By doing this there is a sense of movement and accomplishment in the exchange. It may also establish a basis for further discussion and pull together major ideas, facts and feelings, e.g. 'A number of good points have been made about rules for the classroom. Let's take a few minutes to go over them and write them on the board.'

Primary empathy reflects content and feelings in order to show that you understand the speaker's experience, and that allows the speaker to evaluate their feelings after hearing them expressed by someone else. The basic formula for this is: 'You feel [state feeling] because [state content]', e.g. 'It's upsetting when someone doesn't let you tell your side of the story.'

Advanced empathy, by contrast, is a deeper reflection of content and feeling to achieve greater understanding, e.g. 'I get the sense that you are really angry about what was said, but I am wondering if you also feel a little hurt by it?'

Active listening intentionally focuses on who you are listening to, whether in a group or one-on-one, to understand what they are saying. As the listener, you should be able to repeat – in your own words – what they have said, to their satisfaction. This does not mean you agree with, but rather that you understand, what they are saying.

NEURO–LINGUISTIC PROGRAMMING

Linking to the ability to actively listen is the notion of being able to understand and 'read' how people are reacting to any form of communication or situation. Interestingly, the notion of Neuro-Linguistic Programming (NLP) may help with the ability to 'read' how people are reacting within a given situation, and thus what course to follow to achieve the best outcome. NLP was advocated in the mid-1970s by a linguist (Grinder) and a mathematician (Bandler) (Bandler and Grinder, 1990) who had strong interests in:

- successful people
- psychology
- language
- computer programming.

It is difficult to define NLP because those who started it and who are involved in it use such vague and ambiguous language that it means different things to different people. While it is difficult to find a consistent description of NLP among those who claim to be experts at it, one metaphor keeps recurring. Neuro-Linguistic Programming claims to help people change by teaching them to programme their brains. Furthermore, consciously or unconsciously, it relies heavily upon the following:

1. The notion of the unconscious mind as constantly influencing conscious thought and action
2. Metaphorical behaviour and speech, especially building upon the methods used in Freud's *Interpretation of Dreams* (1911)
3. Hypnotherapy as developed by Milton Erickson (2002).

A common thread in Neuro-Linguistic Programming is the emphasis on teaching a variety of communication and persuasion skills and using self-hypnosis to motivate and change oneself. NLP is said to be the study of the structure of *subjective* experience, but a great deal of attention seems to be paid to observing *behaviour* and teaching people how to read 'body language'. I am not aware of signalling my feelings because the message is coming from my subconscious mind, so how might we test these kinds of claims? Probably the answer is that we can't test them with any degree of reliability and there is no empirical evidence to back up the claim. Sitting cross-armed at a meeting may not mean that someone is 'blocking you out' or 'getting defensive'. They might just be cold or have a backache, or simply feel comfortable sitting that way. It is dangerous to read too much into non-verbal behaviour. Finally, NLP claims that each of us has a Primary Representational System (PRS), i.e. a tendency to think in specific modes (visual, auditory, kinaesthetic, olfactory or gustatory). A person's PRS can be determined by words the person tends to use or by the direction of one's eye movements. Supposedly, a therapist will have a better rapport with a client if they have a matching PRS. None of this has been supported by the scientific literature.

The BAGEL Model (Dilts, 2006) specifies the five elements (in mnemonic form) purportedly comprising the behavioural cues that indicate an individual's internal processes. The BAGEL Model is predicated on the notion that internal processes are subjectively represented in sensory terms (visual, auditory, kinaesthetic, and least likely, olfactory and gustatory):

*   Body posture (e.g. leaning back, head upwards and shallow breathing indicates visual representation)
*   Accessing cues (e.g. fluctuating voice tone and tempo indicate auditory representation)
*   Gestures (e.g. gesturing below the neck indicates kinaesthetic representation)
*   Eye movements (see eye accessing cues and the representational systems below)
*   Language patterns (specifically sensory-based, e.g. 'I see!', 'Sounds right!' or 'I feel that …').

Most of the cues we already know about and use within a meeting situation. A leader can tell when members of the meeting have started to lose interest because they fidget or fiddle with their pen – the worst-case scenario would be that the person goes to sleep. However, the eye-accessing cues of NLP (see Figure 7.6), normally outlined for the naturally right-handed person, are interesting and mainly unused. They are the core for NLP training exercises and involve learning to calibrate eye movement patterns with internal representations. According to NLP developers, this core tenet loosely relates to the VAK guidelines below:

- **Visual:** eyes up to left or right according to dominant hemisphere access; high or shallow breathing; muscle tension in neck; high pitched/nasal voice tone; phrases such as 'I can imagine the big picture'
- **Auditory:** eyes left or right; even breathing from diaphragm; even or rhythmic muscle tension; clear mid-range voice tone, sometimes tapping or whistling; phrases such as 'Let's tone down the discussion'
- **Kinaesthetic:** eyes down left or right; belly breathing and sighing; relaxed musculature; slow voice tone with long pauses; phrases such as 'I can grasp a hold of it'; 'I feel that …'.

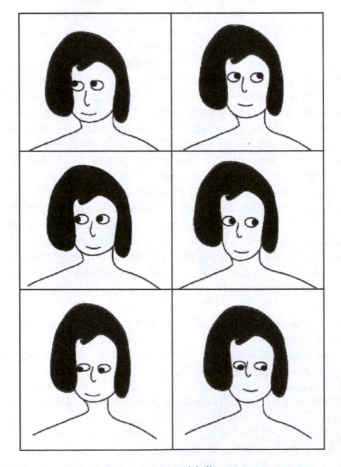

Figure 7.6   Verbal/auditory/kinaesthetic guidelines

NLP theory explains this breathing and mental processing according to the varying levels of chemical composition in the blood that affects the brain. 'Visual' people tend to be fast visual thinkers and can seem untrustworthy to 'kinaesthetic' thinkers because thinking by feeling is inherently slow. So by using judgements from your style compass (Figure 5.1), together with observing others, you can become an effective leader, although most effective leaders would say that they continue to learn as leaders and are open to new situations and new opportunities. Some authors use internal verbal/auditory/kinaesthetic strategies to categorise people within a thinking strategy or learning styles framework, e.g. that there exist visual, kinaesthetic or auditory types of manager. Certainly it is worth being aware of this, but without empirical evidence it is difficult to say, with any degree of certainty, that it is an effective practice.

These communication techniques offer valuable insight into advancing your leadership skills when dealing with patients, relatives and staff in your team or outside agencies.

LEADERSHIP, COMMUNICATION AND MOTIVATION

As a leader, it is important to consider the importance of how communication can assist you in team building, coherence and maturity to develop quality patient care and change improvements. Kjellström et al. (2017) undertook qualitative research in Sweden concerning health care professionals' motivation, and found that when their individual goals aligned with organisational goals and reforms, patient-centred health care improvements occured. This is important for leaders to translate improvements by integrating with the values and drives of staff and encouraging collaboration, participation, professional autonomy and structured reflection.

The concept of motivation is complex and relates to a desire or a need to behave or act in a certain way and can be affected intrinsically or extrinsically. As you might expect there are numerous theories of motivation, where each are either explaining the same concept using different words or offering a new theory; it is said that there are as many motivational theories as there are scholars that studied and continue to study them. Motivational theories can be clustered into three broad categories:

1. Needs, Growth or Actualisation Motivation theories
2. Hedonic or Pleasure Motivational theories
3. Cognitive or Need-to-Know Motivational theories.

Maslow's Hierarchy of Needs is an example of *Needs, Growth or Actualisation-*based theories. Maslow proposed that there were five hierarchical steps relating to the various needs of the individual. Each step must be fulfilled before the next step can be addressed. This model is represented as a triangle and the five needs are as follows:

- Self-Actualisation
- Esteem
- Social
- Safety
- Physiological.

As each need from the bottom is met, the one above becomes a motivator. So as hunger and thirst (Physiological) are met, security and safety become paramount and so on. This model has been further adapted to seven steps to include conitive and aesthetic needs before Self-Actualisation; see Maslow's Hierarchy of Needs (1943) on the book's website; www.businessballs.com/maslowhierar chyofneeds7.pdf

Maslow's Hierarchy of Needs (1943) has been criticised and modified by various critics. As a model it did not appear to hold true for many of the Jewish people in Nazi concentration camps where their physiological needs were not met but they were still motivated by their belongingness (social) needs.

Another example is McGregor's Theory X, Theory Y and Theory Z theories. McGregor in the 1980s proposed various assumptions about how individuals are motivated. He highlighted that Theory X assumes that individuals are lazy and self-centred in nature, lack ambition and will avoid work activity. Managers who prefer Theory X assumptions utilise a more authoritarian style and one-way communication. The use of threats and disciplinary action is more common. McGregor compared this to a more positive set of beliefs: Theory Y, which assumes individuals prefer to be involved in the work they do, seeking responsibility and a need for creativity and engagement in their work. Managers who prefer Theory Y assumptions utilise a more participative style of management and prefer multiple communication. There is a more developmental and liberating culture where performance management is favoured. Theory Z relates to Ouchi's (1981) work and is seen in the nature of Japanese cultures that reflect a tradition of lifelong employment. It assumes that people enjoy interaction, interdependence and use of reasoning, and thus managers' behaviours need to play to these aspects of work life.

Herzberg's Two Factor Motivation Theory is an example of *Hedonic or Pleasure* theories where praise underpins the way people behave. Herzberg discovered from his research that certain factors are related to job satisfaction or dissatisfaction. These were *not* opposites of each other. Trying to address dissatisfaction factors would not lead to satisfaction. If you want to motivate a team and lead them to improved performance, you need to eliminate job dissatisfaction and then focus on the satisfaction factors.

However, critics note that there is only an assumption between satisfaction and performance which has not been proved (see Table 7.1).

Table 7.1 Satisfaction and dissatisfaction factors

Factors for Satisfaction 'Motivating' factors	Factors for Dissatisfaction 'Hygiene' factors
Achievement	Company policies
Recognition	Supervision
The work itself	Relationship with supervisor and peers
Advancement	Work conditions
Growth	Salary
	Status
	Security

Source: www.mindtools.com/pages/article/herzberg-motivators-hygiene-factors.htm

David McClelland (1984) identified four motivational needs:

1. Need for achievement
2. Need for power
3. Need for affiliation
4. Need for avoidance.

His iceberg model depicts knowledge and skills (what you do) above the waterline, and then below the waterline there are opionons and values (what you think), and at a deeper level there are qualities and driving factors (what you want) reflected.

Victor Vroom's Expectancy Theory is an example of a *Cognitive or Need to Know* Motivational Theory. Vroom (1964) focused on outcomes rather than on needs like Maslow (1987) or Herzberg (1966). This theory states that the employee's motivation is an outcome of how much an individual wants a reward (Valence), the assessment of the effort will lead to expected performance (Expectancy) and the belief that the performance will lead to reward (Instrumentality). Expectancy is influenced by factors such as the possession of appropriate skills for performing the job, the availability of the right resources, the availability of crucial information, and getting the required support for completing the job. Instrumentality is the faith that if you perform well, then a valid outcome will be there. So, the expectancy theory concentrates on the following three relationships:

- **Effort–performance relationship** This assesses the likelihood that the individual's effort will be recognised in his performance appraisal.
- **Performance–reward relationship** This talks about the extent to which the employee believes that getting a superior performance appraisal leads to organisational rewards.
- **Rewards–personal goals relationship** This is all about the attractiveness or appeal of the potential reward to the individual.

Vroom was of the view that employees consciously decide whether to perform or not at the job. This decision solely depended on the employee's motivation level which in turn depended on three factors of expectancy, valence and instrumentality.

The advantages of 'Expectancy' theory are:

- It is based on the self-interest of the individual who wants to achieve maximum satisfaction and to minimise dissatisfaction.
- It stresses the expectations and perception; what is real and actual is immaterial.
- It emphasises rewards or pay-offs.
- It focuses on psychological extravagance where the final objective of the individual is to attain maximum pleasure and least pain.

However, again this theory is not without its critics as it is thought to be too idealistic and reward is not directly correlated with performance in many organisations. It is related to other parameters also such as position, effort, responsibility, education, etc.

Landsberg (2003) described an eclectic motivational theory and leadership as leading to a 'VICTORY Model' which reflects the relationship between self-motivation and the motivation of others. Neuro-Linguistic Programming (NLP) and the mastery of motivation model encompass the following themes:

- Vision
- Impetus (money, power, respect)
- Confidence
- Taking the plunge
- Observing outcomes
- Responding to feedback
- You.

This motivational model clearly supports the newer focus of the leadership activity of coaching and mentoring staff in the workplace. Porter-O'Grady and Malloch (2018: 404–6) raise the importance of coaching, mentoring and emotional intelligence (EI) for the twenty-first century and recognise these as advancing leadership skills and behaviours (see Chapter 10 for a further discussion). Within the health industry this is particularly important in supporting non-hierarchical multidisciplinary teams and in the context of clinical supervision.

Together with the need for effective verbal and non-verbal communication we must ensure that all paper and electronic records are now maintained correctly to validate the care given in whatever setting. Leaders should consider the importance of communication and reflect on how they can strive for better communication with all stakeholders in health care.

Summary of Key Points

- **Describe various forms of communication networks and their effects in clinical practice** Here we examined the notion of chain, wheel and all channel communication, recognising that these are models that depict the phenomena of effective communication.
- **Discuss the importance of effective communication and the 6Cs in the context of 'Leading Change, Adding Value'** NHS England postulated the notion of six elements of compassion in clinical practice and effective communication is one of the main components; together with this we have seen that the 'Leading Change, Adding Value' model can also be adapted and used by all those involved in clinical care and decision making.
- **Discuss the importance of effective communication** Without effective communication it has been shown that nobody would know what they were supposed to do within a given situation.
- **Consider the benefits of therapeutic communication, active listening and Neuro-Linguistic Programming** This is an essential tool of caring, as without it we may not really hear what our patients/clients are telling us. On occasion we know that even though someone is telling us that everything is OK there is something about the way they say it that indicates this isn't really the case.
- **Explore communication, leadership and motivational theory and its place in the clinical area** Motivational theory must be recognised in the clinical area, because without motivation people will not work to achieve the common aims of clinical care.

ONLINE RESOURCES

For online resources, including SAGE journal articles, weblinks and videos, visit the book's website: https://study.sagepub.com/barr4e.

FURTHER READING

Bach, S. and Grant, A. (2009) *Communication and Interpersonal Skills for Nurses* (Transforming Nursing Practice Series). Exeter: Learning Matters.

Bavister, S. and Vickers, A. (2004) *Teach Yourself NLP*. London: Teach Yourself.

Burton, K. and Ready, R. (2010) *Neuro-Linguistic Programming (NLP) for Dummies* (2nd edn). Oxford: Wiley.

Cassedy, P. (2010) *First Steps in Clinical Supervision: A Guide for Healthcare Professionals*. Maidenhead: McGraw-Hill/Open University Press.

Fiske, J. (2010) *Introduction to Communication Studies* (3rd edn). London: Routledge.

Pierce, J.R. (2010) *An Introduction to Information Theory, Symbols, Signals and Noise* (2nd edn). New York: Dover.

8 PROBLEM SOLVING

Chapter Contents

Learning Outcomes

By the end of this chapter you will have had the opportunity to:

- Discuss the concept of problem solving
- Critically review the models of problem solving
- Critically examine the theory and skills associated with decision making
- Critically explore the importance of clinical decision making and research within the context of problem solving for health care practice

INTRODUCTION

Health care practitioners spend a good proportion of their clinical and management time involved in dealing with patient needs and problems as well as professional decision making. Leadership therefore involves the need to have experience and skills in problem solving and effective decision making. Having examined the team, it is prudent to now focus on some of the relevant theoretical perspectives associated with problem solving and decision making both for the health care professional and from a patient perspective. The chapter will offer viable solutions and explore the clinical decision-making process. Problem solving in practice is seen as important in the context of evidence-based health care (Van Aken and Berends, 2018: 4). Muir (2004) noted the significance of clinical decision making, its effect on patient health care and the impact on the health care professional. Due to the complexity of health care, and the constant need to keep up to date, the professional is faced with a multitude of problems that require their attention. Professional accountability in the context of clinical governance and evidence-based care (Chapter 12) has also made health care professionals aware of the need to understand the nature of problems and the need to recognise the rationale for the professional judgements they make (Muir Gray, 2007; NMC, 2018b).

Goodwin (2014: 46) suggests that as the culture of managerialism has risen in the NHS, accountability is laced throughout professional practice and linked to autonomous practice and decision making. This is at its clearest in the codes of practice produced by professional bodies such as the General Medical Council (GMC), the Health and Care Professionals Council (HCPC) and the Nursing and Midwifery Council (NMC). These regulatory bodies dictate the standards to which each practitioner should conform and against which their performance may be evaluated.

WHAT IS PROBLEM SOLVING?

Problem solving is a key management skill that involves complex cognitive processes. It was VanGundy (1988: 3) who noted that a problem could be defined as 'any situation in which a gap is perceived to exist between what is and what should be'. On the other hand, Armstrong (1990) noted ambitiously that there were no real problems – only opportunities.

Activity

What do you think?

Think about a recent problem you have faced and decide which of the above ideas fits the situation in your view.

Although Armstrong offered a useful 'glass half-full' perspective it is not always true for certain life events. For instance, when the King family took their child with a brain tumour out of hospital in 2014 to Spain for proton therapy treatment, which UK doctors thought inappropriate. The Hampshire police became involved and the father was taken into custody. The media reversed their perspective of this being a criminal event to one where the family were pursuing the opportunities for treatment they thought was in the best interests of their child. In 2018 it was reported by Hardy (2018) that Asha is now eight, plays football rides a tricycle and is in remission.

Problem solving and decision making are often seen as the same activity. Problem solving assumes a fuller analysis of issues than pure decision-making issues because it relies on trying to discover the root cause of the problem. Decision making, however, may not address these issues in-depth and this can mean that the process will not take the same amount of time and energy (Tappen et al., 2004; Whitehead et al., 2009). As can be seen, the larger fish really does not stand a chance of getting into the bottle; the seahorses know this to be a fact but can do nothing to dissuade the larger fish from his task.

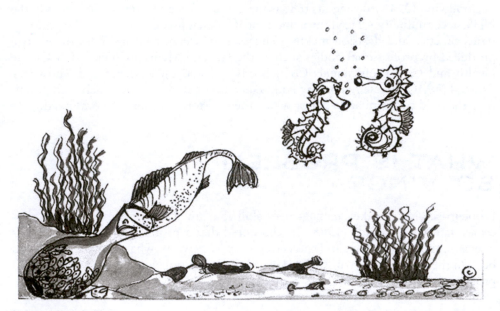

Source: Sue Saillet

In some of the literature you may find that decision making involves problem solving while in others decision making is seen as part of problem solving. For the purposes of this chapter, we will assume the latter model. Neither is wrong but is simply a different perception of the link between the two concepts. Huber (2014) identifies a tripartite relationship between problem solving, decision making and critical analysis. The reality of focusing in on problems may present a negative aspect of our professional work, so care is needed to balance this leadership activity with a proactive stance that seeks solutions to potential problems. Problem redefinition is often helpful in seeing an issue from a number of perspectives.

PROBLEM MANAGEMENT

Problem management can be considered using the main fourfold organisational management approaches:

- Classical Management
- Human Relations
- Systems
- Contingency.

The scientific (Classical Management) approach, where the need for optimum productivity is sought in an organisation, will relate to how problem management influences the goal. The Human Relations approach focuses on the impact and implications of work-based problems on people and the importance of their human values. A Systems approach highlights the impact and implications of problem management on the interdependency of relationships within an organisation. Finally, a combination of these ideas is seen in the Contingency approach (Barr and Dowding, 2016: 63–4). It was VanGundy (1988) who suggested that success in problem management relied on two elements: the approaches used and the nature of the problem.

The notion of successful problem solving relates to how organisations or individuals address the following issues:

- Recognition of the nature of the problem
- Assessing the intelligence, implications and impact concerning the problem
- Identifying the success criteria in problem solving
- Decision making for solution generation
- Communicating solutions.

Simon (1977) identified decision making as 'management itself'. He was also concerned with how decisions are made and how problem solving could be improved. This has real relevance for the health care industry if leaders are to learn how to do things better and smarter. The novice practitioner often looks for the 'quick fix' idea to solve a problem, using a 'blueprint' approach, whereas the effective leader uses a reflective approach, considering the wider perspectives or implications. Robotham and Frost (2005) highlight the work of Benner (1984) and describe the proficient practitioner as someone who perceives situations as wholes rather than in terms of specific aspects.

TRADITIONAL AND CONTEMPORARY APPROACHES TO PROBLEM SOLVING

Traditionally, problem solving and decision making used a rational model as a basis. One perspective, known as the 'Economic Man' approach, has underpinning assumptions that rely on two notions:

- That individuals are all working towards the same organisational goals
- Rationally, that they use the best methods to achieve these goals.

This model has been criticised because of the unrealistic nature of its assumptions. There is another approach to compare with the 'Economic Man', which is based on the real or actual behaviour of the problem solvers/decision makers (Cyert and March, 1963; Simon, 1994). Linstead et al. (2004) highlight the differences between 'Economic Man' and the more realistic 'Administrative Man' (Table 8.1).

In recent years feminist writings have rejected this patriarchal approach as being politically incorrect and 'man' would be replaced with 'person'. Either way, leaders of both sexes need to understand the nature of problem solving.

Table 8.1   Economic vs Administrative Man

Economic Man	Administrative Man (Simon, 1960; Cyert and March, 1963)
Rational approach	Solves problems that are 'good enough'
Complete knowledge of the problem	Complete knowledge not possible, knowledge is always fragmented
Complete list of possible choices	
Decisions based on maximising effect	Impossible to predict accurate consequences due to their futuristic nature
	Choice is usually from few alternatives
	Choice is based mainly on satisfying

THE TYPES OF PROBLEMS

In straightforward terms, there are two types of problems. First, there are the *simple* or *bounded* problems that face us every day and are fairly easy to solve in terms of the time and energy spent on them. Second, there are more *complex* problems that need a good deal of our time and often create internal and external tensions. There are many ways in which health care professionals manage the problems they face. It is often much easier to try and position a problem in the 'simple' category, particularly when we face a new situation where we think a quick solution is desirable and valued by others. It is, therefore, easy to jump to conclusions about the type of complexity of some problems.

Ackoff (1993 [1981]) and Ackoff and Greenburg (2008) described simple or bounded problems as difficulties or hard problems with clear boundaries (Figure 8.1). The more complex ones were referred to as 'soft, messy problems'. These messy problems are unbounded (Figure 8.2), connected to mess or chaos theory. There is uncertainty and there are no straightforward answers to these problems (Table 8.2). It is all too easy to try and solve messy problems quickly, like simple problems, without really thinking what the real problem is all about and who the problem concerns. The real trick is to recognise the type of problem, the stages for solving it, and how to make the process look and feel simple. Leaders unconsciously select an approach in managing problems that is most closely related to their personal leadership style. There is a continuum of approaches related to problem solving from a rational approach to a more creative approach. Both approaches have their place, depending on the situation being dealt with.

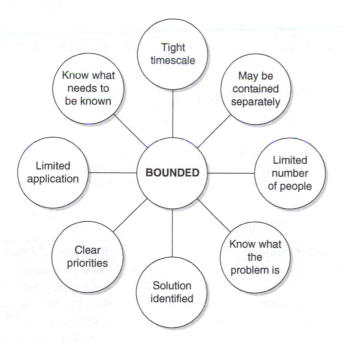

Figure 8.1   Bounded problems

Source: The Open University, 1996 © The Open University. Reproduced with kind permission

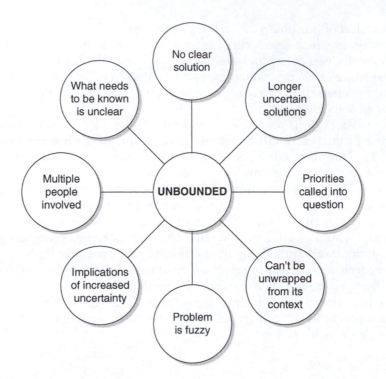

Figure 8.2   Unbounded problems

Source: The Open University, 1996 © The Open University. Reproduced with kind permission

SCIENTIFIC RATIONAL APPROACH

It has generally been accepted in the *rational approach* that there are several stages to problem solving that may help us to understand the concept. Marquis and Huston (2006: 71) illustrate a more traditional Problem-solving Seven Step

Table 8.2   Hard and soft problems

Hard Problems or Difficulties	'Soft, Messy' Problems
One clear problem	Complex problem
One clear solution	No one clear solution
Know what needs to be done	Answer can be one of many
Clear methods for working out solution	Uncertainty about the problem
Problem is structured	No obvious way of working it out
	Problem is unstructured

Source: Ackoff (1981)

Model. This can be compared to the handy Six Is model depicted by Stott (1992) (Table 8.3), which emphasises the need to involve relevant people when making decisions.

These stages seem like a useful way of logically looking at problems, but it must be said again that human minds do not always work in such a rational, sequential and logical fashion. We do not always work out solutions in a one-to-seven step process. We may look at any of these steps and move through various stages at the same time when dealing with complex problems. However, this traditional problem-solving approach is useful to see some of the elements involved and to have some memorable structure to work with. Indeed, this type of problem-solving approach has been modified to a four-stage process and utilised as the Nursing or Health Visiting Process in addressing the needs and problems of our patients/clients. Midwifery does not have a named midwifery management process because most of their women/clients are not generally seen as having problems but are undergoing normal physiological changes during pregnancy and childbirth.

Table 8.3 Traditional v Six Is framework

Traditional Problem-Solving Process	Six Is: A Framework for a Staged Problem Solving
1. Identify the problem	1. Identify: Try to understand the problem and its causes
2. Gather data to identify cause and consequences	2. Isolate: Separate the details of the problem and further define the criteria for successful solution
3. Explore the range of alternative solutions	3. Involve: Involve necessary and helpful people
4. Review the range of alternative solutions against evaluation criteria	4. Investigate: A range of viable solutions and evaluate their application to the problem
5. Select a solution	5. Implement: Decide, act and communicate a decision
6. Implement	6. Inquire: Ask about the effectiveness of the decision and reflect on the process for future learning
7. Review success	

Source: adapted from Stott (1992: 206)

There are also some three-stage problem-solving models that offer the simplest way of approaching problem solving (Table 8.4).

Table 8.4   Simon (1977) v VanGundy (1988)

Simon (1977)	VanGundy (1988)
Intelligence	Problem analysis and redefinition
Design	Idea generation
Choice	Idea evaluation and selection

INTELLIGENCE OR PROBLEM ANALYSIS

As stated earlier, there are a variety of problems – from simple to more complex ones. There are lots of problems facing health care professionals on an hourly basis which are dealt with quickly and intuitively because the solutions are clear. For more complex problems several problem-solving frameworks may be useful. The Six Sigma problem-solving and decision-making statistical model is another scientific approach (Pyzdek and Keller, 2014). It was developed by Motorola in the 1980s and is a quality model like TQM (see Chapter 12). Huber (2014: 76) notes that the model is 'error-free' and one decision-making application may be in the activity of hospital discharge planning. It is a complex model, in some respects, but Ackoff (1981) indeed felt that there was a need to look for different approaches when dealing with messy problems.

From these rational frameworks, there is more emphasis on analysing the type of problem presented, rather than reaching a quick solution. It is also important to look at who should be involved with the problem analysis as there may be many stakeholders in the context of the problem and the impact of the solutions (Stott, 1992). Stakeholders may be those who have an interest in the problem and workable solutions due to two factors: relevance and expertise.

The problem/solutions may have relevant implications for known stakeholders. Stakeholder analysis or mapping is a useful technique to consider, perhaps through an organisational value chain approach. Porter's (1985) 'value chain' considers a collection of processes to deliver a product or service. For example, these relate to primary and support activities in a hospital:

Primary activities may relate to:

- Admission
- Care
- Discharge
- Marketing/sales
- Other services – such as ambulances, referral to other centres, health promotion materials.

Secondary activities may relate to:

- Hospital administration: Executive, HR etc.
- Information services

- Diagnostic and other therapeutic services
- Other support systems; catering, cleaning, CSSD, linen, portering etc.

This value chain can also be extended to cross health care sectors from primary to secondary to tertiary care. Stakeholders in all these processes need to be considered.

One simple stakeholder analysis tool (see Table 8.5) may help you to think about the variety of stakeholders in the decision making.

Table 8.5 Stakeholder analysis tool

Stakeholder Interest ↑	Influence of Stakeholders ⟶	
	Keep completely informed (inform)	Manage most thoroughly (involve)
	Regular minimum contact (monitor)	Anticipate and meet needs (consult)

Other stakeholders who may not be directly affected may have expertise in supporting the decision making, so it makes sense to think about the wider group. For example, a team of community health professionals are aware of an isolated group of new mothers and their babies in a rural area, who have difficulty accessing the health centre/GP provision in the city. The team leader wants to explore the problem with relevant stakeholders such as the new mothers, the GP, the midwifery and health visiting team, social workers and the voluntary sector. It may not be possible to get all these people together physically, but if they can set up a communication network they will be able to explore the issues and reach a range of choices for a solution. The team leader may well engage with other stakeholders who can help because of their expertise, e.g. a financial expert, charity organiser or legal representative.

In some instances, stakeholders may be very few. For example, there may be time to work through health care goals and therapies with just you and your patient/client. Other cases may involve working through the problems with a variety of other professionals and the required quality of the solutions may arise out of a period of reflection and collaboration with others. It is useful, therefore, to identify who might own or be affected by the problem, or even be affected by any solution proposed: these are the problem owners. Remember, then, that the *problem itself* needs to be analysed, redefined, and separated from the *symptoms*.

A staged approach to problem solving may offer guidance for complex issues and help you to resist coming up with a *quick fix* solution that has no value in the long term. However, this notion of a staged process to finding successful solutions is still not without its difficulties – or debate – as the approach remains based on the notion of several assumptions that:

- the problem-solving process is a rational one
- there are no conflicting objectives within the process
- there is perfect knowledge which can be shared
- all viable solutions and consequences will be acknowledged.

ROLE OF THE CREATIVE/ INTUITIVE APPROACH IN PROBLEM SOLVING

Against the backdrop of the debate concerning the scientific approach is the value put on the creative or intuitive approach. The illustration confirms the intuitive approach of hiding from the predator (sea lion).

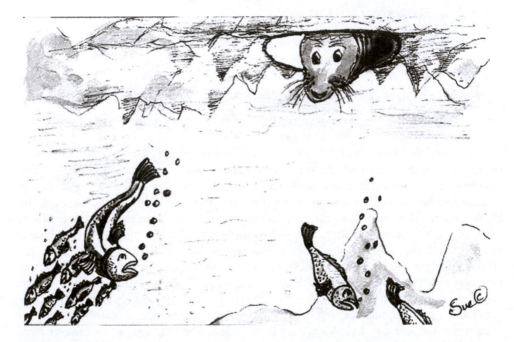

Benner and Tanner (1987) signalled that intuition relates to being able to understand phenomena without any rationale. McCutcheon and Pincombe (2001) used grounded theory to collect data from 262 Registered Nurses, to explore their perceptions of intuition and its impact on practice; they concluded that it is not some mystical power that appears from nowhere but is a product of the synergy that occurs because of several factors. It could, therefore, be said that intuition is a linear deductive process (Agor, 1986) and 'The act or faculty of knowing or sensing without the use of rational processes; immediate cognition' (Wordnik, n.d.). More recently, Green (2012), using contemporary neurophysiology research and the philosophy of Jacques Maritain and Yves R. Simon, claimed that intuition, particularly nursing intuition, is a valid form of knowledge today.

I can think of many instances where intuition has played a major part in caring. One example was when working in the recovery unit of an operating theatre and a patient was ready to go back to the ward, but there was just something about her condition that I didn't like. I didn't know what it was but when she was seen by the anaesthetist he said she was developing heart block. On another occasion

Activity

Can you recall any problems you faced in the last month and relevant decisions you made where you were not aware of why you made them?

I remember dealing with a daughter whose father was terminally ill. When she asked whether it was advisable if she went home for a short rest, I decided to encourage her to stay a while longer. She was present when her father died about an hour and a half later and was pleased she had remained with him. Intuition has been linked with firsthand experiences influenced by prior patterns of knowledge. Having experience in dealing with many people who have died in your care, there are physiological and psychological patterns of events that are not always easily internalised or communicated to others.

Another view on intuition is one of heuristics, or rules of thumb, whereby substantial amounts of stored knowledge are bypassed using procedural shortcuts. Many think that this is really about common sense but people, ill health and health are complex issues.

Intuition is often used to solve problems at a subconscious rather than a conscious level (Buckingham and Adams, 2000). Indeed, the work of de Bono (1990) and others has enabled more creative problem-solving approaches to become accepted, and allows for fresh idea generation, lateral thinking and innovation, especially where the complexity of the problem may be overwhelming to the team. Creative approaches are often used in leadership courses for health care professionals.

IDEA GENERATION OR DESIGN

There are a vast number of management tools that can help in unpicking a complex problem in more detail. These tools can be shared among any of the problem stakeholders at any part of the process. VanGundy (1988) provides a wealth of ideas for problem-solving techniques:

- **PEST/STEP:** (Political, Economic, Societal and Technological context) analysis of problem.
- **Six honest serving men:** Kipling (1902), *The Elephant's Child*:

  I keep six honest serving-men:

  (They taught me all I knew)

  *Their names are **What** and **Where** and **When***

  *And **How** and **Why** and **Who**.*

I send them over land and sea,

I send them east and west;

But after they have worked for me,

I give them all a rest.

I let them rest from nine till five.

For I am busy then,

As well as breakfast, lunch, and tea,

For they are hungry men:

But different folk have different views:

I know a person small–

She keeps ten million serving-men,

Who get no rest at all!

She sends 'em abroad on her own affairs,

From the second she opens her eyes–

One million Hows, two million Wheres,

And seven million Whys!

- **Why method**
  - The problem statement is written down and the team is asked to keep asking 'Why?' to the responses to get to the root of the problem.

- **Input and output framework**
  - The input and output factors are uncovered to review the contributing elements and results on a situation.

- **Cause and effect or Fishbone** (Ishikawa, 1985)
  - The cause and effect factors are uncovered to review a situation. An Ishikawa analysis can use brainstorming to identify plausible causes or effects of an issue. The fishbone may involve looking at elements such as man, materials, 'mother nature', machines, measurements and methods related to a problem (www.mindtools.com/pages/article/newTMC_03.htm).

- **Thought-showering or thought-writing,** which can use a verbal or written word method.
- **Checklists**

- **Six Thinking Hats** (de Bono, 1990), where six coloured hats (with specific characteristics) can be used for individuals in a group to allow them to abandon their own personalities.
- **Six Action Shoes** (de Bono, 1990) is a similar approach to the above, but allows people to have two personalities/roles.
- **Metaphors or analogies** can allow you to see the problem in another context, such as a game, an animal, event or a journey.
- **Visualisation** may help in providing a reflective internal environment in thinking through a problem.
- **Reversals** are where problem statements are made, and the wording is reversed. For example:

  o   How to deal with relatives of patients parking, when there are limited spaces, can become how to provide relatives of patients with available parking spaces. This could lead to more provision of park and ride facilities where there is ample parking provision.

- **Superheroes and heroines** is where a hero or heroine is seen as the problem solver and you are asked to identify how they might see the situation.

Activity

Some of these ideas may be useful within your work teams and others may be useful in helping patients to work through their own problems.

Which of these do you think lends itself to patient support?.

You may have thought of a superhero-type person, the one you can always go to when you have a problem at work, the one who will offer suggestions while not making you feel small for asking for help. There may also be a person who looks on the good side all the time, looking for positives. I remember being on placement with a Sister who was always on my back, to the extent that I used to look at the duty rota to see if I was on with her. If I was, I would consider throwing a 'sicky'. I didn't, and a colleague pointed out that although I had another six weeks on placement it could be broken down into 30 days, and as I only worked with her once or twice every five days, that was only another six to ten shifts I had to do with her. That made it all far more acceptable to me, so I survived! Clearly, reflection on the situation made sure that I would not inflict a similar experience on students when I became a Sister.

'GROUPTHINK'

Caution must be taken when involving groups of people in identifying problems and solutions. Janis (1982) identified that when groups of people come together to make decisions they are more likely to conform to the majority decision because they do not feel comfortable being an outsider; this means less creative solutions may be offered up. This 'groupthink' is the result of group pressure which prevents members testing the reality and using their individual judgement to decide whether something is good or not. The outward signs of 'groupthink' present themselves in diverse ways; members of the group may be less likely to challenge the judgement of the majority as they don't want to be seen to be rocking the boat. Also, when suggestions within the group are asked for, there is reluctance to voice ideas. Janis further suggests that the following are key characteristics of 'groupthink':

- Illusion of invulnerability
- Belief in integrity of the group
- Negative views of competitors
- Sanctity of agreement
- Erecting a protective shield.

The consequences that flow from 'groupthink' are synonymous with those of poor decision-making processes and ultimately could affect patient care. Snell (2009) undertook a quantitative correlation study using a survey method to identify how job stress, conflict and ambiguity affected 'groupthink' in nursing in two acute hospitals. His research showed that the low to moderate incidence of these factors helped explain the low incidence of 'groupthink' in the organizations. As leaders need to bring out a diversity of ideas to address problem solving, they should perhaps work towards counterbalancing the possibility of 'groupthink' within their team.

CHOICE AND DECISION MAKING

The skill of decision making, within the context of health care, alludes to the presence of natural cognitive and learnt abilities. We learn to make decisions in our early childhood days through identifying how to connect with the environment; we learn to deal with more complex decisions as we develop through to adulthood and even into the role of health care professional.

Activity

Have you ever had an experience where you felt something was wrong with a patient during your training but didn't know what decision to make about that feeling?

I well remember a time when I was a very junior nurse on my first surgical placement during my first week. I had completed a task and noticed that the last patient in the ward didn't look very well. I didn't feel I had enough knowledge of what could be wrong to decide about his care. I was unsure what I should do but when the staff nurse told me to go on my break a few minutes later I made the decision to mention my concerns to her. The decision-making process took place but I have little recollection of the formality of recognising the various stages in a conscious manner. The staff nurse responded by going to see him and when I returned from my break she told me that he had unfortunately passed away (this episode took place prior to the introduction of Cardio Pulmonary Resuscitation in the 1960s).

Interestingly McCallum et al. (2013) explored the awareness of student nurses when caring for patients who were deteriorating and their ability to take decisions to refer on for medical support. Student nurses' skills in managing patients whose condition is deteriorating may be limited, and it was noted that learning and using 'Early Warning Signs (EWS)' scoring systems is not helpful in developing student nurses' decision-making skills. These findings concur with a study by Cooper et al. (2010) with a focus on student nurses which noted consistency with research undertaken with qualified nurses. One plausible reason for this may be the dissonance between early warning scoring systems and decision-making theory involving information processing, professional judgement and intuition. McCallum et al. (2013) indicated that EWS tools can deskill the student experience and development of their own problem-solving and decision-making skills, which involves getting to know each patient and their changing condition.

DEFINITIONS OF DECISION MAKING AND RESEARCH

There are many definitions associated with decision making. A Google search (www.google.co.uk) reflects these inconsistencies and uncovers the link with dealing with finite human and other resources, psychology, law and sporting events (Table 8.6).

Table 8.6 Definitions of decision making

The act of making your mind up about something (www.wordreference.com/definition/decision).
A decision is the commitment to irrevocably allocate valuable resources. A decision is a commitment to act. Action is therefore the irrevocable allocation of valuable resources (https://en.wikipedia.org/wiki/Decision).
A formal, written judgement or verdict (www.nfa.futures.org/basicnet/glossary.aspx).

Decision making may be a systematic and sequential process of making choices from several alternatives and putting that choice into action (Lancaster, 1999). Porter-O'Grady and Malloch (2018: 599) stated that in decision making it is the quality of the information rather than whether there is enough information to make a decision and act; if the pusuit of information is sought for too long then the time for effective action could be missed. Ellis and Bach (2015: 27) also distinguish between effective and ineffective health care team decision making where the former is featured by:

- Consensus
- General agreement
- Acceptability
- Toleration of dissenters
- Acceptance of diverse views.

Linstead et al. (2004: 489) noted that it could be regarded as a commitment to a course of action, rather than the action itself. An example of deciding could be when a nurse decides to administer a specific dose of a drug from the range that has been prescribed, e.g. if one or two tablets are ordered then the nurse must decide how many to give. It is not necessarily their visible action that constitutes the first stage of the decision-making process but the cognitive activity prior to this.

It is useful to see further development where multi-agency decision making is critical. JESIP (Joint Emergency Services Interoperability Principles, 2018a; 2018b) was a two-year programme from 2012 to 2014 to improve the way the Police, Fire & Rescue and Ambulance services worked together when responding to major multi-agency incidents. Much-needed practical guidance to help improve multi-agency responses resulted. A standard approach to multi-agency working, along with training and awareness, is now in place for organisations to train their staff. They have produced a shared model of decision making.

The Manchester Arena terrorist attack in 2017 required such a broad collaborative response to emergency decisions and major trauma events, and the Kerslake Report (Kerslake, 2018) highlights the lessons learnt from such an emergency; it is worthy of reading and identifying what impact it makes on you professionally as well as personally.

The importance of decision making is thus critical to everyday health care work. It is about giving patients/clients the best care to meet their needs. Bucknall (2000) undertook an observational study of decision making among critical care nurses in Australia and found that they made, on average, patient care decisions every 30 seconds. The three main decision-making areas were:

- intervening – to modify the patient situation
- communicative – to give or receive information
- evaluative – to review patient data to evaluate their status.

Nibblelink and Brewer (2018) undertook a literature review and found that acute care nurses employed a variety of decision-making factors and processes and informally identified experienced nurses to be important resources for decision making. They also highlighted that acute care nurses faced difficulties in using evidence in nursing practice. Experienced nurses bring a broad range of previous patient encounters to their practice, influencing the intuitive, unconscious processes that facilitate their decision making. Using naturalistic decision making as a conceptual framework to guide research may help with understanding how to better support less experienced nurses' decision making for enhanced patient outcomes. These clinical examples show how critical decision making is within the sphere of everyday health care, and often relate to critical episodes and patient outcomes. Table 8.7 gives you a comparison of how some management theorists have classified problem and decision types.

Table 8.7 Problem/decision types

Drucker (1989)	Simon (1980)	Stott and Walker (1995)
Simple or generic decisions – decisions are based on using principles	Programmed	Standard Crisis
Unique or complex	Non-programmed (novel, unstructured, consequential)	Deep (involving the generation of alternatives)

There are similarities between all these ideas sets but Stott and Walker (1995) appear to offer a little more relevance in the real world of health care with their inclusion of crisis decisions. It was Stott (1992: 203) who highlighted that not all decisions are of equal importance, and thus will involve a greater or lesser time commitment, the differing skills needed, who might be involved and what resources you may need:

- Standard decisions are those we make on an everyday basis and tend to be repetitive. Solutions are usually found by rules of thumb, procedures or policy, e.g. deciding to offer patients or relatives tea when you encounter them in stages of emotional upset.
- Crisis decisions arise from unexpected situations and need an immediate response with little or no time to negotiate and plan with others. A quick, precise response is required, e.g. in the case of severe haemorrhage or other life-threatening situations.
- Deep decisions require more intense planning, reflection and consideration. They may concern forward planning as part of change management and often incur debate, disagreement and conflict. They require a substantial amount of time and networking with a range of people, e.g. you may encounter a patient with complex needs who requires a greater understanding of their lifestyle and attitudes to health. At other times a case conference will need to be called to make decisions with several health care professionals as well as the patient and carers.

Visit the book's website to complete an activity relating to decision making.

There may be a need to use a variety of skills to solve problems – logical thinking, intuition or trial and error – depending on the type or the context of the specific problem. The kind of management skills and styles you have may affect the outcome of the solution and decisions made. Vroom and Yetton (1973) identified unique styles of problem solvers depending on their position on a management-style continuum. The style of problem solving will depend on who and how other people are involved in the problem-solving process (Table 8.8).

Table 8.8   Types of decision makers (Vroom and Yetton, 1973)

A1	Solve problems and make decisions using the available information
A11	Get information from subordinates and solve problems themselves
C1	Share problems with individual subordinates, generate solutions, then make their own decisions
C11	Share problems with subordinate groups, generate suggestions, then make their own decisions
G11	Share problems with subordinate groups, generate ideas, and come to a consensus on a solution

The quality of decision making may depend upon a variety of factors. Vroom and Yetton (1973; 1973) noted the following:

- Values and personal beliefs
- Life experience
- Individual preference
- Willingness to take risks
- 'Our' way of thinking
- Critical, collegial culture.

Buchanan and Badham (2008) concurred with these ideas but noted important principles for being considered a successful political decision maker. These were to be able to develop liaisons, appear conservative, clear the air, ally with power, use trade-offs effectively, strike when the iron is hot, ape the chameleon, limit communication, involve research, and know when to withdraw.

Activity

What do you make of these principles?

How could you apply them in your everyday work?

At first sight the principles appear to be interesting, but they may in part represent a double-edged sword. They imply networking is essential but there is a need to be careful and wary of the power within the environment and keep on the right side of it. Good decision making is therefore seen to be about awareness of the environment, learning from past experiences, wanting and forcing things to happen, and looking for new ways to solve problems while possibly taking risks.

APPLICATION OF RESEARCH

Doherty and Doherty (2005) looked at patients' preference for involvement in clinical decision making using an interpretative phenomenology/triangulated approach. They noted the continuum scale from full patient decision making to health care professional with full decision-making rights. The researchers conducted semi-structured interviews of 20 patients in one British Acute Trust; there were equal numbers of medical and post-surgical patients, and nine men and 11 women. Seventeen of the group were over 60 and the youngest was 18. The researchers categorised the patients into active, collaborative and passive, based on their responses (Table 8.9).

Table 8.9 Active vs collaborative vs passive role of the patient

Active Role of Patient	Collaborative Role of Patient	Passive Role of Patient
• Active decision-making role 15% (three) medical and 5% (one) surgical; 10% (two) noted the importance of personal autonomy, e.g. requesting the GP to prescribe steroids. However, they did not know about their discharge plans. • Patient knowledge The surgical patient felt he disagreed with his surgeon's opinion that he needed more surgery but he consented based on the fact that he wasn't asked for his opinion. • Communication issues Concern noted regarding the need for better communication.	• Shared decision-making role 40% (eight); believed they could make their own opinion but still required professional knowledge to help in decision making. • Specific barriers: one noted pain was a barrier to taking an active role; one noted Doctor interpersonal skills; two noted limited opportunity for being involved; one noted there were 'too many on the ward round'. 'Sometimes I find the doctors talk to the nurse and they don't consult you. You're the last one to know.'	• Passive role 40% (eight) – mainly because they felt 'Doctors had greater knowledge of illness' than they did. Some felt they were powerless.

These are interesting, patient-focused results as most of our research has related to health care professionals dealing with their own problems and decisions. However, more research may be needed concerning patients' roles in this activity. From these results it is suggested that most of the research participants experienced a paternalistic health service and never thought to challenge it.

Activity

How will this research change your practice?

You may have considered becoming a better patient advocate. You need to think about the perceived powerlessness of your patients and how you can help to avoid their passive role developing. This could be achieved by ensuring that the patient is made fully cognisant of the facts about their treatment, and any alternatives there might be, in order that they have an involvement in the clinical decision-making process. It is important that, whatever your discipline, your patients/clients can use informed consent for any treatment or intervention offered.

Summary of Key Points

This chapter has briefly looked at various aspects of problem-solving and decision-making theory in order to meet the identified learning outcomes. These were to:

- **Discuss the concept of problem solving** Only a small number of the many theories have been explored, but it was noted that problem solving is a key leadership skill that involves cognitive processes.
- **Critically review the models of problem solving** Traditional and contemporary approaches to problem solving were addressed, highlighting the notion that there is more than one way to solve problems.
- **Critically examine the theory and skills associated with decision making** Here we examined two models of problem solving, the traditional and the 'Six Is', together with comparing the three-stage models offered by Simon (1977) and VanGundy (1988). Value chain and stakeholder analysis were explored to consider the influence and interests of others in decion making.
- **Critically explore the importance of clinical decision making within the context of problem solving for health care practice** Clinical decision making was explored by the examination of research to support the need for multi-agency collaboration as well as patient involvement in the process.

ONLINE RESOURCES

For online resources, including SAGE journal articles, weblinks and videos, visit the book's website: https://study.sagepub.com/barr4e.

FURTHER READING

Dowding, D. and Thompson, C. (2004) Using decision trees to aid decision-making in nursing, *Nursing Times*, *100* (21): 36–9 (accessed 5 June 2011).

Dowding, D. and Thompson, C. (2004) Using judgement to improve accuracy in decision making, *Nursing Times*, *100* (22): 42 (accessed 8 May 2011).

Higgins, J. (2006) *Creative Problem-solving Techniques: The Handbook of New Ideas for Business* (rev. edn). Florida: New Management Publishing Company.

Thompson, C. and Dowding, D. (2002) 'Decision Analysis', in C. Thompson and D. Dowding (eds), *Clinical Decision-making and Judgment in Nursing*. Edinburgh: Churchill Livingstone.

9 ETHICAL, LEGAL AND PROFESSIONAL ASPECTS IN LEADERSHIP

Chapter Contents

Learning Outcomes

By the end of this chapter you will have had the opportunity to:

- Discuss ethics in the context of health care leadership
- Explore ethical principles, models, rules and frameworks
- Identify the importance of accountability in legal and professional contexts

INTRODUCTION

An important aspect of health care leadership is the ethical, legal and professional issues underpinning the relevant activities and expectations of the role. It is useful to have knowledge of these topics for all health care professionals. In the most simplistic of forms the notion of ethical standards can be embodied in the biblical phrase 'do as you would be done by', noted by Charles Kingsley (1863) in *The Water-Babies*.

This chapter will explore a range of principles and theories related to ethics highlighting key issues with regard to patients and provide an overview on the importance of legal and professional accountability.

ETHICAL ISSUES IN HEALTH CARE

Hawley (2007: 4) defined ethics as the 'study of people's moral behaviour'. Morality implies the difference between right and wrong or good and bad. So, truth telling as an example is morally good and right. Ethics is the study of what our conduct and actions *ought to be* (rather than what they are) with respect to others, the environment and ourselves. It is sometimes difficult to separate out ethics and legal issues. In health care, there have been several incidents where leadership morality has been questioned, e.g. the Tuskegee experiment in the USA from 1932 to 1972 into the treatment of syphilis, where 400 African American men with the disease were persuaded to forgo the penicillin treatment and be part of the control group. They were unaware of their rights and there was no informed consent. In New Zealand at the National Women's Centre an 'experiment' with women who had 'cervical cancer in situ' was undertaken between 1966 and 1987. Again, two groups were created with those having treatment and those that were not given the correct care. It was called 'The Unfortunate Experiment'. More recent ethical scandals in the UK relate to the 2001 Bristol Royal Infirmary Heart Inquiry into events between 1984 and 1995, where babies and children requiring cardiac surgery were not provided with the correct standards care and consequently died. This was not because of research experimentation but a poor organisational culture. The Kennedy Inquiry (2001) found staff shortages, a lack of leadership, an 'old boy's culture' among doctors, a lax approach to safety, secrecy about doctors' performance, a lack of monitoring by management, and a lack of leadership, accountability and teamwork. The scandal resulted in cardiac surgeons leading efforts to publish more data on the performance of doctors and hospitals. Other scandals have occurred and the Francis Inquiry (2013) into poor care has been one of the most recent. Northouse (2016: 337) notes that ethics is central to leadership because of the influence and authority which goes with it. Ethical dilemmas are also faced daily by clinical staff. Haddad (1992: 46) defines an ethical dilemma as a novel, complex and ambiguous problem that does not lend itself to programmed or routine problem solving for which a precedent has been set. In other words, ethical dilemmas are forms of 'messy' problems.

PRINCIPLES FOR ETHICAL HEALTH CARE LEADERSHIP

It is useful to explore the underpinning theoretical ideas and models for leading ethically. Beauchamp and Childress (2013) explore the four ethical principles in healthcare:

- **Respect for autonomy** relates to respecting an individual's right to making their own decisions. It moves against the notion of health care paternalism where the health professional 'knows best'.
- **Non-maleficence** relates to the notion of 'doing no harm' and the duty of care and action to avoid actual harm as well as the risk of harm.
- **Justice** refers to the expectations of society which are fair and right. Equity and equality are at the centre of this principle.
- **Beneficence** relates to health care plans and actions which are aimed at being good for the well-being of patients. This may be compromised by available resources.

These relate to healthcare leadership and are linked to the ethical leadership model.
   Marquis and Huston (2017: 88) expanded on these principles and highlighted the following:

Autonomy   Promotes self-determination and freedom of choice

Beneficence   Actions are taken to promote good

Non-maleficence   Actions are taken to avoid harm

Paternalism   One individual assumes the right to make decisions for another

Utility   The good of the many outweighs the wants or needs of individuals

Justice   Seeks fairness, believes 'equals' are treated equally and 'unequals' treated according to their differences

Veracity   Obliged to tell the truth

Fidelity   Need to keep promises

Confidentiality   Privileged information must be kept private.

CRITICAL APPROACHES TO ETHICAL DECISION MAKING

Several ethical theories may need to be considered when making clinical or leadership decisions:

- Deontological or duty-based theories (Kant, 1774-1804) emphasise what people do rather than the consequences. This relates to:

  o doing the right thing
  o doing it because it's the right thing to do
  o not doing wrong things
  o avoiding actions because they are wrong.

- Utilitarian or teleological theories (Bentham 1748-1832) emphasise the goal of actions and consequences.
- Postmodernism ethical theories highlight the following:

  o Virtue ethics, which concerns an individual's moral behaviour (McDowell, 1979; Hursthouse, 1999)
  o Care ethics, which concerns what makes an action morally right or wrong; initially developed through the feminist movement (Gilligan, 1977; Noddings, 2013).

The theories above are considered as Western in the philosophical approaches. This is often seen as different from Eastern world traditions which have evolved through the influence of cultural and health beliefs. The principles of Eastern ethical principles are said to be:

- harmony
- respect
- hospitality
- modesty
- balance.

(Hawley, 2007: 103)

Leadership involves decision making and therefore it is useful to realise the importance of ethics as the decisions will affect the lives of others in the team, the health care organisation, and the patients that are being served. Zydziunaite et al. (2010) identified, through a systematic literature review in Scandinavia, that there were three levels of ethical decision making within leadership:

- **Institutional**: related to the organisation
- **Political**: related to the organisation's management
- **Local**: professional expertise.

It was also recognised that record keeping in any of the above decision-making levels is seen in the context of professional and ethical standards of practice and within a legal framework. The ethical issues concern:

- **Integrity** The quality of possessing and steadfastly adhering to high moral principles or professional standards
- **Truth** Something that corresponds to fact or reality

- **Respect** Consideration or thoughtfulness
- **Confidentiality** Being entrusted with somebody's personal or private matters
- **Consent** To give permission or approval for something to happen
- **Informed decision making** Based on proper knowledge and understanding of a situation or subject.

There are a number of ethical decision-making frameworks from simple to complex. The IDEA Ethical Decision-Making process proposed by Daniels and Sabin (2002), and adapted by Gibson et al. (2005), is one which is fairly simple in its approach:

1. Identify the issues
2. Determine the relevant ethical principles
3. Explore the options
4. Act.

This model highlights the importance of exploring various perspectives and options before undertaking any rash decision-making actions.

HEALTH EQUITY AND HEALTH EQUALITY

Equity concerns fairness, impartiality and treating like cases alike. It is concerned with treating patients and clients equally when they are in similar situations. Health equality is seen as the condition of being equal and concerns the removal of disadvantage. Health inequality relates to differences in health experience and outcomes between different population groups; health inequity relates to differences in opportunities for different population groups, which result in unequal:

- life chances
- access to health services
- access to nutritious food
- access to adequate housing, etc.

NHS England's (2017) *Next Steps: The Five Years Forward Review* particularly noted the need to improve access to GP services. The target was that by 2018 40% of the country would benefit from extended access to GP appointments at evenings and weekends. By March 2019 this will extend to 100% of the country. It is hoped to improve access to cancer, mental health, urgent care and maternity services.

Buck and Jabbal (2014), through The King's Fund and the Joseph Rowntree Foundation, proposed a 'poverty-focused' NHS through a public health, system leadership and culture approach, e.g. deprived children and young people in Derbyshire were targeted through the development of care being offered nearer to their home or school, increasing access mainly through health visitors and school nurses.

Darzi (2018: 5) points to the issue of inequities of access to services. There has been a serious decline in the number of people receiving state-funded social care, putting more responsibility onto informal carers and leaving many without the support they need. It is also noted that timeliness on everything from ambulance responses to access to A&E to getting a GP appointment has deteriorated:

> The stress on the whole system – primary and community services, acute care and social care – is vividly illustrated by the significant increase in delayed transfers of care over the period (which is even starker when we consider those medically fit for discharge). Finally, there are also signs of rationing in terms of access to new and innovative treatments as NHS patients are denied care that is at the scientific and technological frontier. (Darzi, 2018: 5)

Activity

There are several words above associated with equity. Jot down what your thoughts are about the notion of equity and professional commitment to address this issue in your area of practice.

The notion of equity sparks off the health inequalities debate, and why some people have better treatment and care than others due to their postcode, their ethnicity, age or other social determinants. Professional commitment to equitable health care highlights an awareness of health inequalities and a need to look for opportunities to address these through innovative projects. Wickware (2018) notes the restrictions on GPs in London for surgery referrals, including hip and knee replacements. The restrictions have come as part of a review of eight surgical procedures, which aims to standardise how people are referred for surgery across the 32 CCGs in London. Therefore, inequity of referral across the country will be evident. Leadership and innovation is an important feature of modernising the health service to bring in better service delivery that is more responsive to the needs of the public.

ACCOUNTABILITY

Accountability within the health service is influenced by employment, criminal, civil and professional action. Legal and ethical issues are therefore important professional considerations. It is interesting to note that health care professionals, once held in high esteem, are now less trusted and are held to account more than before, as cases where individuals who have abused their autonomy for personal satisfaction and criminal activities have become more visible. The health care industry is also facing the ethical problem of trying to meet infinite demand with finite resources. Financial, physical and human resources are being allocated on a priority basis. This had been the case previously but there is now more openness.

The implications for these points are that ethical considerations form a vital component of health care management.

Legal issues stem from the statutes and the law of the land. As a health care professional, you should be aware of the legal controls surrounding your practice. Professional negligence in health care concerns any form of malpractice. Malpractice is the failure of a professional with a body of knowledge to act in what is considered a reasonable and prudent manner. This would imply a manner expected of the average health care professional in that discipline, based on expected judgements, foresight, intelligence and skill. Health care professionals hold their own personal liability concerning practice. Fletcher and Buka (1999: 53) identify that it is a professional code of conduct that will enable a judge to decide whether a practitioner was acting within the expectations of their profession. This point is known as the Bolam Test from a notable legal test case (Bolam *v* Friern Hospital Management Committee, 1957). Issues such as the position of trust afforded to the professional and the action taken to protect patients' or clients' best interests will be of interest in the eyes of the law.

Employers have no legal right, within a contract of employment, to ask you to account for your professional action. They could, however, bring a disciplinary case against you if you failed to account for care which was deemed poor, and this could thus lead to unemployment. It is only when there is a legal inquiry (criminal or civil) that a health professional may need to go to a court of law, e.g. child protection, murder or assault/harm cases, and account for their actions. In legal inquiries, the health professional may have to account for any breach in their 'duty to care'.

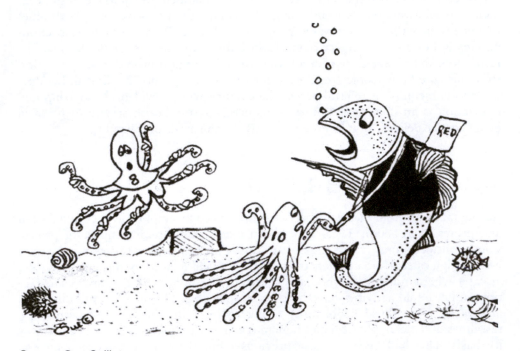

Source: Sue Saillet

The GMC, NMC or HCPC may also ask professionals to account for their actions but they have no statutory right to force an account. They can, however, through their disciplinary procedures make certain decisions concerning registration. The NMC (2017d) identified that nurses and midwives had an obligation to raise and escalate concerns and provide information regarding 'whistleblowing'.

The image above depicts a fish whistleblowing and giving a 'red card' for unacceptable behaviour.

Activity

Make a note of any recent clinical problems where you felt ethics played a part.

It may be that you have thought about resuscitation decisions made in your area or decisions about withholding medical treatment for certain groups of people such as the elderly, those with a disability, or those who have problems considered to be self-inflicted. You may have identified that screening for certain abnormalities may also pose ethical decisions.

Whilst the 6Cs address the philosophy of patient care, the NMC (2017b) states that 'Professionalism means something to everyone who works as a nurse or midwife' and describes what professionalism looks like in everyday practice through the application of The Code (NMC, 2018b; 2015). It recognises that professionalism has four key elements and defines these as:

1. Definition of what professionalism is, and its purpose
2. Description of attributes that demonstrate professionalism
3. Description of organisational and environmental factors to support and enable professional practice and behaviours
4. Description of individual responsibilities to support and enable professional practice and behaviours.

By adopting both the 6Cs and Enabling Professionalism principles the foundation of the profession will be strengthened, and the public will know what to expect whenever and wherever they meet them. To maintain professionalism all actions must be underpinned by the Code (NMC, 2018b; 2015a) highlighted in the following table.

Table 9.1 Professionalism and the Code

Being Accountable (Practise effectively)	Being a leader (Promote professionalism and trust)
• Problem solving • Able to challenge • Reflective • Evidence based	• Autonomous • A coordinator • Honest • Innovative • System thinking

(Continued)

Table 9.1   (Continued)

Being an advocate (Prioritise people)	Being competent (Preserve safety)
• Emotionally competent • Resilient • Impartial • Compassionate	• Technically competent • Critically thinking • Inquiring

Source: NMC (2017b) *Enabling Professionalism in Nursing and Midwifery Practice.* Available at www. nmc.org.uk/globalassets/sitedocuments/other-publications/enabling-professionalism.pdf

As role models, leaders should be exemplary in their conduct and accurate in their communication and record keeping. Leaders should abide by their professional ethical rules.

Activity: Case Scenario

Using ethics and your professional code as a basis for decision making consider the following scenario.

A 37-year-old gentleman arrives at a Walk-In centre at 16.30 hours complaining of acute abdominal pain. His English is poor, and he is in a poor state of dress:

   Q1.What are your initial clinical actions and why?

   Q2.Would these actions be the same if the gentleman stated he was on holiday from Tunisia?

   Q3.What are the ethical issues you may wish to consider?

Initially, you will assess his condition as with any clinical situation – you cannot withhold care but must 'act in his best interests'. The Code of Ethics surrounding your practice and duty of care is governed by your relevant council (NMC; HCPC; GMC) which recognises the importance of arranging an interpreter as soon as possible to ensure informed consent and that continuing care is relevant. However, you will also need to liaise with the finance department to ascertain if he will be required to pay for his care; for those currently inside the EU there are reciprocal arrangements in place for care provision, but for non-EU residents this is not the case. Clearly, when the UK has left the EU you will need to readdress this issue.

CONFIDENTIALITY

The need for continued vigilance to maintain confidentiality is an important ethical rule in health care. This means that relevant health information concerning patients should not be disclosed to others, even after the patient dies. The DH's (2003) *Confidentiality: NHS Code of Practice* notes that 'patient information is generally held under legal and ethical obligations of confidentiality. Information provided in confidence should not be used or disclosed in a form that might identify a patient without their consent. There are a number of important exceptions to this rule but it applies in most circumstances. This Code is based on current legal requirements and professional best practice. This will assist organisations in implementing the recommendations of the Mid Staffordshire NHS Foundation Trust Public Inquiry relating to records management and transparency.

INFORMED CONSENT

Informed consent underpins the principle of autonomy as an ethical rule. Clinically, for patients, this autonomy requires information on their condition, the choices that may be available regarding treatment, and the risks and benefits of these treatments. However, patient autonomy will depend on their mental capacity to make reasoned decisions without external pressure. Fry and Johnstone (2008) highlight that above all else, consent means patients exercising their will to decide, understanding the information given and given help to understand, with no coercion. Busquets and Caïs (2017) undertook an interpretive designed piece of research with 20 seriously ill patients in Spain. They found patients had serious difficulty obtaining and then understanding the information offered to them at the moment when they were being asked to sign informed consent documents. They were also critical of the consent documents, which they considered were treated as a mere formality; some even felt they had been coerced to sign. They concluded that in good professional practice, health professionals need to provide patients with whatever medical information will help them reorganise their lives to manage their illness. Communicative skills are needed to help patients understand their situation and that are attuned to any particular fragility and vulnerability of an ill person.

RECORD KEEPING

The importance of documentation will grow in the future as the culture of litigation increases and health care expectations rise. Paper records are beginning to be over-taken by computerised records so that, while previously there was a need to retain records of care delivered for some time before they were destroyed, this will become a thing of the past as giant computer mainframes store information electronically. NHS Digital now has a legal responsibility to collect data about NHS and social care services. However, patients can now choose not to have their information shared or used for any purpose beyond providing their treatment or care. The *Records Management Code of Practice for Health and Social Care* (Information Government Alliance/DH, 2016) is a guide to the practice of managing records. This Code is relevant to organisations that work within, or under contract to, NHS organisations in England. It also includes public health functions in Local Authorities and Adult Social Care where there is joint care provided within the NHS. There is a drive towards more standardised formats within electronic records. NICE supports record-keeping guidance for doctors (Academy of Medical Royal Colleges, 2008). The RCN (2017) also provides the following advice:

- Records should be completed at the time or as soon as possible after the event.
- All records must be signed, timed and dated if handwritten.
- If digital, they must be traceable to the person who provided the care that is being documented.
- Ensure that it is up to date in the use of electronic systems in your place of work, including security, confidentiality and appropriate usage.
- Records must be completed accurately and without any falsification and provide information about the care given as well as arrangements for future and ongoing care.
- Jargon and speculation should be avoided.
- When possible, the person in your care should be involved in the record keeping and should be able to understand what the records say.
- Records should be readable when photocopied or scanned.
- In the rare case of needing to alter a record, the original entry must remain visible (draw a single line through the record) and the new entry must be signed, timed and dated.
- Records must be stored securely and should only be destroyed following your local policy.

Record keeping can be delegated to health care assistants (HCAs), assistant practitioners (APs) and nursing students so that they can document care. As with any delegated activity, the nurse needs to ensure that the HCA, AP or student is sufficiently competent to undertake the activity and that it is in the patient's best interests for record keeping being delegated. Supervision and a countersignature are required until the HCA, AP or student is deemed competent at keeping records. Registered nurses should only countersign if they have witnessed the activity or can validate that it took place. Care is obviously needed with medical acronyms to avoid misunderstanding.

Patient records form a large part of any serious incident investigations, especially when the incident is directly related to patient care. The process by which an incident is investigated is often known as a root-cause analysis (RCA). Records help to establish, for example, what happened and when, what actions were taken, why those actions were taken, and who was informed about this incident. Investigations are difficult to complete when this information has not been recorded. Incomplete records not only imply that inadequate care was given, but also make it difficult for the root cause of the incident to be established and solutions to be put in place to address this. It is obviously important that accurate records of care are kept if one is to maintain registration and practise safely.

In light of the legislation that allows patients to access their own medical records, health care professionals need to consider a less paternalistic approach to this professional activity. Working with patients and family to document planned care, interventions and evaluation is essential. It requires a cultural change in this professional activity. So much documenting of health care activity is not seen as a partnership with patients.

Activity: Case Scenario

Ethical dilemma:

> In the community, some patient records are kept in the patient's home; however, in hospital, it feels inappropriate for patients and staff to discuss records. Observation and medicine charts are kept at the bedside but there is a notion that these 'belong to the nurses' and should not be explored or discussed as a true partnership. Medical records are kept in a separate trolley. Patients and families often struggle to know the 'planned medical clinical plan' or nursing care plans (agreed or not) in some NHS Trusts.

Discuss with a colleague how you might improve record communication and good partnerships with patients/families.

Medical or nursing records and plans in the NHS could be better shared. They often appear to change daily for some patients depending on individual registrar and consultant visits, which leads to patients and families becoming unclear about these and falling under the paternalistic approach. Private health care is less paternalistic and diagnostic tests and discharge letters are shared with patients.

PROTECTING THE VULNERABLE

All leaders need to be aware of key ethical dilemmas not only in their own area of clinical practice but also within the wider sphere of health care. There is a need to understand that each ethical dilemma health care case is individual and specific to the patient and family. The ethics around protecting the vulnerable remain enshrined in health care but are complex and multifaceted, depending on local arrangements for ethical decision making.

The main ethical dilemmas in health care concern the following:

- Reproduction, contraception, abortion and pregnancy
- Safeguarding children and those with learning disabilities
- Death and dying
- Organ donation
- Mental health issues.

Activity: Case Scenario

Consider the following scenario.

Mrs Brown has recently experienced a stroke, has left-sided hemiplegia and has a low mood and is very labile. She is being nursed in a rehabilitation unit. One day, you note that the physiotherapist is encouraging her to move from the chair back to the bed. However, Mrs Brown appears exhausted and tells the physiotherapist that 'it is all too much' and wants help with getting back into bed. The physiotherapist responds by saying, 'I think you could at least try standing up and straightening your left leg.' Mrs Brown attempts to do this but cannot straighten her leg. She then bursts into tears about the activities requested.

Q1.**What do you think are the ethical issues involved?**

Q2.**What actions would you feel are appropriate at this stage?**

The physiotherapist may see her encouragement of independent mobility as being of beneficence, i.e. doing good in the long term. However, it could be seen by the observer that this was not ethical encouragement but maleficence which resulted in upsetting a tired and depressed lady. It could also be said that Mrs Brown's autonomy and consent to therapy were being challenged and had a kinder response been made by the physiotherapist it would perhaps have resulted in a compromise. The notion of justice and society's expectations and fairness in health care can be questioned in the realm of elder and mental healthcare where there may be too few staff and resources to give quality, patient-centred care. From an observer's point of view, you might consider suggesting to the physiotherapist that you both help to get Mrs Brown back into bed for a rest and a cup of tea. You might also have a conversation with the physiotherapist that you would perhaps try again when Mrs Brown is less tired later in the day.

RESOURCE ALLOCATION

The allocation of health care resources can only be made within budget limits and it is the health service that decides this. When health services are limited, some might argue that these should be focused on those people who lead a healthy lifestyle as it is more cost effective. On the other hand, more compassion may be needed for those people who have had less life opportunities in life as others (Barr, 2007).

Health care resource allocation is decided at several levels: not just government, regional CCGs, Trust and other health care organisations, but also at other micro department or team levels. The ethical principle of justice is a subject for debate in relation to fairness and the right to health care. Cost-benefit, cost-effectiveness and life quality are key ethical concerns in the debate on resource allocation.

OTHER LEGAL ISSUES

Legal issues are obviously important in leading out in any health care organisation and ignorance of the law does not carry weight for any health care professional. Health care law, however, is complex and involves criminal law, Human Rights law, contract and property law, tort law and family law (Herring 2012:2). Ethical and professional considerations in health care are bound up intrinsically in the many statute Acts, policies and guidelines already highlighted in other chapters.

A recent legal issue affecting health care which is worth mentioning here is the General Data Protection Regulation (GDPR) (Regulation (EU) 2016/679). This is a regulation by which the European Parliament, the Council of the European Union and the European Commission intend to strengthen and unify data protection for all individuals within the European Union (EU). With respect to health data protection this involves the process of protecting data and the relationship between the collection and dissemination of the data and technology, the public perception and expectation of privacy, and the political and legal underpinnings surrounding those data. For patients as well as health care employees and all UK individuals, there are now eight rights that have impacted on all organisations and UK citizens:

1. The right to be informed. Personal data held have to be:

    - concise, transparent, intelligible and easily accessible
    - written in clear and plain language, particularly if addressed to a child
    - free of charge.

2. The right of access

    - Access should be provided in an electronic format if the request is made electronically.

3. The right to rectification

    - Individuals are entitled to have their personal data rectified if inaccurate or incomplete and a response to rectification request must be within one month if not deemed complex. Third parties must be informed where possible if the personal data are also disclosed to them.

4. The right to erasure

    - The right to be 'forgotten', or right to erasure, means there must be procedures in place for removing or deleting personal data easily and securely where there is no compelling reason for possession and continued processing of data.

5. The right to restrict processing

    • Individuals have the right to 'block' or restrict the processing of personal data.

6. The right to data portability

    • The right to data portability allows individuals to obtain and reuse their personal data across different services for their own purposes.

7. The right to object

    • The right to object means individuals have the right to object to direct marketing (including profiling), processing based on legitimate interest, and purposes of scientific/historical research and statistics, in which case you must stop processing personal data immediately and at any time, with no exemptions or grounds to refuse, free of charge.

8. The right to related automated decision – making and profiling

    • If any processing operations constitute automated decision making including profiling, individuals have the right not to be subject to a decision and must be able to obtain human intervention, express their point of view, and obtain an explanation of the decision and challenge it.

The power of individual rights over organised health industry organisations has yet to be tested as this came into force in May 2018. All those in a leadership role need to consider how this Act impacts on that role.

The complexity of law, ethics and professionalism is ever-changing and is in response to the current moral expectations in society. It is inherent in the leadership role that we are aware of the implications in every decision we make. Health care sustainability is essential for the future and poor decision making can ultimately mean we bear the cost in human, economic and environmental terms.

Summary of Key Points

• **Discuss ethics in the context of health care leadership** It is vital that health care leaders recognise the importance of ethics in their role. Being an exemplary ethical role model is key to excellent patient services.

• **Explore ethical principles, models, rules and frameworks** It is vital that health care leaders are aware of various ethical perspectives, principles, rules and frameworks to become effective and accountable in health care.

• **Identify the importance of accountability in legal and professional contexts** Accountability in all aspects and levels of health care depends on ethical practice. Legal, professional, employment and therapeutic accountability set out to protect patients with respect to confidentiality, consent and record keeping. Health care leaders need to be aware of vulnerability in the public domain and the complexity of resource allocation and other legal issues.

ONLINE RESOURCES

For online resources, including SAGE journal articles, weblinks and videos, visit the book's website: https://study.sagepub.com/barr4e.

FURTHER READING

Avery, G. (2013) *Law and Ethics in Nursing and Healthcare: An Introduction*. University of Essex: Sage.

Griffith, R. and Tengnah, C. (2016) *Law and Professional Issues in Nursing* (4th edition). Exeter: Learning Matters.

Woodman, W., Roche, S., McArthur, M. and Moore, T. (2018) Child protection practitioners: involving children in decision making, *Child and Family Social Work*, 23 (3): 475–84.

10 MANAGING CONFLICT

Chapter Contents

Learning Outcomes

By the end of this chapter, you will have had the opportunity to:

- Discuss the concept of conflict
- Critically review a range of models associated with conflict management
- Critically explore the importance of conflict management within the context of problem solving
- Recognise the importance of cultural diversity on leadership during conflict

INTRODUCTION

This chapter explores the notion of conflict management within the context of health care. Conflict involves discord and friction brought about by differences in ideas, values or feelings between two or more people (Forsyth, 2010). Each of us has our own values that form our thinking, behaviour and motivation; so not surprisingly when we meet and work with others we find they have different perspectives from ours. This may then give rise to conflict in any given situation, so managing conflict effectively requires many qualities and skills for effective patient care. Conflict is not necessarily a terrible thing; if you think back to the discussion related to group formation (see Chapter 5) the second stage, *storming*, is all about conflict as the group settles to become effective (or not) as they begin to work together, and as such is an inescapable part of team working. Where there are vast numbers of people with differing backgrounds interacting with each other daily, conflict is an expected occurrence; together with this we must consider the demands being put on the health service due to the competitiveness of diverse groups for scarce health service resources. Results of conflict may be poor team behaviour, time wasting, poor productivity, absenteeism, stress and ill health. Leadership, therefore, must be interested in managing conflict; leaders must try to foresee as well as make sense of conflict situations, and plan solutions before patient care is compromised. McElhaney (1996, cited in Valentine, 2001) identified that probably about 20% (about one day a week) of managerial time is spent dealing with conflict.

THE CONCEPT OF CONFLICT

In the twentieth century, conflict was considered in a negative light. In terms of organisational life, it was even thought to highlight poor leadership and as being dysfunctional to the objectives of an organisation. Everything was meant to run smoothly and harmoniously and so conflict was pushed underground or accepted passively. Buchanan and Huczynski (2017: 702) suggested that conflict was a state of mind perceived by the parties involved. There has been debate concerning whether conflict within organisations is harmful. Tjosvold (2008) argued that conflict was an inevitable aspect of all organisations, but if properly managed he believed it provided better ways of working by combining the energies of different team members who used their experience and knowledge to generate innovative ideas. In his view, conflict was essential to successful teamwork and organisational effectiveness; therefore, it should be welcomed and managed appropriately. By contrast, De Dreu and Weingart (2003) felt that conflict was always detrimental, and research that supported the beneficial aspects of workplace conflict was weak. They felt that organisations had to make efforts to manage conflict, not because it had positive effects but to minimise its negative consequences. An example of clinical conflict can be seen in the research by Pecanac and Schwarze (2018). They found that interventions which improve understanding of each profession's responsibilities may be helpful to reduce intra-team conflict in the ICU.

Activity

Think about a recent episode where you experienced a conflict situation:

- Write down ten words that come to mind when you think about this situation.
- Look back on your ten words.
- Would you say they are negative or positive words?

Conflict is now seen as neither bad nor good, so you may have written both negative- and the odd positive-sounding word. Good conflict management can bring about organisational growth whereas poor conflict management can bring about destruction. The other side of the argument is that 'well managed conflict' can be energising and vitalise forces that produce constructive group life, which is more of a positive, pluralistic approach and can result in a win–win situation (Handy, 1985; Covey, 2004; Cemi et al., 2012). Figure 10.1 reflects how conflict can affect the performance of an organisation both positively and negatively. On a more positive note, Chan et al. (2014: 943) note that constructive conflict can inspire innovations and creative strategies to address challenging issues, and improve teamwork, patient care delivery and outcomes.

Within clinical practice there are always elements of conflict due to the nature of professional roles and responsibilities. Pecanac and Schwarze (2018) undertook research regarding decision making about the use of Post Operative Life Sustaining Treatment in the Intensive Care Unit (ICU) between nurses and surgeons. A concept analysis using an evolutionary approach was undertaken by Almost (2006) concerning conflict in nursing environments. She found that conflict was a multidimensional notion with both detrimental and beneficial effects. The antecedents to the concept related to individual and organisational issues as well as interpersonal relationships.

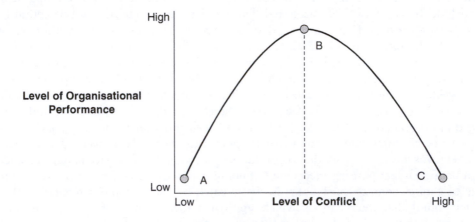

Figure 10.1   Conflict and organisational performance

LEVELS OF CONFLICT

It is useful to understand the three levels of conflict when leading teams in health care. These levels are:

- Intrapersonal
- Interpersonal
- Intergroup.

A good leader should acknowledge these as different but also recognise how to attempt to manage conflict competently.

INTRAPERSONAL CONFLICT

This takes place *within* an individual who may have difficulty in managing their contradictory felt needs or wants. It may involve role conflict or confusion, or it may be about balancing work and home life. Discord and unhappiness might occur before the situation is resolved. It is valuable to turn these internalised felt needs and wants into expressed needs. This can be achieved through self-awareness, and peer and leadership support.

INTERPERSONAL CONFLICT

This takes place between two or more people with different values and beliefs. It is becoming a significant issue in health care where the conflict may bring about bullying and harassment, causing discontent, stress and grievance. Farrell (2001) identifies the phenomena of 'horizontal violence' in nursing where some nurses are left squashed and deflated by more powerful members of their own profession; as is depicted in the cartoon, the more powerful fish is defending or deflating the small fish whilst fending off or harassing the swordfish.

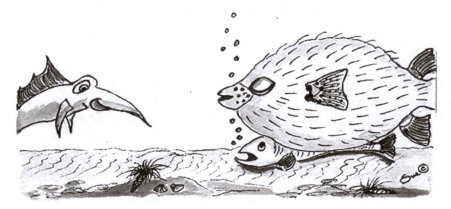

Source: Sue Saillet

INTERGROUP CONFLICT

This takes place between two or more groups, departments or organisations. This kind of conflict may be the result of jealousies about others receiving more resources, recognition or favourable rewards.

Activity

Jot down any examples of these three types of conflict you have experienced as a health care professional.

From a personal perspective, my own intrapersonal conflict example relates to the dislike of driving to work and back along the motorway with lots of roadworks. I try and leave home very early or later to avoid the rush hours. Recent interpersonal conflict related to confronting staff workload in a team, when one member was not happy helping another member of the team, because they felt they had enough to do. Last week, I experienced intergroup conflict when the teachers on the post-registration programmes felt the teachers on the pre-registration programmes got the first choice of classrooms in the university building. It sounds as though I have had a very difficult time but really, I see it as everyday working life; however, it can cause stress and disruption if not dealt with effectively.

STAGES OF GROUP LIFE AND CONFLICT

How conflict emerges is important, because if leaders can identify the initial stages they can deal with them appropriately. Indeed, in terms of developing a team (see Chapter 5), the principles of leadership are related to two main ideas:

- Diagnosis of the group stage
- Intervening to help 'move the group on'.

It is interesting to relate the stages of group development and where these fit with emerging conflict. As discussed in Chapter 5, Tuckman's (1965) notion of a natural sequence for small groups offers a straightforward way of identifying with group life.

Activity

Have you ever experienced ALL five stages described by Tuckman?

I have experienced these working as a theatre sister in an operating department where all the required instrumentation was available. Storming arose when we had new members in the team who were uncertain of the expectations in order that both the surgeon and anaesthetist had all they needed to ensure a safe and positive outcome for the patient care. Eventually they became assimilated in the team and we functioned efficiently again. Whilst there are many different models relating to conflict, it is important to remember that they are just a simple representation of a complex situation. You may find yourself preferring one model to another or using an eclectic approach to leadership during conflict.

CAUSES OF CONFLICT

The causes of conflict might have nothing to do with the work situation but may be associated, as briefly suggested above, with individual differences and possibly relate more specifically to differences in ideology and personal objectives. Conflict can arise or a variety of reasons. These can generally be grouped under the following headings:

- Hidden agendas
- Finite resources
- Departmentalisation and specialisation
- Work design
- Role overlap
- Unfair situations.

HIDDEN AGENDAS

The ward sister had been told in July that her rehabilitation ward would close in October and the staff would be relocated to another ward area. She had also been told that she must not discuss this with the staff as they would be duly informed at the beginning of September, when plans are in place. Staff are becoming concerned that the ward sister is reluctant to discuss any staffing issues. Rumours, from an unknown source, are starting to emerge that the ward will be closed. As might be expected the level of 'chatter' around this situation is escalating and putting the ward sister in a difficult position. Managerially it might have been better if either nobody knew, or everyone had been told what was proposed. The stress levels could have been reduced if the closure plan had been presented and the staff would have had time to accept the situation.

FINITE RESOURCES

A medical ward and a medical admissions unit (MAU) would like to send a few members of staff on a clinical update. Due to the turnover of patients in the MAU, staff numbers have been curtailed. All NHS staff are aware of the current problems of financing professional development, but if they are informed about the potential time frames for possible inclusion on courses they are invariably more accepting of the situation.

DEPARTMENTALISATION AND SPECIALISATION

A renal ward is introducing a new outreach service into the community. Selected staff will be supporting patients and district nurses in keeping patients at home as much as possible. Some of the senior staff will continue with their inpatient work but those chosen will be given a new title of 'renal specialist'. For the effects of this to be reduced there need to be very clear criteria for the selection of staff being transferered to the outreach facility (qualifications, roles, responsibilities etc.) so that everyone can appreciate their position in the team.

WORK DESIGN

The general surgical theatre nursing staff have been divided into two teams and their theatre coverage has been allocated between the two theatres. One team, however, appears to complete their elective work by 4:30 p.m. while the other team are faced with elective work until 5:30 p.m. Using emotional intelligence the staff who have completed their list might go to those in the other theatre to see if they could relieve someone for a short break, start to wash down the 'scrubroom' or offer some other help.

ROLE OVERLAP

The district nurse has been sent a referral from the hospital to visit a patient. When she gets to the patient's house, the Macmillan nurse is there already, and the district nurse feels that she will not be required. Here, there is confusion about the complexity of community roles and an overlap of role expectations. This scenario highlights they need for effective communication with the patient, their family and community services, regarding discharge planning.

UNFAIR SITUATIONS

The night staff in a clinical area cannot gain access to educational updates while on duty. They have to try and 'fit their professional development' sessions in and around their working hours, which often means they get to the sessions after only a couple of hours' sleep or in the middle of their annual leave. The day staff can get to their updates for these sessions during their working time. Some employers can put on formal update sessions in the evening prior to a duty shift, in order to accommodate and address this problem.

SYMPTOMS OF CONFLICT OR COLLISION

From the above examples conflict can be a result of the multiple competing demands we have in health care. Leadership is required to help deal with past, present and even anticipated conflict situations. There are underpinning symptoms of conflict; these can help us to identify situations before the conflict becomes too oppressive.

These symptoms are:

- Territorial issues
- Poor communication – laterally or vertically
- Intergroup jealousy
- Interpersonal friction (personalities)
- Escalation of arbitration
- Increasing rules, norms and myths
- Evidence of low morale.

Activity

Make some notes of these symptoms related to the following:

- Your past work-life experience
- Your current work-life situation
- Potential future work-life issues.

You will probably recognise that these symptoms are a feature in all work-life experiences. These symptoms may culminate in increasing sickness/absence and ultimately clinical staff retention. When pursuing new positions, you may need to critically question why a vacancy has occurred and why the position looks so glamorous. Being aware of 'staff turnover' in that clinical area may influence how you see your application. This should form part of your SWOT analysis. You must also understand how the organisational culture deals with symptoms of conflict when people are joining or leaving a workplace. You will need to get a sense of the quality of leadership, past and present, together with histories of conflict, so that you are fully aware of the environment you are applying to work in.

CONSEQUENCES OF CONFLICT

Almost (2006) noted that the consequences of conflict related to those highlighted in Figure 10.2. From these ideas you can identify both positive and negative outcomes, but unless it is managed effectively, negativity can dominate the situation.

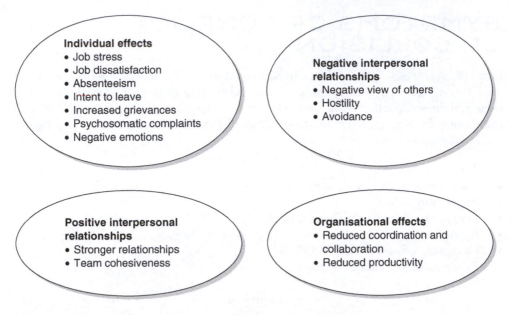

Figure 10.2   Consequences of conflict (Almost, 2006)

Unresolved conflict in the workplace has been linked to miscommunication or a lack of communication by leaders and managers which can then result in confusion over role expectations, a refusal to cooperate, poor quality output, missed deadlines, increased stress, decreased collaboration, and a lack of willingness for the team to problem solve. I am sure you can think of many other effects as the list can go on for some length.

MANAGEMENT OF CONFLICT

Marquis and Huston (2017: 560–1) suggest that the manager must examine the problem central to the conflict before deciding whether to intervene or not. If they decide to handle a conflict crisis when it occurs, they must also have thought about what the outcome would be if they did nothing. However, later they may decide to address the problem by identifying the root cause of the conflict before deciding whether to do anything about it. They go on to describe six stages of conflict as being:

- **Latent Conflict** implying the existence of antecedent conditions, e.g. short of staff, rapid change, but is often hidden or 'bubbling under the surface'
- **Perceived Conflict** usually involves issues and roles; if addressed the problem could be resolved at this stage
- **Felt Conflict** when emotionalised, e.g. hostility, fear, anger
- **Manifest Conflict** is sometimes called Overt Conflict, where action is taken, and the reaction may be withdrawal from the situation or to seek conflict resolution

- **Conflict Resolution** is often influenced by culture, gender, age, power, position, and upbringing
- **Conflict Aftermath** occurs after all episodes of conflict, whether it is positive or negative in its outcome.

Interestingly the notion of the 6Cs (see Figure 10.3) may also be used for decision making where the 6Cs become:

- Construct a clear picture
- Compile a list of things to do
- Collect information
- Compare all alternatives
- Consider what could go wrong
- Commit to the decision. (www.fgbt.org)

In this way you can be assured that all 'angles' of the problem have been considered before any action is taken, thereby ensuring that time and resources are not wasted during the actual execution of the task.

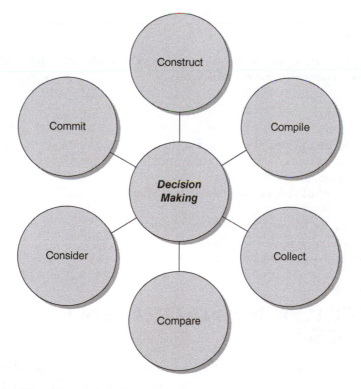

Figure 10.3   The 6Cs of decision making

(*Source*: Full Gospel Businessman's Training, 2014)

The Royal College of Nursing (RCN) (2005) highlighted that most people experience negative and positive colleague relationships. They note the importance of good working relationships and support within teams, and have produced an excellent tool to explore relationships on an individual and team basis through observable behaviours. You might like to follow the link provided to this tool, which is based on a self-awareness exercise, in the Useful Weblinks section for this chapter on the book's website.

The resource on the book's website focuses on five aspects of leadership:

- Creating a friendly atmosphere (Qs 1 and 3)
- Helping everyone to feel part of the team (Qs 4 and 6)
- Looking after colleagues (Qs 5, 7 and 9)
- Showing appreciation of the work that people do (Qs 1, 2, 10, 13, 14 and 15)
- Demonstrating respect and consideration (Qs 8, 11, 12, 14, 15 and 16).

Obviously you will have scored well here as we always have a better perception of ourselves than maybe others do! Now try to think about negative behaviours in the workplace and tick whether you have had any experience of these.

Activity

Go through the issues in the resource on the book's website and discuss with a colleague the bullying or harassment examples.

Bullying normally involves overt or covert behaviour to another individual who cannot defend themselves effectively and involves an imbalance of power (RCN, 2005). This power may involve status, information, knowledge, skill, access to resources or social position.

Three types of bullying behaviours are identified as:

- Downward bullying (superior to subordinate)
- Horizontal bullying (between peers)
- Upward bullying (subordinate to superior).

CONFLICT MANAGEMENT STYLES

Individuals respond to conflict in diverse ways – look back at the Johari Window (see Chapter 1) and the learning styles activity (see Chapter 11) to see where you differ from your colleagues as it is clear from the comparisons that you will react differently in a conflict situation; some may like to argue the point whilst others are accepting of the situation. There are thought to be several styles of conflict management which people use in organisations. Blake and Mouton's (1985) grid for differentiating conflict management styles along two axes stems from their 1960s model, and relates to people's motivation in two dimensions:

- Concern for production
- Concern for people.

Thomas (1976) reshaped this model and focused on:

- the desire to satisfy one's own concern
- the desire to satisfy others' concern

while Rahim (2011) relabelled the dimensions more simply:

- Concern for self
- Concern for others.

Five styles of conflict management have been identified that reflect a degree of how well conflict can be managed. They are based on levels of assertiveness and cooperativeness. The model which depicts these styles along the two axes can be seen in Figure 10.4.

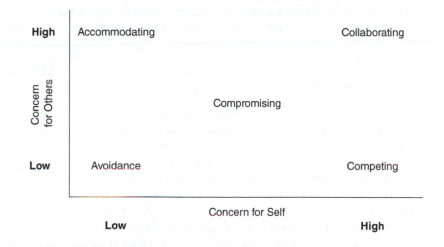

Figure 10.4   Conflict styles

Source: adapted from Thomas, 1976 and Rahim, 1983

AVOIDANCE

Seen as a passive activity where there is a withdrawal from a tricky situation. Complaints are ignored and there is a closure put on open discussion. This reflects a lack of concern for a healthy team life where problems are largely unresolved, and conflict persists.

COMPETING

Seen where power is used to dominate the situation for self-interest and ignores the needs of the team. This is generally a win–lose situation, and the style reflects a high concern for self but low concern for others in the team; often there is the perception that one person's success is directly related to another's failure.

ACCOMMODATING

Seen as a style to minimise differences as an obliging act and there is surrender to the stronger party. This reflects a low concern for one's self but a high concern for others in the team. Team members demonstrating this style are often quick to give in to avoid any conflict. They also may have difficulty in communicating their concerns openly and directly to the perceived leader.

COMPROMISING

Seen where there is negotiation and an attempt to meet on middle ground so that all sides win. This reflects a moderate degree of concern for one's self and team life, and as such is the best alternative in order to get a team to agree on the way forward.

COLLABORATING

This involves exploring and examining each of the differences to find a solution that is acceptable and of benefit to all involved. Openness and exchanges of information with effective communication and problem solving are evident. This style reflects a high concern for one's self and the team, and is an optimal approach as it attempts to take everyone's concerns into considerstion, and often has the best long-term results.

It would appear that the research points to both positive and negative conflict management styles. However, Thomas (1977) indicated that there were occasions when each of the conflict management styles would be required and may be active. Barzey (2005: 62) notes the importance of being aware of behaviour that causes problems, and suggests that 'difficult' people elicit negative behaviours to gain control over situations. She sees the following difficult behaviour types:

- **Complainers** They are quick to find problems but offer no solutions
- **Negatives** Refuse to involve themselves in change
- **Insecure** They throw tantrums and are critical of others
- **Bull in a china shop** They are always right and must win, stamping all over others
- **Know it alls** They are usually valuable to the team but give off a superior attitude and override others

- **Timidly pleasant** They are quiet and pleasant but often unresponsive to requests for help
- **Passive-aggressive** They are indecisive in not wanting to disappoint others
- **Oblivious** They have little regard for the way they come across.

Activity

Do you think we categorise people into these typologies?

Are these behaviours difficult to cope with?

It is important that these behaviours are real, but care should be taken not to stereotype individuals. These behaviours happen because of circumstances, and indeed may have developed to protect individuals from their external world because of past experiences. It is very difficult to change these behaviours overnight. A philosophy for overcoming future conflict in a team may relate to the following points:

- Having participative and supportive leadership for a trusting and respecting climate
- Clarifying higher order goals, objectives, roles and standards
- Knowing when to confront, how to diffuse aggression and reduce the risk of aggression
- Paying careful attention to Human Resources policies and procedures
- Focusing on problematical systems and processes (rather than individuals)
- Attempting to use initiative/innovation to overcome resource limitations and use of non-monetary rewards
- Paying attention to the factors affecting group dynamics.

In terms of effective strategies to handle conflict, Barzey (2005) suggests that to prevent the escalation of any conflict situation, the following actions may prove useful:

- Keep calm
- Remain positive
- Protect privacy
- Be direct and objective
- Address the problem not the person
- Maintain eye contact and be aware of body language
- Be aware of the tone of your voice
- Know when to involve a third party such as your line manager or Human Resources.

Hartman and Crume (2014), using a survey methodology with student nurses concerning team conflict, recommended the importance of designing a framework for conflict competency in nursing programmes. Enhancing conflict competency could be considered a key skill related to EI and leadership development (Waite and McKinney, 2014).

CULTURAL INFLUENCES

The method of conflict management by individual leaders may be influenced by their own cultural background. Hofsted (1980) used a cross-cultural study to identify cultural similarities and differences between 116,000 employees in a large multinational company. He identified four cultural dimensions that could affect conflict management, and mapped out 40 cultures into eight categories according to the following dimensions:

- Power distance (PD)
- Uncertainty avoidance (UA)
- Individualism–collectivism (IC)
- Masculinity–femininity (MF)

POWER DISTANCE (PD)

This related to the degree to which inequality of power was accepted by the culture. Like intergroup conflict this can be the result of jealousies towards others who are receiving more resources, recognition or favourable rewards. Argentina and Spain ranked as high-power cultures where leaders were expected to use their full power over subordinates, resulting in low mutual trust and a preference for leaders to be more directive to avoid disharmony. Australia and Canada ranked as low power cultures, where a more collegial relationship existed with mutual trust being demonstrated.

UNCERTAINTY AVOIDANCE (UA)

This dimension related to the extent to which each culture encouraged or discouraged risk taking. Japan, Iran and Turkey were high on uncertainty avoidance and disliked ambiguity and risk taking. Hong Kong and Taiwan were low uncertainty avoidance cultures.

INDIVIDUALISM– COLLECTIVISM (IC)

Britain and the USA were individualistic cultures as opposed to collectivist cultures such as the Philippines and Singapore, which required loyalty to the family and wider social structures.

MASCULINITY–FEMININITY (MF)

Some cultures, such as those of Italy and South Africa, were considered masculine, with an emphasis on material possessions such as money, status and ambition. In contrast, in feminine countries such as Scandinavia and Holland, emphasis was placed on the environment, quality of life and caring with greater equality between the sexes. The eight cultures and their typologies were defined as outlined in Table 10.1.

Table 10.1 Cultural typologies

1	More developed Latin e.g. Belgium, France, Argentina, Brazil, Spain	↑PD, UA and individualism Medium masculinity
2	Less developed Latin e.g. Columbia, Mexico, Chile, Yugoslavia, Portugal	↑PD and UA Individualism Mostly masculine
3	More developed Asian e.g. Japan	Medium PD and individualism ↑ UA High masculinity
4	Less developed Asian e.g. Pakistan, Taiwan, Thailand, Hong Kong, India, Philippines, Singapore	↑PD UA, individualism Medium masculinity
5	Near Eastern e.g. Greece, Iran and Turkey	↑PD and UA ↑ individualism Medium masculinity
6	Germanic e.g. Austria, Israel, Germany, Switzerland, South Africa, Italy	↑PD ↑ UA medium individualism High masculinity
7	Anglo e.g. Australia, Canada, Britain, Ireland, New Zealand, USA	↑PD and low to medium UA High individualism High masculinity
8	Nordic e.g. Denmark, Finland, Netherlands, Norway, Sweden	↑PD and low to medium UA Medium individualism Low masculinity

What are your thoughts on this research forty years or so on? Do you think each culture based on a country can be simplistically broken down like this or do you think that the gender, age or social class of individuals as well as the growth of multiculturalism negates these ideas when we think about dealing with conflict?

Despite the question, it appears that the way leaders manage conflict has probably been influenced by the nurturing culture in which they have been socialised, and the work by Hofsted offers some explanation of the diversity in the way people manage and lead their teams.

CONFLICT RESOLUTION

So how do we resolve conflicts? If I could answer this question with any degree of confidence, then the world would be a peaceful place. We must always consider the 'other person's' point of view and decide where the points of collaboration and agreement can be met and exactly what the sticking points are. Becoming aware of your own responses to conflict is an important part of becoming an effective leader. In Chapter 11 we will examine Emotional Intelligence, which again looks at how we interact with others and how other might assume we behave.

Activity

Think of a situation where you wanted the floor to open up and swallow you, where you felt you needed to get out of the situation quickly:

- Why did you want to go?
- What happened when you left?
- How did the situation get resolved?

- Conflict is often person centred, so it is useful to separate the people from the problem. Often, we attribute the problem to a person or a group of people which tends to cloud our vision in determining a solution; hence problems in teams are attributed to a *personality clash*. Was it this that led you to try and leave the situation?
- Maybe you offered a solution 'as you saw it' rather than 'as they saw it' which was rejected as your team members didn't want to give in to your ideas, but perhaps after you left they thought about it and went with your suggestion. West (2012: 190) tells the story of his two daughters fighting over an orange; he cut it in half and gave them half each but watching them afterwards he noted one wanted the zest whilst the other wanted juice. Had he taken the time to find out what the real problem was they could easily have had more zest or more juice rather than wasting the bit they didn't need. Within teams we need to delve into the underlying causes of the conflict rather than focusing on the individual positions of the combatants.
- As a leader we need to be inventive to come up with mutually acceptable solutions through negotiation. If your conflict was about workload, try to find a way of evaluating the solution to demonstrate that it is fair to everyone to some degree.

Clearly conflict is something we must live with to some degree and something we must deal with. If we are part of a team that has a 'difficult' member, rather than ignoring them we should listen to their issues (however thoughtless we might think they are) and attempt to coach that person by setting targets to improve their interpersonal skills; if you encourage the whole team to take responsibility for engaging that person as a valued member of the team, they should become more effective as a team member.

Constant kindness can accomplish much. As the sun makes the snow melt, kindness causes misunderstanding, mistrust, and hostility to evaporate. (Schweitzer, n.d.)

Summary of Key Points

This chapter has examined various aspects of managing conflict to meet the identified learning outcomes. These were to:

- **Discuss the concept of conflict** Here we explored the negative and positive perceptions of conflict and its importance to organisational performance.
- **Critically review a range of models associated with conflict management** Models that underpin conflict levels, conflict causes, and conflict management were offered in the context of the leadership role in developing positive collegial relationships and recognising negative behaviours in the team.
- **Critically explore the importance of conflict management within the context of problem solving** Conflict management styles were positioned against concern for self and others in dealing with problems faced by leaders in health care.
- **Recognise the importance of cultural diversity on leadership during conflict** Here four cultural dimensions that could affect conflict management were discussed.

ONLINE RESOURCES

For online resources, including SAGE journal articles, weblinks and videos, visit the book's website: https://study.sagepub.com/barr4e.

FURTHER READING

Almost, J., Doran, D. and Hall, L. (2010) Antecedents and consequences of intra-group conflict amongst nurses, *Journal of Nursing Management*, 18 (8): 981–92.

Brinkert, R. (2010) A literature review of conflict causes, costs, benefits, and interventions in nursing, *Journal of Nursing Management*, 18: 145–56.

Cox, K.B. (2001) The effects of unit morale and interpersonal relations on conflict in the nursing unit, *Journal of Advanced Nursing*, 35 (1): 17–25.

O'Grady, T.P. (2003) Conflict management special, part 2, *Nursing Management*, 34 (10): 34–40.

11 EMOTIONAL INTELLIGENCE

Chapter Contents

Learning Outcomes

By the end of this chapter you will have had the opportunity to:

- Discuss the notion of EI
- List a variety of preferred learning styles
- Identify your preferred learning style
- Critique the value of EI in complex team-working situations
- Define the emergence and value of positive psychology in leadership
- Discuss the notion of neuro-leadership in the workplace

INTRODUCTION

An estimated 40 per cent of all managers, in general, fail in the first 18 months on the job (Carnes et al., 2004), with costs both to the organisation and to individuals being significant. There is, therefore, a need for innovative approaches that will improve the success rate of clinical leaders in the health industry and have better outcomes for quality patient care. Shanta and Connolly (2013: 174) noted the importance for nurses to understand their own emotions and those of others within a complex health service, but this rightly applies to all those who care for others. Indeed, Rankin (2013: 2719) notes that 'being compassionate involves a significant degree of emotional expression'. Most leaders develop their personal essence, based on education, experience, mental intelligence, EI and the ability to form meaningful relationships. When I first heard of the concept of EI I thought it was a 'fad', but after reading about it further I realised that it has been around for at least the last two decades and is gaining in popularity.

As long ago as the 1920s Thorndike was discussing social intelligence which he said was the ability to act wisely in human relations, and in doing so he popularised the notion of Intelligence Quotient (IQ) being a crucial factor in the ability to learn (Thorndike, 1932). Current theory indicates that one should not only take on the idea of IQ but also recognise EI as being a significant part of the effective leader's toolkit. Many of the skills grouped together under the heading of EI appear to be innate. Interestingly some scholars argue that the causal significance of EI has been overstated due to the lack of evidence supporting the relationship between EI and workplace success (Vitello-Cicciu, 2002).

The historical timeline can be outlined as it developed from the early 1990s (Table 11.1).

Table 11.1 A historical timeline of emotional intelligence

1990–1993	The 1990s saw the first sustained development of the concept of EI. An editorial in the journal *Intelligence* argued for the existence of an EI as an actual intelligence (Mayer et al., 1990; Mayer and Salovey, 1993; Salovey and Mayer, 1990); also, further foundations of EI were developed, particularly in the brain sciences (Damasio, 1994).
1995–1997	Goleman, a science journalist, published *EI* which became a world-wide bestseller and was widely copied. *Time* magazine used the term 'EQ' on its cover, and a variety of personality scales were published under the name of EI (Bar-On, 1997; Cooper and Q-Metrics, 1996–1997; Goleman, 1995).
1998–present	Several refinements to the concept of EI took place, along with the introduction of new measures of the concept of EI; a growing number of peer-reviewed research articles on the topic became available.

It is now generally accepted that emotions as well as logic govern the way we act, learn and function throughout our lives. Emotions motivate us and affect the ways in which we make decisions and govern our actions. Goleman (1995) reminds us that we have two minds: a rational mind that thinks things through and an emotional one that feels; both these 'minds' store memories which will ultimately influence our responses within any given situation. The effective leader should be aware of the preferred learning styles of their subordinates and be empathetic to these when directing them in their work, to get the best from the workers in reaching the overall goals of the organisation. This chapter will attempt to clarify the concept of EI, and indicate how it 'fits' with current health care practice and how it can help to create an effective, efficient and successful team culture, thereby impacting on quality care delivery.

THE CONCEPT OF EI

Gardner (1983) suggests that psychologists have identified a variety of intelligences over the years which can be grouped into three clusters: abstract, concrete and social. *Abstract Intelligence* is an ability to understand and manipulate verbal and mathematical symbols while *Concrete Intelligence* is deemed to be the ability to understand and manipulate objects. *Social Intelligence* is the ability to understand and relate to people; it is here that EI has its roots.

DEFINITIONS

EI – The capacity to be aware of, control, and express one's emotions, and to handle interpersonal relationships judiciously and empathetically.

'EI is the key to both personal and professional success'

Emotional Quotient – The level of a person's EI, often as represented by a score in a standardised test.

'her emotional quotient was below average'

English Oxford Living Dictionaries (2018)

The phrase EI, or its alternative Emotional Quotient (EQ), has become ubiquitous as the concept has spread across the world, being recognised in many languages as well as situations where some religious scholars within Christianity, Judaism, Islam, Hinduism, and Buddhism identify that the concept of EI resonates with outlooks in their own faith. Similarly, the concept has been embraced by educators, in the form of modules in *social and emotional learning* (SEL) incorporated in training programmes.

Perhaps the biggest surprise is the impact of EI in the world of business, particularly in the areas of leadership and employee development. Today, companies worldwide routinely look through the lens of EI in hiring, promoting and developing their employees, and find that those identified at mid-career as having high leadership potential were far stronger in EI competencies than were their less-promising peers (Goleman, 2018). Lee (2017) discusses the impact this has when applied in health service employment, highlighting that public service workers require higher levels of EI because their work is focused on a service to the public, and their various roles may lead to greater levels of burnout. Whilst her research was conducted in the

USA it is not unreasonable to consider that there is a similar impact on stress and burnout in any public service institution. She uses the headings, highlighted by Wong and Law (2002: 243–74), *emotional self-awareness, emotional other-awareness* and *emotion regulation* as a basis for investigation.

Within each of these elements there are characteristics that include being aware of oneself and allowing oneself to respond more appropriately to a given situation. People having high emotional other-awareness tend to be talented in recognising others' emotional reactions and thus produce an empathetic response to them; they may appear warm and genuine, whereas those not possessing these skills may come over as being impolite or diffident. They also claim that EI can be used effectively in problem solving because both positive moods and emotions enable more flexibility in future planning, so making the most of wider opportunities. In addition, Salovey et al. (2004: 15) claim that a good/positive mood is also very useful in creative thinking. Mayer et al. (2001: 234) identified EI as 'the ability to recognize the meaning and emotions and to use them as a basis for reasoning and problem solving'. EI must support clinical judgements and thus effective patient-care outcomes in health care. Shanta and Connolly (2013: 174) conclude that EI is a crucial component in the ability to provide holistic care in the wider context of patients, colleagues and themselves.

So EI is based on a long history of research into human behaviour and social psychology. Goleman's (1995) 'corporate' approach focuses on personality traits that imply people with a high EI are ambitious, enthusiastic and committed to achieving their goals. Emotional labour plays a large part, not only in leadership but also in patient care. Smith (2011: 1) talks of 'making little things big', i.e. the things that mean so much to a patient like brushing hair, cleaning teeth or ensuring the hearing aid is worn and working. These tasks are often left to carers/health care assistants and may be thought of as *menial* tasks; they are not 'nurse jobs' and are part of the carers' role. However, they are elements of true nursing that are not in the care plan or documented in any way and yet are a vital component of emotional labour. Similarly, it is important for the paramedic, doctor, occupational therapist or anyone involved with the patient journey to be aware that all tasks are vital to that patient. There is a saying that 'if something isn't on the chart then it didn't happen'. Indeed, this is a view taken by lawyers defending any service personnel for any reason. In conclusion, emotional labour may be invisible when you consider this point: it is this element of care that is embodied in *Leading Change, Adding Value* (NHS England, 2016).

Assanova and McGuire (2009) cite Hein (2003) who offers a differing perspective to EI with more of a focus in line with his social perspective of this, and suggests it is the innate potential to feel, use, communicate, recognise, remember, learn from, manage and understand emotions. He goes on to say that Goleman and others suggest that EI is the ability to feel good about doing whatever you are told, ordered, forced, convinced or expected to do. It is the ability to keep doing it regardless of the personal or professional success or the level of stress or pressure you are put under. It is the ability to find ways to cope with your stress and thus keep doing it, regardless of your actual sincere desire to do it. In other words, EI is the ability to keep doing it despite all your negative feelings – even feelings which may be coming from your conscience. It is, therefore, the ability to go against your feelings and not feel your emotional pain or discomfort. It is the ability not to listen to your conscience or your own inner voice, but to listen instead to external voices which tell you to study, achieve, perform, run, jump, buy, sell, shoot, kill (as depicted in the cartoon). An emotionally intelligent leader, then, is one who can persuade others to do the same thing and make them feel sufficiently good about it that they want to wake up in the morning and keep doing it.

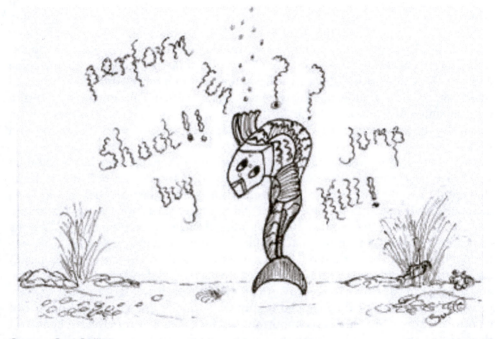

Source: Sue Saillet

Boylan and Loughrey (2007) suggest that during the training of students, time should be given to developing skills in EI through experiential workshops. It has been proposed by Pau and Croucher (2003), in their research among dental under-graduates, that stress is related to their level of EI; health care leaders would there-fore benefit from skill development in this area. Littlejohn (2012) highlights the emotional scarring from stress and conflict in the workplace, particularly in the acute sector, where patient turnover is constant and with now more highly depend-ent patients. She advocates for more training in EI to reduce workplace stress and enhance resilliance and problem-solving skills, thereby helping to prevent more risks to patients and provide better quality care. McMullen (2003) also suggests that to foster a self-directed adult learning culture, leaders need to be emotionally intelligent themselves and encourage an atmosphere of respect and honesty. In line with this,

Akerjordet and Severinsson (2010) explored the state of science of EI related to nursing leadership and concluded that, despite controversy, nurse leaders need to have an in-depth knowledge of EI as it could contribute to improved professional identity and evidence-based nursing; these findings could be extrapolated to include other health care professionals.

Activity

Think of a situation where there were difficulties in interacting with a patient.

Now imagine you are that patient in the middle of this situation.

- What difficulties could you have with the interaction with the professional?
- What feelings do you have concerning this interaction?
- How would you like this tricky situation to be resolved?
- How well do you think the health professional has dealt with your feelings?

Often when we interact with a patient who appears difficult it is because of a previous poor experience or they may be just plain frightened by the whole illness scenario. Many times, we take on board the feelings and findings of others when we are going to care for the patient who appears difficult. It is, of course, much better to formulate your own opinion when you meet with the patient. I can remember many occasions where I was in this situation. Having talked to both colleagues and the patient, it was quite clear that for some reason my colleagues and the patient had not 'hit it off'. I found the patient was fearful of their proposed surgery and needed reassurance – we got on perfectly well. Many complaints in the NHS occur because health care professionals use advoidance strategies when there are difficult relationships between staff and patients.

In the context of the 6Cs and the need for value-based practice and compassionate care for patients, Rankin (2013) undertook a longitudinal quantitative study with 307 student nurse applicants and found that there was a positive relationship between EI and practice performance, academic performance and retention. Although the study only went so far, further research was recommended to promote the notion of a more positive link between EI and compassionate care. EI applies not only to patient relationships but also to students' experiences in their placement areas and staff relationships in general. For undergraduates it can be daunting to find they have been allocated a placement where the person in charge is said to be very regimented but then find them to be a quite amiable person – I have often found this to be the case through the years; it is therefore best practice not to listen to another person's account of the person in charge. Ward sisters will be concerned about the care of their patients, students, staff, patients' relatives and the MDT, whereas students may only have concern for 'getting the best' out of the learning situation; this is similar in all aspects of care delivery regardless of your discipline. We must accept that we cannot always 'get on' with everyone, but if we adapt our approaches we should be able to get the best out of people most of the time. I would like to think my approach – of putting myself in the other person's shoes – appears to work.

As a leader it is desirable that you are aware of the emotions of others and reflect on this in the context of how people perceive they can learn from the situation facing them. As a health care professional, understanding the differing preferred learning styles of individual patients, their relatives and members of the multidisciplinary team is essential.

PREFERRED LEARNING STYLES

We all have a preferred way of learning, and if we are to subscribe to the notion of EI, then as a leader we need to allow for learner and patient/client differences in their learning styles. As we learned in Chapter 2 the MBTI test highlighted our differing qualities in terms of personality, but to be an effective leader we should consider ways of learning in terms of our own preferred style and that of others to be an effective team. According to Honey and Mumford (1982) there are four main learning styles (Activist; Reflector; Theorist; Pragmatist), each of which exhibits its own features. An examination of these styles reveals a range of characteristics attaching to each:

- **Activists:**
    o   Are 'hands-on' learners
    o   Get fully involved in new experiences
    o   Are open-minded and enthusiastic
    o   Will 'try anything once'
    o   Revel in crisis management, i.e. 'fire fighting'
    o   Get bored by detail
    o   Act first and consider the implications later.

- **Reflectors:**
    o   Are 'tell me' learners
    o   Prefer to stand back and observe
    o   Look at all the angles and implications
    o   'Chew it over' before reaching conclusions
    o   Take a back seat in meetings and discussions
    o   View the situation from different angles
    o   Enjoy watching others and will listen to their views before offering their own.

- **Theorists:**
    o   Are 'convince me' learners
    o   Like to think problems through logically, step by step

- o   Assimilate disparate facts into complex and logically sound theories
- o   Rigorously question assumptions and conclusions
- o   Don't allow their feelings to influence decisions
- o   Are uncomfortable with subjectivity and creative thinking.

- **Pragmatists:**

- o   Are 'show me' learners
- o   Are keen to try out new ideas to see if they work
- o   Like concepts that can be applied to their job
- o   Tend to be impatient with lengthy discussions and are practical and down to earth
- o   Emphasise expediency – 'the end justifies the means'. (Adapted from Mumford, 1997)

However, based on these preferences, different activities are likely to produce different responses and have implications not only for team management but also for therapeutic patient care. There are many different learning style tests that can be undertaken to help you understand the diverse ways people learn. If we are to be emotionally intelligent we must allow for these differences.

Activity

Many people use a combination of learning styles, whereas others learn best by using just one. Want to know your learning style? You're just 20 questions away from finding out!

Take the following test to see what kind of preferred learning style you have: www.educationplanner.org/students/self-assessments/learning-styles-quiz.shtml (See Table 11.2 for explanations of the three learning styles.)

Table 11.2   Learning styles

Learning Style of Team Member	Example of Preferred Activity
Visual	You prefer using images, pictures, colours and maps to organise information and communicate with others. You can easily visualise objects, plans and outcomes in your mind's eye. You also have good spatial sense which gives you a good sense of direction.
Auditory	You like to work with sound and music. Certain music invokes strong emotions. You notice the music playing in the background of movies, TV shows and other media. You often find yourself humming or tapping a song or jingle, or a theme or jingle pops into your head without prompting.
Tactile	Making up about 5% of the population, tactile and kinesthetic learners absorb information best by doing, experiencing, touching, moving or being active in some way, and enjoy feeling, discovery and action.

I tend to be Visual (45%), Auditory (25%) and Tactile (30%) so I learn by seeing and doing rather than hearing; the description of how I might behave in the learning situation is scarily accurate! My colleague is Visual (40%), (Auditory 35%) and Tactile (25%) so more of a listener than me, but we complement each other well when working together.

You may find you fit into several categories, as we do, or that you have a dominant style with far less use of the others; what is important is that you recognise there is no 'right' mix and your preferred styles are not fixed. You can develop your ability in less dominant styles as well as further developing the styles you already use; when you demonstrate EI you will recognise that as a leader you will need to adjust your approach to teaching or getting others to see your point of view. All these styles come back to the fact that we need to recognise different approaches both in ourselves and others because throughout your career you will be teaching colleagues, patients and their relatives about their conditions or treatment. In terms of effective health education there is little point in giving a pamphlet to someone who prefers the auditory learning style without talking them through it.

Activity

How do you remember a telephone number?

Try saying it aloud as though you are giving it to another person. Perhaps you will remember it in groups made up of three numbers (123 456 789) or groups of two numbers (12 34 56 78 9). Interestingly, I remember my house phone number in groups of two but my mobile in groups of three; I am not sure how to explain this, but it does demonstrate that we think differently depending on the situation.

Using multiple learning styles and 'multiple intelligences' for learning is a relatively innovative approach; it is an approach that educators have only recently started to recognise. Traditional schooling uses mainly linguistic and logical teaching methods and a limited range of learning and teaching techniques. Many schools still rely on classroom and book-based teaching, much repetition, and pressured exams for reinforcement and review, i.e. theorist, reflector styles. A result is that we often label those who use visual and auditory learning styles as 'bright'. Those who use less favoured learning styles (tactile) often find themselves in lower streamed classes, with various not-so-complimentary labels and sometimes lower-quality teaching. This can create both positive and negative spirals which reinforce the belief that one is 'smart' or 'dumb'. By recognising and understanding your own learning styles, you can use techniques better suited to you which, in turn, will improve the speed and quality of your learning; it will also make learning in the workplace more meaningful. So, in much the same way as teachers can use their knowledge of preferred learning styles in the classroom, to enhance the student learning experience by presenting information to the learner in diverse ways, the effective leader can use these skills in the workplace in order to achieve the desired outcomes.

Your preferred learning style(s) can have more influence than you may realise by guiding the way you learn, and changing the way you internally represent experiences, the way you recall information, and even the words you choose. Research shows us that each learning style uses various parts of the brain. By involving more of the brain during learning, we remember more of what we learn. Researchers using brain-imaging technologies have been able to find out the key areas of the brain responsible for each learning style. For example, the styles described by Fleming (2010) may also be called:

- **Visual** The occipital lobes at the back of the brain manage the visual sense; both the occipital and parietal lobes manage spatial orientation
- **Aural** The temporal lobes handle aural content; the right temporal lobe is especially important for music
- **Verbal** The temporal and frontal lobes manage this, especially two specialised areas called Broca's and Wernicke's areas (in the left hemisphere of these two lobes)
- **Physical** The cerebellum and the motor cortex (at the back of the frontal lobe) handle much of our physical movement.

In some literature you will also see the following styles referred to:

- **Logical** The parietal lobes, especially the left side, drive our logical thinking
- **Social** The frontal and temporal lobes handle much of our social activities; the limbic system also influences both the social and solitary styles and has a lot to do with emotions, moods and aggression
- **Solitary** The frontal and parietal lobes, and the limbic system, are also active with this style.

Being aware of these factors will mean that the effective leader will be able to get the most out of their workforce.

In this way, to fit with the above theories, clinical effective leaders would attend first to the social conditions that foster good team working by ensuring there is a stable, cohesive team; they can then logically provide the team with a clear direction for improving patient care through confident self-directed practice by individual members of the team. They also need to ensure that work practices empower the team rather than impede the work. Where necessary they will adapt and support organisational structures and systems so that the support and necessary resources are available to complete the task. They arrange for (or provide themselves) expert coaching to help their team take full advantage of the situation. The leader will do all these things in their own way by using the behavioural/learning style and strategies that they have found have worked best in the past. The one thing that makes them stand out from the 'not so effective' leader is that they can adapt their style as they recognise the need to from the reaction of others.

THE VALUE OF EI IN COMPLEX TEAM WORKING

Within teams there are individuals who work and think in diverse ways, each benefiting the overall progress of project work. Belbin (2015) notes differing roles taken on within the team structure and how each of these enhances or detracts from the team's effectiveness. Similarly, it can be argued that if the leader of a team knows about the best ways people work or take instruction, they can ensure that the team is effective in the way it works.

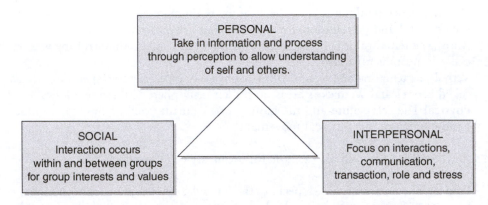

Figure 11.1   Representation of King's (1981) Interacting Systems Theory

Shanta and Connolly (2013) linked EI in nursing practice to King's *Interacting Systems Theory* (Figure 11.1) which has a focus on the dynamic interactions of humans through three interacting systems: personal, interpersonal and social realms. Knowing how people work and think can ensure you get the best out of them. One manager I have worked with asked a member of staff to sort out an issue. This member of staff reacts like a chicken whenever she is asked to do anything; you can watch her ruffling up her feathers as she thinks through what might be required and what she feels she will not be able to achieve. A few well-chosen words to 'smooth' her feathers and she happily leaves to complete the task. Another member of staff was approached with the same issue by the manager who only had to say: 'I have had this idea ...'. The staff member said 'OK' and the next time the manager saw her the idea had been taken up and successfully planned out. For yet another member of staff who was passed the idea from the manager, the response would be 'Oh that's interesting' but nothing further would be done. This member of staff requires a direct list of actions: first, do this; second, do that; third, do the other, and so on to attempt to complete the task.

As effective leaders we need to be flexible; one manager I knew preferred the direct, ordered chain of acts approach as it worked for her, assumed that it would work for everyone and consistently used that approach; this links loosely to two of the elements of King's model (Personal and Interpersonal) that allow for information to be processed but also include information about about the role and the stress that may be perceived, though with limited social considerations. In doing this she could alienate new employees as they did not feel valued, and this interpersonal approach allowed no recognition of the skills and experience they had which would allow them to deal with the issue in their own way. I found that part of my (hidden) role was to let each new staff member know that it was just the manager's way and not directed at them personally.

Kite and Kay (2012) highlight that EI is linked to better situational outcomes by linking intellect and the emotional awareness to manage ourselves and our relationships better. They note ten characteristics of emotionally intelligent people and less emotionally intelligent people (Table 11.3).

Table 11.3 Characteristics of EI people and less EI people (Kite and Kay, 2012)

EI people	Less EI people
1. Continually striving for personal development	• Assuming that something good will turn up
2. Unrelenting commitment to support others' interests	• See things with their own eyes
3. Clarity of intentions	• Are imprecise about their goals
4. Sustaining positive values	• Follow the crowd before they follow their conscience
5. Listening and observation	• Reject the opinion of those they perceive to lack authority
6. Objectivity	• Don't want to believe they can change themselves or others
7. Challenging the status quo	• Put status before authority
8. Taking the longer view	• React on impulse not thought
9. Converting negative inclinations into positive thoughts	• Are pessimistic in the face of change
10. Nurturing the team	• Communicate what they think people want to hear

Activity

The debate about whether there are two types of people can be too simplistic and the issue of context is perhaps more important.

Can you suggest two recent clinical situations when you have behaved in a 'less EI' mode and another occasion when your behaviour was more EI mature?

Maybe the notion of a polarised status of people suggested by Kite and Kay is a long way from the truth; you may also find that when reflecting on your own styles as in a force-field analysis you exhibit elements of both behaviours but a dominance towards one side or the other. To develop professionally it is useful to identify where you stand on the EI/less EI scale so that you can work to reduce any 'less EI' traits. The idea that individuals can behave differently in specific situations is likely and must be recognised as well as strategies that can then be changed with a situation to be effective.

Considering styles of leadership alongside EI we can see that transactional leaders tend to be serious, value one-way communication, use emotional management, and often delay gratification. Transformational leaders value empathy and two-way communication; they tend to be friendly and use empathy to motivate staff. So, taking these different approaches into account will lead to effective team working. Clearly there is still a place for the more traditional leadership approaches in patient care, particularly within emergency care when the end goal is one of patient safety. The engaged leader with emotional competence should be able to use their knowledge to help members of their team identify and reach their personal destiny; this type of leadership plays on the cognitive and behavioural knowledge and skills linked to the notion of neuropsychology.

POSITIVE PSYCHOLOGY

'Positive Psychology' (PP) is a term summarised as the study of positive emotion, positive character and positive institutions (Seligman, 2011). This emerging science is based on the premise that we are capable of happiness, life satisfaction and optimal performance by devoting our efforts to cultivating our strengths. Two main concepts are identified:

- **Expressing gratitude** This has surprisingly wide-ranging benefits for both the recipient and the person conveying appreciation.
- **Identifying and augmenting your signature strengths** This is a far more effective strategy to accomplish life satisfaction (authentic happiness) than exploring and trying to improve your weaknesses.

Considering these two elements the successful leader will use praise and then thank the workforce when a task has been completed effectively. However, an overzealous commendation may appear false but demonstrating 'thanks for a job well done' will enhance the way the team works together and give the team members a sense of pride. By using its unique individual strengths, the team is also more likely to achieve positive and timely outcomes. There are said to be four pillars of PP which are outlined in Table 11.4.

By being aware of these 'pillars' the effective leader can utilise the strengths of each member of the team to achieve the goals of the organisation. This adds to the value of good leadership. In terms of clinical health care professional leaders, this means moving from a *blame culture* to a *lessons learned* climate.

Table 11.4 The four pillars of Positive Psychology

Positive Emotion	Find a realistic perspective on catastrophic thoughts
Meaning	Humans want to belong to something bigger
Positive Relationship	Celebrate together when something good happens
Positive Accomplishment	Mastery; competence; achievement

Activity

How would you assess the overall EI of your team, e.g. with respect to:

- Near misses?
- Medication errors?
- Poor compliance to manual handling procedures?

There is a 'lessons learnt' climate (circle appropriately):

Strongly Agree   Agree   Neutral Disagree   Strongly Disagree

NEURO-LEADERSHIP

Linked to PP is the notion of neuro-leadership which refers to the application of findings from neuroscience to the field of leadership. It is an emerging field of study focused on bringing neuro-scientific knowledge into the areas of leadership development, management training, change management, education, consulting and coaching. It provides a new scientific framework for understanding and therefore enhancing the practice of leading others. An enhanced understanding of how the brain works has been able to shed light on ways those leaders can:

- enhance their thinking
- strengthen their ability to influence others
- help staff successfully work through change.

Rock et al. (2009: 1) suggested that understanding the neuroscience of engagement is more than just an interesting discussion; it will open insights for leaders to more accurately and effectively predict, measure and improve employee engagement across all types of organisations.

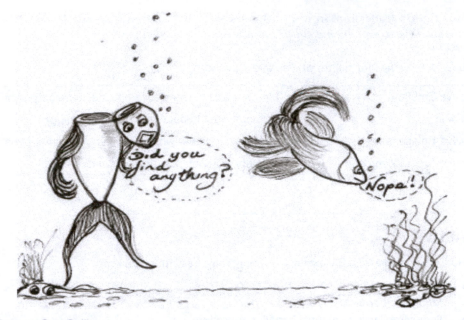

Source: Sue Saillet

At first glance you might think that the fish on the right is looking in the wrong place for the missing brain; however, he may be running away from the situation and making a throwaway comment over his shoulder having found nothing when he investigated the empty head.

When considering the strengths and weaknesses of the team leader and the team overall, Rock (2008) suggested five SCARF domains (Status, Certainty, Autonomy, Relationships and Fairness):

- **Status**   Individual's self-perceived importance in relation to others
- **Certainty**   Ability to predict the future
- **Autonomy**   Individual's perception regarding their sense of control over events
- **Relatedness**   Safety with others, of being associated with an in-group
- **Fairness**   The perception of fairness in the way people are treated.

Each element identified in this model will have an effect on leadership success and so help health care professional leaders to positively influence the environment and drive the workforce forward in a constructive manner.

Activity

- Assess these issues considering the strengths and weaknesses of people in your team.
- Do you jointly believe that EI leads to a better environment and better patient care?

Overall it can be seen from the literature that EI has almost as many followers as it has critics. Neuro-leadership is also not without its critics; it has been questioned whether having scientific brain data to back up what is commonly believed adds any value. Yet advocates suggest that neuro-leadership provides a scientific basis and language to management studies that managers and leaders can relate to. Further, it is believed that the relatively young field of neuro-leadership will continue to reveal new insights into how to lead effectively. It could be concluded that awareness of EI and PP can be of significant use if working in a health care arena where to be 'tuned in' to patients' and clients' feelings may well enhance treatment. Similarly, the notion of neuro-leadership will complement EI by supporting meaningful team leadership.

Summary of Key Points

This chapter has briefly looked at various aspects of EI to meet the identified learning outcomes. These were:

- **Discuss the notion of EI** While EI is not a new phenomenon, it can clearly be seen to be of benefit within the overall management of effective team working.
- **List a variety of preferred learning styles** Here we examined the notion of a variety of learning styles that can be recognised and used by the effective leader.
- **Identify your preferred learning style** Through examining our own preferred learning style we can appreciate how different people may react in given situations and how these learning styles may benefit patient/client care.
- **Critique the value of EI in complex team working situations** EI can be used to provide a good stable base for the team to work from. It is also strongly linked to compassionate care.
- **Define the emergence and value of positive psychology in leadership** Positive psychology in leadership is said to aid the organisation in becoming a positive place to work, thus leading to a happier and more cohesive workforce.
- **Discuss the notion of neuro-leadership in the workplace** Valuing the workforce and developing a method by which all leadership strands are brought together are vital in the role of the effective leader.

ONLINE RESOURCES

For online resources, including SAGE journal articles, weblinks and videos, visit the book's website: https://study.sagepub.com/barr4e.

FURTHER READING

Bellack, J.P. (1999) EI: a missing ingredient?, *Journal of Nurse Education*, *38* (1): 3–4.

Chapman, M. (2005) The positive psychology of EI and coaching, *Competency and EI*, Winter 2005/06, *13* (2).

de Mio, R.R. (2002) On defining virtual EI, *ECIS 2002*, June, Gdansk, Poland.

Harmes, P.D. and Credé, M. (2010) EI and transformational and transactional leadership: a meta-analysis, *Journal of Leadership & Organizational Studies*, *17*: 5.

Kong, F. (2017) The validity of the Wong and Law EI Scale in a Chinese sample: tests of measurement invariance and latent mean differences across gender and age, *Science Direct*. Available at www.sciencedirect.com/science/article/pii/S0191886917302751 (accessed 5 April 2018).

Senge, P., Hamilton, H. and Kania, J. (2015) *The Dawn of Whole System Leadership*. Stanford Social Innovation Review. Available at https://ssir.org/articles/entry/the_dawn_of_system_leadership (accessed 8 February 2018).

Skinner, C. and Spurgeon, P. (2005) Valuing empathy and EI in health leadership: a study of empathy, leadership behaviour and outcome effectiveness, *Health Services Management Research*, *18*: 1–12.

PART 3

THE ORGANISATION

12 THEORY OF ORGANISATIONAL LIFE

Chapter Contents

Learning Outcomes

By the end of this chapter you will have had the opportunity to:

- Understand the importance of the overall organisation
- Discuss the importance of strategy, structures and systems within the organisation

(Continued)

(Continued)

- Critically explore the notion of organisational culture
- Reflect on the nature of organisational roles
- Critically examine professional responsibility and accountability as well as the notions of authority and delegation
- Develop an overview of Human Resource processes in organisations

INTRODUCTION

Over the last few chapters, you will have been encouraged to examine the individual as a leader and within the dynamics of the team. For you to be effective within an organisation, whatever your status, it is useful to scrutinise the structure, culture and management strategies of the organisation and its top leadership. The health economy has diverse types of organisations: some lie within the 'not for profit' public sector, some organisations are run 'for profit', and some organisations are a combination of both models, such as General Practice; others are run through charity finance and the public purse, e.g. hospices or establishments for serious long-term conditions. This chapter will attempt to unravel the theoretical aspects of organisational life for you to learn more about the context in which health care delivery operates.

WHAT IS THE PURPOSE OF AN ORGANISATION?

Organisations can be a simple, collective group of people such as in a small General Practice or they can be more complex, reflected as enterprising entities like the National Health Service (NHS). Organisations are integral to our social, cultural, political, economic, technological and physical environment. Sullivan and Garland (2013: 309) define an organisation as a 'collection of people working together under a defined structure to achieve predetermined outcomes using financial, human and material resources'. An organisation can more precisely be defined as:

A social unit of people, systematically structured and managed to meet a need or to pursue collective goals. (www.businessdictionary.com/definition/organization.html)

Activity

Do you feel these ideas reflect the health organisation in which you work?

If so how do they apply to the following?

- The NHS
- Private hospitals
- Residential care homes
- Live-in carer/nursing provision
- General Practice
- St John's Ambulance/Red Cross.

You might have thought that the purposes listed above relate well to the current NHS even as it faces its biggest challenges since its inception in 1948. They may also hold true for the other health care organisations listed but smaller businesses are more focused on their goals and it may be argued are better able to care for their staff. However, it could also be argued that the ability to ensure humane treatment of NHS employees is compromised due to the pressures of throughput and dependency. Similarly, in these times of change the influence of Brexit and the reduction in work visas has been detrimental to the recruitment of some staff. The UK government has now lifted the restrictions related to the numbers of people entering the UK from Europe and further afield, but continues to attempt to 'grow' UK staff from within the current population (Blackpool Teaching Hospitals, 2015). Both these strategies appear to be failing (The King's Fund, 2018), possibly due to the 'growing time' being between three and seven years, and thus it can be said that this strategy should have been put into effect three to seven years ago. The effects of the reduction in overseas staffing may vary according to which area you are currently working in and the philosophy of the employer, but discussions emanating from the North Staffordshire debacle (Francis, 2013) indicate that consideration of NHS employees comes low on the hierarchy of business needs.

The NHS is a statutory organisation that is governed by statute in the UK and steered under the direction of the government party in power. Over the last fifty years or so, the NHS has been driven by the following policy issues:

- The introduction of market-based mechanisms to allocate and distribute its finite resources to meet ever-growing health needs and demands
- 'Contracting out' of some of the peripheral services to the private sector
- Notions of private initiatives to support the fixed budget of the NHS.

This is not so very different for any other international health care organisation across the developed market economy; therefore, these have been a way of dealing with the complexity and increased demands placed on health care provision today. The study of organisational life is a specific discipline that is pertinent for leadership and requires knowledge from the social sciences, psychology, economics and possibly political science. Leaders need to have an awareness of how their own organisation works and the extent of its effectiveness and success. Initially leaders, but with the input of ALL members of staff, need to be able to steer the organisation towards this, on a continuous basis, whether that organisation is a small team, a clinical ward, a directorate, an NHS Trust, or even the entire NHS.

Generally, organisational models are classified as functional, product/service based (divisional) or a matrix structure. Functional organisations are traditional business hierarchies in which tasks are grouped by functional area, such as sales, administration, and production, engineering and customer services. Functional models are most effective in a business where routine processes are performed on time or where there are just a few products or service lines. The function of any health care service is to provide safe, effective, robust care to members of the community it serves. Most health care providers function in a hierarchical organisation that has a mission statement reflecting the high quality of care it wishes to offer. However, these are often seen as particularly service based (urology, oncology) and thus often have a matrix structure to deal with the complexity. For an organisation to be regarded as effective and efficient, many elements must be coordinated and managed, which means that leadership is vital. The McKinsey 7 'S' model (Peters and Waterman, 2004: 9) suggests the elements required are:

- Strategy
- Style
- Structure
- Systems
- Skills
- Staff.

Leavitt's (1965, 1978) simple model (People; Structure; Technology; Task) helps leaders to reflect on the interdependency of organisational matrix elements. These interdependent elements are crucial, and a good leader should be able to recognise the importance of all of them, especially when it is thought that the organisation is becoming less effective and efficient.

The Weisbord (1976) Six Organisational Model (Figure 12.1) offers another perspective but highlights the crucial importance of leadership.

Activity

Write down what you think about the strengths of these three models.

It is useful here to note the importance of structure, strategy and systems in all three models. Although other elements are relevant they have been covered elsewhere in this book.

ORGANISATIONAL STRATEGY

The concept of strategy is complex because it has various meanings. It could be 'a general plan of action that describes resource allocation and other activities for

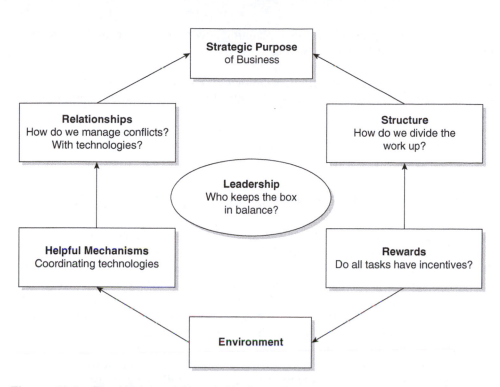

Figure 12.1 The Weisbord (1976) Six Organisational Model

dealing with the environment and helping the organization attain its goals and achieve the vision' (Daft, 2017: 411). Doherty et al. (2014) state that it is clearly concerned with identifying the aim of the organisation and the specific related actions to achieve it. Indeed, Mintzberg et al. (2003) noted it could also be used to mean:

- a plan
- a position
- a pattern of behaviour
- a perspective.

These ideas illustrate that a strategy is not always considered as rationally and pro-actively planned. Leadership requires strategic thinking; what does this mean for clinical leadership? Strategic decisions are based on the values, beliefs and expectations of those in power in an organisation. Clinical leaders need to be aware not only of their own power base but also that there is no single way of thinking strategically. Organisational strategy involves strategic analysis, strategic choice and implementation. The basis of strategic analysis should come from a review of the organisational mission and goals followed by internal and external analysis. Iles and Sutherland (2001) point to several external and internal analysis tools that can be used in health care, particularly when planning new developments and as a form of project management for clinical change:

- **PEST** (Political, Environmental, Sociological, Technological factors)
- **PESTELI** (including features above but also Ecological, Legislative and Industry factors)
- **SWOT** (Strengths, Weaknesses, Opportunities and Threats)
- **Process modelling** (e.g. a 'patient journey').

VISION, MISSION AND GOALS

We need to examine the need for such things as 'Vision Statements' as in many organisations the statement is published but nobody could tell you what it says. Nameki (1992, cited in Doherty et al., 2014: 315) suggested that any chance for a shared sense of vision between managers and staff was undermined by recruiting leaders from the private sector. This led Doherty et al. (2014: 314–19) to suggest the notion of a conversational approach to leadership where there is a need for continuity or a proven need for change. Health care organisations do need to set annual goals and objectives that can be regularly measured or evaluated.

In terms of mission statements, these formal statements communicate the vision of the organisation. They are usually brief and cover the following areas:

- The purpose of the organisation
- The strategic intent
- Policies and standards
- Organisational values.

Activity

- Has your Health Trust communicated their mission to you?
- Try to find out where this is and check whether you feel it represents what is happening in your health industry.
- What about your own clinical area – do you have an identified mission statement?
- Does it need revising?
- Do your team members know about it?

The mission statement is often found on an organisation's web page; this is a broad statement of core purpose and should not be confused with the vision (ambitious desire) although the two work together (Daft, 2017). 'Visions' grow and change whereas 'missions' provide a core basis from which visions are created. The goals, objectives and future are there for public scrutiny. Policies, procedures and guidance can be found on the organisational intranet. These should be accessed as they include information pertinent to the smooth running of the organisation and are used as a benchmark by which to assess quality of delivery when the organisation is being inspected.

LEADERSHIP AND HEALTH POLICY

Health policy is a rational strategic plan to distribute scarce resources. There are two main economic issues concerning the health service industry in all countries:

- Rising expectations and demands for health care – infinite demand
- Finite resources to deal with these needs, demands and wants.

Health policy reflects how political leaders shape the distribution of these finite health funds and resources to deal with the presenting infinite health service demands. Policy also denotes the strength of belongingness within a society to achieve solutions and a commitment to trying new ways of coping with the under-lying issues.

Palfrey (2000) suggests health policy is therefore about:

- a desire to improve people's quality of life
- an attempt to improve a nation
- a perceived need to reduce costs/save money
- a perceived need to stabilise expenditure but improve the standard of services
- a practical concern to retain power/authority.

Not all countries' governments have the same commitment to health care as each other and the amount of money put into a system varies widely across the world. However, a higher percentage of funding to a health system does not necessarily equate to healthier populations. New health policy focuses on changing and challenging the status quo. This can relate to the following:

- Changes to the perception of health needs
- Changes to health care structures and systems
- Changes to health care processes
- Changes to roles and responsibilities
- Changes to power bases.

Health policy can be explored through International, National and Local perspectives.

INTERNATIONAL POLICY

It could be said that the World Health Organization (WHO) leads on health issue policy. They defined health policy thus:

> Health policy refers to decisions, plans, and actions that are undertaken to achieve specific health care goals within a society. An explicit health policy can achieve several things: it defines a vision for the future which in turn helps to establish targets and points of reference for the short and medium term. It outlines priorities and the expected roles of differing groups; and it builds consensus and informs people. (www.who.int/topics/health_policy/en/)

Griffiths (2014: 163) identifies that due to world ageing populations, lifestyle-related disease and environmental issues, public health concerns are increasing on a global basis. The United Nations (2000) set out eight Millennium Development Goals (MDGs) for 2015. In 2015, there were mixed results and world leaders further agreed 17 Sustainable Development Goals (SDGs) under the United Nations Agenda 2030. Health leaderships across the world are thus facing huge challenges to put policy into practice for better health outcomes.

More international policy which has been relevant to UK health policy development includes:

- The European Convention on Human Rights (ECHR) – The 1998 Human Rights Act (UK)
- The European Equality Directives – The 2010 Equality Act (UK)

NATIONAL POLICY

National health policy making is now related to the NHS Constitution (DHSC, 2015) and there are relevant, overarching UK Acts pertaining to health, e.g. the Health and Social Care Act 2012, the Mental Health Units (Use of Force) Act 2018, the Mental Capacity Act 2005 and the Children Acts 1989 and 2004 as well as the broader NICE Guidelines – to name but a few. There are also the main policies from the professional statutory regulatory bodies. In the UK these are the General Medical Council (GMC), the Nursing and Midwifery Council (NMC) and the Health and Care Professions Council (HCPC), and they have a public protection role through their standards and practice codes for their members involved in care.

Initially, you might think that it has little to do with you but think on ... what about that patient who might be developing signs that they could be a danger to themself or others? Should they be assessed for Deprivation of Liberty Safeguards (DoLS) or should we consider a Mental Capacity assessment? It is the staff at the 'coalface' who will initiate these assessments in line with local health policy.

Activity

- Go to the NICE website at www.nice.org.uk/guidance/CG138, which identifies your responsibilities as a health care student or qualified professional.
- Read section 1.2.
- Discuss how these guidelines are put into practice with a colleague.
- How does this apply to you locally in practice?

LOCAL POLICY

All health organisations develop their own local policies in light of international, national and regional legislation and directives; these should be reviewed regularly and may relate to DNACPR (do not attempt cardiopulmonary resuscitation) directives and care pathways as well as policies relating to human resourcing, finance and marketing.

INVOLVEMENT IN THE DECISION-MAKING AND LOCAL POLICY-MAKING PROCESS

There are four main stages that staff teams, at all levels, can get involved with. Leaders could make their teams aware of these areas and the need for utilising evidence or research-based information.

- **Agenda setting** – problem identification and recognition of issues for policy
- **Communicating the development of health care options by appraisal** – setting of alternatives, forecasting, cost-benefit analysis
- **Helping in choosing policy and its implementation** – in line with the vision and mission statements for the organisation
- **Evaluation and review of policy** – Are we meeting the requirements of the organisation?

ORGANISATIONAL CULTURE

Daft (2017: 428) reminds us that organisational culture is powerful because it affects the company's performance for better or for worse. He reminds us that a shifting environment will call for new values and fresh approaches to doing business. When a company culture fits the needs of the external environment and company strategy, employees can create a successful organisation.

Cultures are affected by:

- the past
- the climate of the present
- the involved technology
- the type of work
- the aims
- the kind of people who work there.

Activity

Can you make some notes about the culture in your own clinical area, paying attention to these aspects?

The hospice area I work in has a relatively short past; it has only been around for about thirty years, is a well-respected and valued organisation in the community, and its foundations lie in the charity that started it and contributes to its maintenance today. The current climate is one of expansion: a day centre, hospice at home and new hospice provision in another city and town reflect a changing organisation. The technology involved is one of palliation, medication, doctoring, nursing and allied health care, inpatient technology of beds, mattresses and home comforts, as well as therapeutic alternatives such as counselling, aromatherapy and reflexology. The type of work is generally of a slower pace than in an acute hospital. There is very little rushing around. Work centres on drug rounds, medical rounds, meals and choices that the patients make – be it activities such as bathing, talking with visitors or other patients, and a range of activities in the day centre. The aim of the hospice is to provide palliative care for those who have a progressive, deteriorating health condition. The kind of people who work there must be particularly able to cope with the difficulties of bereavement, but also be active in rehabilitation skills to empower patients to take as much control of their lives as possible. There is kindness and caring in the staff I have seen that is in-built, and they demonstrate care throughout the whole organisation, be they doctors, nurses, catering staff or volunteers – almost as though they are all potential 'hospice customers'.

An organisation's culture is important in the way it influences the process of socialisation for team members and shapes organisational behaviour. French and Bell (1990: 19) have modelled organisational culture on the structure of an iceberg, where there are formal (above the sea) and informal (below the sea) aspects of the organisation (Figure 12.2).

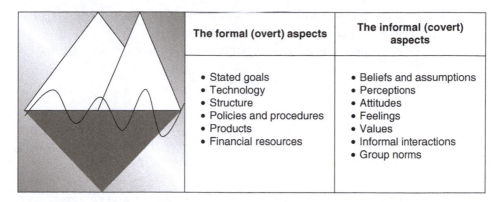

	The formal (overt) aspects	The informal (covert) aspects
	• Stated goals • Technology • Structure • Policies and procedures • Products • Financial resources	• Beliefs and assumptions • Perceptions • Attitudes • Feelings • Values • Informal interactions • Group norms

Figure 12.2 Formal (above the sea) and informal (below the sea) aspects of an organisation

There are many models of types of organisational cultures. We will reflect on three models of organisational culture (Handy, 1985; Schein, 1985; Johnson and Scholes, 1989). Handy (1985) identified four types of organisational culture (Figure 12.3).

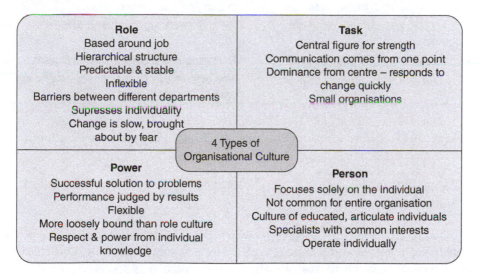

Figure 12.3 Types of organisational cultures

Source: Adapted from Handy, C.B. (1993) *Understanding Organisations* (4th edn). Oxford: Oxford University Press

Activity

Can you give an example of each of these types that may be seen in health care?

- The NHS may be a role culture
- Small project teams may be working in a task culture
- Research teams, high dependency, theatres or educational units may have a power culture
- Consultancy may be one of person culture.

Another model of culture types is from Schein (1985), who identified two continuums. One is not better than the other; they are simply different. Schein noted that leadership should be seen in context and in the culture of that context highlighting the relationship between leadership and culture formation (Table 12.1).

Table 12.1   Schein's (1985) relationship between leadership and culture formation

←	→
Operate independently	Ideas valued from older, wiser and higher status individuals
Ideas valued from any individual	
People are responsible, motivated and capable of governing themselves	People are capable of loyalty and discipline in carrying out directions
Conflict is OK and can be sorted out through groups	Relationships are lineal and vertical
Group members will care for each other	Everyone has a place in the organisation
	The organisation is responsible for taking care of its members

Schein (2017) further identifies three distinct levels in organisational cultures:

- Artifacts and Behaviours
- Espoused Values
- Assumptions.

The three levels refer to the degree to which the diverse cultural phenomena are visible to the observer and will be recognised by new employees in a short space of time. I remember going to visit an organisation when they were preparing for a long-service award ceremony; coming from the NHS where long service meant twenty five or more years I was amazed to find that within this organisation it meant five years and over! However, everyone clearly though this was a great achievement.

Artifacts include any tangible, overt or verbally identifiable elements in any organisation. Architecture, furniture, dress code, office jokes, all exemplify organisational artifacts. Artifacts are the visible elements in a culture and they can be recognised by people who are not part of the culture.

Espoused values are the organisation's stated values and rules of behaviour. It is how the members represent the organisation both to themselves and to others. This is often expressed in official philosophies and public statements of identity. It can sometimes often be a projection for the future of what the members hope to become. Examples of this would be employee professionalism, or a 'family first' mantra. Shared basic assumptions are the deeply embedded, taken-for-granted behaviours which are usually unconscious, but constitute the essence of culture. Schein describes six ways to observe culture as being:

- *Regular behaviours*: ways members greet one another, dress, lunch/coffee breaks, treatment of older members
- *Norms*: how hard one works in the organisation, weekend work, work taken home
- *Dominant values:* 'customers are number one', high quality products, travel style, importance of family
- *Philosophy*: overall views of employees, community relationships/partnerships, profit motive
- *Rules*: managing time, getting along with co-workers, supervisor relationships, fringe benefit management, gender relationships
- *Feeling or climate*: physical layout, level of trust among workers, attitudes towards customers, safety/security, dominant feelings

(Schein, 2017: 123)

The third model is that highlighted by Johnson and Scholes (1989) (Figure 12.4). It is one of an organisational cultural web, which portrays the complexity of organisation culture in reflecting how the different components all influence each other.

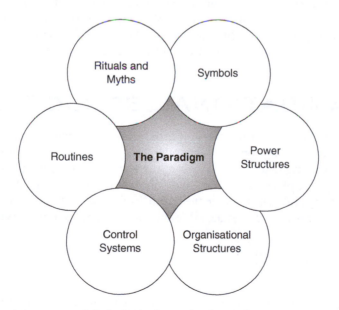

Figure 12.4   Johnson and Scholes's Organisational Cultural Web (1989)

Activity

Can you write five words about each of the components seen in the web and your organisation?

You may have thought about many elements within your practice area. Coming from a nursing background my thoughts are:

- *Rituals and myths*: community staff using newspaper as a barrier to infestation
- *Symbols*: wearing a uniform
- *Power structures*: visibility of Ward Sisters, Charge Nurses or Advanced Practitioners
- *Organisational structures*: salary bandings, Agenda for Change structures
- *Control systems*: appraisals, Personal Development Reviews
- *Routines*: bathing and dressing everyone before 11 a.m.; Health Visitors to leave the office and commence visiting homes starting late morning.

At the most basic ideology of culture there are shared standards defining acceptable behaviours in the NHS that can be visible or invisible (Daft, 2017: 429–30). To 'fit' the culture it is vital that we take note of the 'norms' in terms of the expectations of the sector we are employed in (which can include such things as piercings, tatoos, hairstyle, uniform or manner of dress where no uniform is required) together with understanding the functioning of the organisation we are joining. It does not matter what level we are employed or our perceived status, the industry is judged from the overall image rather than individuals. Every cog in a wheel is vital; sometimes we feel like we don't matter or have any influence over decisions because we are 'at the bottom' of the organisation. This cannot and should not be further from the truth: we all can voice concerns, offer solutions and gain information.

ORGANISATIONAL STRUCTURE

The way an organisation structures its people or functions is important in order to understand how the communication flows from one organisational area to another. Another perspective concerning structures may be that the way an organisation plans its structure relates to the way it plans to *constrain* and *control* its people. Generally, a hierarchical organisational structure is seen within the health service. Task allocation, supervision and coordination generally are undertaken through the organisational structure.

Activity

Can you briefly draw your own immediate structure within your organisation?

Drucker (1989) suggests that organisational structure should satisfy the following tests:

- The structure should be geared for future performance, *not* on a historical basis.
- The structure should have the minimum number of management levels.
- The structure should reflect *upward training and development* towards the top of the organisation.

TYPES OF STRUCTURES

The most usual structure that is represented is the hierarchical vertical structure (Figure 12.5). This hierarchy can be quite 'flat' but it could also be depicted as a 'tall' hierarchy with many more levels, which is currently true within the NHS. Another structural form may be a cross-functional team under several project managers (Figure 12.6). This is usually seen as a complex matrix form of structure. Smaller matrix forms of project teams may be less hierarchical, such as those community teams who work together depending on the needs of specific patient groups. Generally, however, within the health service most professionals have a hierarchical structure of accountability as well.

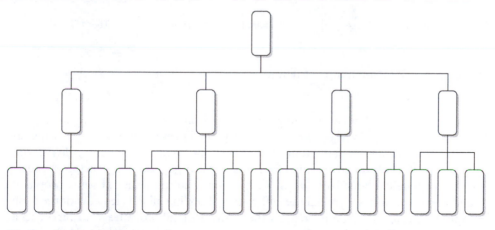

Figure 12.5   Vertical structure

There are many other shapes and forms of structures influenced by international and historical factors. The European Community as an organisation is a highly complex structural entity that bears no resemblance to a hierarchy. However, Leavitt (2005: 2) argues that hierarchies pervade all life, 'in democracies, theocracies, oligarchies, monarchies and autocracies'. He goes on to note that there were even heavenly hierarchies. In rank order these are:

- Seraphim
- Cherubim

- Dominations
- Thrones
- Principalities
- Potentates
- Virtues
- Archangels
- Just plain angels.

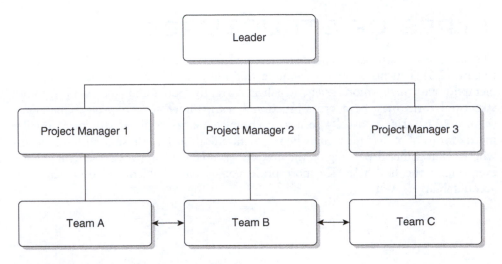

Figure 12.6   Complex matrix structure

He also suggests that human hierarchies were far from being angelic and we do not always like what they do to people and productivity. He goes on to argue that hierarchies are, however, inevitable. Within each level of the hierarchy, job and role descriptions and span of control are essential elements of the organisational structure. Leaders need to recognise the boundaries of job descriptions and the ability of some people to expand these. For others there may be difficulty in fulfilling all the elements of their job description. The span of control reflects the number of subordinates who report to a single supervisor. The 'flat' hierarchy may mean that a supervisor may have a broad span of control whereas a 'tall' hierarchy may reflect a very narrow span of control.

Activity

The organisation you work in has announced plans to change how it is structured to become more efficient whilst being cost effective.

- What do you need to understand to prepare for the changes and ensure that the quality of care offered to patients is not jeopardised and the quality remains high?

Clearly, you would need to know more about the actual plans for the structural change; currently we might think there are too many people within the management team and, by comparison, relatively few people involved with direct patient contact. It is vital to understand the structure of the organisation and the roles of the individual members of the management team before we can make informed decisions related to the proposed changes. Once you fully understand these changes you will be able to form opinions of the efficacy and so be able to offer opinions. We are all able to offer opinions for consideration even though we might think 'they will not make any difference' they just might!

HEALTH SERVICE SYSTEMS

There are many systems within a health care organisation such as the NHS and a variety of ways of looking at the nature of different systems. An organisational system is said to be concerned with flows of processes through the organisational structure (Handy, 1985). The NHS systems could refer to:

- a strategic controlling system
- a marketing system
- a financial system
- an information, research and technology system
- a people management system
- an operational system.

All these systems are interrelated and are as important as each other. Clinical leaders need to recognise these different valuable parts of the organisation and work at networking with different personnel within these systems, so they can seek clarification and advice, as necessary, on a broader scale to help with their own decision making. The relevance of collaboration with the human resource management (HRM) system, however, cannot be overstated. If leaders are responsible for dealing with and influencing people, the skills of the HRM should offer the best support. Intercollaboration between primary, secondary and tertiary systems adds more complexity to understanding how to improve the total patient journey.

ORGANISATIONAL ROLES

In order that an organisation may meet its goals, the work of individual people must be achieved by the variety of roles. Mullins (2016) notes that a 'role' relates to a normal pattern of behaviour linked to a position within the structure of an organisation. Role expectations change and develop from the time someone takes on a new role until they leave that role. Most *health care students* are allocated to clinical placements to learn their professional role during their training, and it is here that they become socialised to their own sphere of work. The learning outcomes, aims and objectives, as laid down by the professional benchmarks, will drive this learning. The management of learning for their professional role is dependent on the learning environments – the place where learners interact with clients, patients and practitioners. Students will then qualify and take their turn in teaching, mentoring and assessing students.

Buckenham (1988) found that the perceptions of students changed during training, in that first-year students thought more about the actual delivery of health care while third-year students thought that the clinical aspects of the job were less important than the effective management aspects. Whatever course you undertake, it appears that many newly qualified practitioners feel unprepared for the management aspect of their roles. Back in 1974, Kramer called this feeling the 'reality shock' where the feeling of dread, terror and fear abounds (Kramer, 1974). Schmalenburg and Kramer (1979) further identified four phases of role transition from student to practitioner:

- **Honeymoon** – finally, the course has been successfully completed and the practitioner has reached their initial aim of qualification.
- **Shock** – suddenly they feel conspicuous in their uniform or new status, and patients expect them to know and understand individual treatments and outcomes and make considered professional judgements.
- **Recovery** – specific practice knowledge is gained (throughout the period of preceptorship) and the practitioner feels more comfortable with their role.
- **Resolution** – efficient practices may lead the practitioner to identify where practice might be improved, and further qualifications might be sought.

It is important that leaders and experienced staff recognise the difficulties that face novice practitioners and help to set up formal and informal support mechanisms. The inclusion of a management and leadership module within pre-registration training gives the newly qualified practitioner an insight into expectations. It is through the exposure to leadership/management knowledge and supervised exposure to practice that new health care professionals can take on leadership roles more effectively. Butler and Hardin-Pierce (2005) note the importance of collaboration between educationalist and service leaders to influence the transition process positively. They recognise the challenges in health care today where there are staff shortages, increased patient acuity and early patient discharges in the acute sector.

The learner, as portrayed in the cartoon, requires support and direction to prevent isolation and bewilderment during the initial period of change and also requires guidance to reach the desired level of confidence; it is vital that the supporters stay in contact rather than move too far away. Whenever you take up a post as a fresh staff member in any of the health care professions, the expectations from your employer will relate to your ability to engage in and maintain exacting standards of health care. There will be an expectation to develop excellent communication skills, both verbal and written. In addition, you are expected to keep yourself up to date with your evidence-base elements of care delivery; however, self-confidence within these

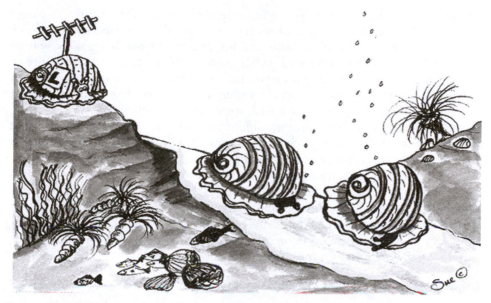

Source: Sue Saillet

expectations may be low at times and it might be difficult for you to recognise the support needed. Feedback on your professional, managerial, educational and administrative skills will help to develop you through a preceptorship and appraisal system. Appraisals are often carried out yearly and a Personal Development Plan (PDP) is agreed between you and your supervisor.

Robinson and Griffiths (2009) in their Scoping Review for the King's Fund explored the impact, facilitation and constraints of preceptorship on clinical practice. Phillips et al. (2015: 118) indicate that transition to newly qualified staff nurse may continue to be difficult for some time. Preceptorship involves supervised practice for a fixed length of time (Gopee and Galloway, 2017: 252) and is dependent on the identified needs of the preceptee, thus it can be of differing lengths of time for different people. The NMC (2016: 6) have indicated that support and guidance from an experienced professional colleague are invaluable for newly qualified nurses, those returning to practice, and for nurses from abroad entering UK practice.

Preceptorship may be a means of improving patient care through workforce retention and development of clinical skills, but more research is needed in these areas. The care delivery expectations of your role will be dependent on the philosophy and culture of the organisation and the health care activities that your course has prepared you for within that context. You will be expected to assess, plan, implement and evaluate care within the standards and philosophy of the organisation. Therefore, it will be important for you to be familiar with policies, procedures and systems that are operationalised in the workplace. There is an expectation that you will contribute to a high standard of care and develop effective relationships at all levels, including those with clients/patients and relatives.

In another part of your role you will be responsible for the care management of a group of patients or clients. However, there should be support from senior colleagues. In your role, your decision-making and problem-solving skills will be applied and tested. You will have to decide on priorities of care and on the use of resources within your control and disposal. The organisation and management of the care of a group of clients/patients is going to be your direct responsibility. In that pursuit you will be expected to cope with some aspects of change as well as being able to delegate, monitor and supervise junior staff who are working in your team. You may also be invited to participate in clinical audit and other activities, which involve collecting information and reviewing care.

There are some expectations that all employers have of their new recruits. Therefore, they have been categorised as general. These include the following behaviours: punctuality, reliability, responsibility, accountability and showing enthusiasm for the post. The importance of authority, accountability, responsibility and delegation is seen within the formal job or role description. This formal contract reflects the ability of the organisation to achieve its mission.

ACCOUNTABILITY, RESPONSIBILITY, AUTHORITY AND DELEGATION

It is useful at this point to distinguish between the terms 'accountability', 'responsibility', 'authority' and 'delegation', and what this means to you and your team in the confines of the organisational structure.

Activity

See if you can define the following:

- Accountability
- Responsibility
- Authority
- Delegation.

It is important to recognise the various definitions of these concepts, which often get confused. Here are some suggested meanings:

- *Accountability* means being able to explain and justify actions or non-actions for a responsibility given to you; this is seen as an important part of a quality system.

- *Responsibility* involves an obligation to perform certain duties or make certain decisions, and having to accept any reprimand from the manager for unsatisfactory performance.
- *Authority* is the right to act or make decisions that legitimises the exercise of power within an organisation.
- *Delegation* means the conferring of a special authority from a higher authority and involves a two-part responsibility; the one to whom authority is delegated becomes responsible to the superior for doing the job, but the superior remains responsible for getting the job done.

Marquis and Huston (2017: 301) give a broad moralistic view of the term when they define accountability as 'Internalised responsibility whereby an individual agrees to be morally responsible for the consequences of his actions'. This definition implies a personal thought process, which is more than just an expectation of a job or a position. Martin (2001) confirms that accountability and responsibility go together. In leading or managing team activities, you may be asked to account for the areas of work for which you are responsible. Accountability is thus more than responsibility. In being accountable, it is now assumed that evidence can be provided for the way the responsibility has been carried out. Accountability within the health service is influenced by professional regulation and civil, employment and criminal law (Table 12.2).

Table 12.2 Features of responsibility, authority and accountability terms

Responsibility	Authority	Accountability
Allocated and accepted	Right to act in areas of given and accepted responsibility	Ability to reflect and evaluate actions/non-actions/decisions
Implies ownership	Levels of authority:	
Implies outcomes		Aids learning for future events
At least a two-way process	• Gathers data/information	
	• Gathers data/information and makes recommendations	
	• Gathers data/information, makes recommendations and initiates action	
	• Informs others how to act/delegates	

We have seen that, over the years, the public's expectations of their health service have been raised. Improved health technology, media coverage and the availability of the internet have meant that the public has had more information on medical and therapeutic advances. Accountability in a civil sense must be seen within this context. The health service is made up of many large organisations where there are numerous people who manage others. The chief executive of a large health Trust is seen to be *accountable* for the total performance and clinical governance of their organisation.

Activity

Why do you think it is important to have a stringent level of accountability in health care?

Patients may not actually know whether they are receiving good or poor care, particularly when they are very ill or disabled. The public have become very aware that they have rights and expectations from their health service; they are now demanding more accountability for public health services especially in light of Francis (2013) and other reviews. Health care professionals work in a very privileged position of trust and need to respect confidences and privacy and use their integrity when managing the care of individuals. The public put a great deal of trust and value in health care personnel when they encounter them in the health service and are often vulnerable when they are in a highly dependent state.

DUTY OF CARE

The concept of 'duty of care' is also important. Cox (2010) in Scrivener et al. (2011) highlights that the law imposes a duty of care on practitioners in circumstances where it is 'reasonably foreseeable' that they may cause harm to patients through their actions or their failure to act. Scrivener et al. also equate the duty of care with responsibility, whatever the task.

Professional accountability on an individual level is laid down within the requirements of each health professional's regulating and registering body, such as the GMC, NMC and HCPC. The term 'professional' is used in this context to convey the notion that health care workers who have a specific qualification which includes registration with a statutory body are expected to display behaviours that are consistent with their specific code of conduct. In this sense, professional behaviour which would be expected of you will include being courteous, non-judgemental, respectful and objective with patients and relatives all the time. In addition to your behaviour, there is also an expectation that your knowledge base and practice will be supported by evidence derived from research and good practice.

Activity

Look at the following dilemma where professional accountability and responsibility feature.

Mr P, a patient in a ward, is very anxious the evening before his operation. The doctor has prescribed Mr P's usual night sedation but unfortunately there is no stock of this drug in the drug trolley for the 10 p.m. drug round.

- What could be done?
- What action should the nurse on duty take, remembering she is accountable for acts of commission and omission?

The nurse could take a reasonable period to try to locate the drug from another ward. If she has no staff to send to look for the drug, she could ask the nurse manager. If the drug was considered 'non-urgent' she may have to decide on whether it could be safely omitted and ordered the next morning or whether it was important enough to contact the duty doctor. Can you think of some 'non-urgent' drugs? Some bowel preparations such as Lactulose may be non-urgent; however, if it is part of the pre-operative preparation it may be considered as vital. As night sedation is important, the nurse should telephone the doctor if the drug cannot be found in the hospital, particularly as it is the night before the operation and it is best practice that the patient has a good night's sleep in preparation for the forthcoming event. The doctor may wish to prescribe something else to ease the patient's anxiety.

EMPLOYMENT ACCOUNTABILITY

Employment accountability is set out under a contract of employment, so all employees will be held accountable to their employing organisation. This is true even for the top person in an organisation, such as the Chief Executive. However, to be held accountable for managing large organisations it is necessary that the top people are effective, so effective delegation is necessary right down the hierarchical line. Registered practitioners are accountable to their line manager for their own actions and the actions of their subordinates in getting the 'job done to the expected standard'. Their subordinates, such as physician's associates or health care assistants, are responsible for doing the job required of them while on duty and will be contractually accountable to the registered practitioner. Students may also be held to account for their 'professional' behaviour to both a university and the NHS Trusts involved, but unless they have an employment contract they will not have a specific line manager. Leaders need to be fully aware of the accountability, responsibility and authority issues that are interrelated with the teams of staff they work with.

HUMAN RESOURCE MANAGEMENT (HRM)

Porter O' Grady and Mallock (2018: 275) note that HRM systems are critical to adjusting and adapting staff behaviours and processes to quality improvement and change. Leaders need to be able to identify the importance of having the right staff to provide health care delivery and how they are formally managed within their employment contract. So, the skills and knowledge are centred around:

- processes of workforce planning
- recruitment and selection
- induction, training and development
- performance management
- employer well-being and support
- outsourcing.

These are all seen within the context of legislation relating to health and safety, equal opportunities, discrimination and rights of the individual. From a leader's perspective, it may be important to end the focus of this chapter on the induction, training and development needs of their team members.

INDUCTION OF NEW STAFF

Induction is seen as an important process in helping inexperienced staff and students settle into the existing culture, such as a clinical environment, to help them understand what is expected of them. It is the first part of a staff development process for new employees and may be closely followed by the period of preceptorship identified earlier. In the health service, important health and safety information needs to be conveyed, such as where the fire alarms are, how the fire alarm system works, and emergency resuscitation and accident procedures. Induction, however, is more than just passing on procedural rules. It is seen as an important part of socialising people into an organisation. Marquis and Huston (2017: 398) even suggest that induction is the first part of the *indoctrination* process and highlight the link with induction, retention and productivity.

Activity

Can you relate to the feelings you had as a newcomer to an established health care team?

It is difficult to try to 'fit' into an already socialised work team and the structure of that organisation. It is, therefore, important that new individuals get a sense of support and friendship when they first join a new team, as well as knowing how to deal with procedural emergencies. Cable and Parsons (2001) found that informal rather than formal types of socialisation had more effect on helping people settle into a new area. Culture is an important aspect in induction. Due to the difficulty of recruiting health care staff, solutions involving recruiting from abroad have meant there have been extra challenges for induction programmes as well. There have been discriminatory stories of the difficulties facing our international recruits who have come in to support our health service. The variations in practice abroad, the language and jargon differences as well as the non-verbal messages that relate to acceptance of staff from abroad, have been barriers to the integration of our internationally trained colleagues. The government (NHS England, 2018d; NMC, 2017c) has issued guidance related to ability in reading, writing, listening and speaking English, together with the adaptation of practice to meet the UK's standard expectations.

TRAINING, DEVELOPMENT AND THE NHS KNOWLEDGE AND SKILLS FRAMEWORK (KSF)

Once staff have been recruited, it is important to value their contribution and motivate them towards achieving a sense of belonging and progression. The Department of Health has produced a framework (DH, 2004) to highlight the variety of levels of skills and knowledge that health care staff reach within the hierarchy of the organisation. It was a complex framework but has been much simplified and now focuses on six dimensions:

- Communication
- Personal and people development
- Health, safety and security
- Service improvement
- Quality
- Equality and diversity.

(www.nhsemployers.org/SimplifiedKSF)

This is a useful framework which can help leaders work with their teams to develop higher order skills and knowledge. The use of regular appraisal, yearly Development and Performance Reviews (DPRs), and training and development plans is essential to help staff move 'upwards' in the organisation. Ultimately this can only enhance better patient care that will fit into the clinical governance perspective of the organisation (Chapter 13).

Summary of Key Points

This chapter has briefly looked at various aspects of organisational life to meet the identified learning outcomes. These were:

- **Understand the importance of the overall organisation** By understanding the organisation in terms of structures and processes you can more easily see an overall picture rather than just a small functioning part.
- **Discuss the importance of strategy, structures and systems within the organisation** From a broad NHS policy to a practice perspective we have seen how the health service sets about achieving its goals. Strategies are vital to cope with the pressures of effective service provision. Varieties of strategies were highlighted to demonstrate organisational direction and its communication through mission statements and policy.
- **Critically explore the notion of organisational culture** This highlighted overt and covert aspects of any organisational climate, be it the NHS or a small team organisation.
- **Reflect on the nature of organisational roles** This involved examining the expectations of staff and students in a health care organisation and the importance of effective leadership in helping people attain their full potential.
- **Critically examine professional responsibility and accountability as well as the notions of authority and delegation** Effective leadership requires an understanding of these aspects in terms of supporting boundary management for team members.
- **Develop an overview of Human Resource processes in organisations** By examining the importance of human resources, leaders should be able to manage effective recruitment and retention strategies. This was looked at in the context of the NHS Knowledge and Skills Framework within the health service.

ONLINE RESOURCES

For online resources, including SAGE journal articles, weblinks and videos, visit the book's website: https://study.sagepub.com/barr4e.

FURTHER READING

Bae, S-H., Farasat, A., Nikolaev, A., Seo, J.Y., Foltz-Ramos, K., Fabry, D. and Castner, J. (2017) Nursing teams: behind the charts, *Journal of Nursing Management*, 25: 354–65.
Department of Health (2005) *A Patient-Led NHS*. London: DH.
Easterby-Smith, M., Burgoyne, J. and Arunjo, L. (1999) *Organisational Learning and the Learning Organisation*. London: Sage.
Schein, E. (1997) *Empowerment, Coercive Persuasion and Organisational Learning: Do They Connect?* Henley on Thames: Henley Management College.
Senge, P.M. (2006) *The Fifth Discipline* (2nd edn). London: Random House Business.

13 QUALITY

Chapter Contents

Learning Outcomes

By the end of this chapter you will have had the opportunity to:

- Identify the importance of quality in the health service for better patient outcomes
- Discuss the historical developments that led to the present quality agenda
- Discuss the importance of clinical governance and audit
- Critically explore the principes of patient safety and human factors in team working in the context of quality health care
- Compare a variety of quality models to inform effective leadership for continuous improvement of health care delivery
- Relate the importance of leadership for professional learning and development

INTRODUCTION

This chapter will examine the concept of quality and how it has developed over time. Overarching health care models such as Total Quality Management (TQM), LEAN and Six Sigma will be highlighted. There will also be a focus on more recent health service quality initiatives, particularly post the Francis Report (2013) which highlighted the NHS's neglect of patient safety and care. The impact of quality and the necessary human factors within the health service will also be examined in the context of how this enhances the overall quality of care delivery to patients/clients.

CONTEMPORARY AND HISTORICAL CONTEXT OF QUALITY MOVEMENT IN HEALTH CARE

The White Paper *A First-Class Service: Quality in the New NHS Health Services* (DH, 1998) demonstrated the commitment of past governments to providing quality health services and its features are still pertinent today, particularly the relevance of the ideas of clinical governance and lifelong learning. It set out a statutory 'duty of quality' for all providers of NHS services. Ten years later, Lord Darzi published *High Quality Care For All: NHS Next Stage Review* (DH, 2008) which proposed a new seven-step framework for quality and included the importance of health care leadership. More recently, Darzi (2018) has written an interim report as the NHS celebrates seventy years, and notes that in the last decade of austerity quality across most areas of the NHS from cancer to trauma, stroke to diabetes, mental health to maternity has been maintained or improved. Patient safety has also improved, and progress has been seen in social care. There are, however, challenges of equity and access to services. The NHS (2014) *Five Year Forward View* (FYFV) had a focus on a shift towards more prevention and integration of NHS systems across sectors. Sir Bruce Keogh (2017) noted the challenges of demand, supply and equity for the future of UK health care, and the NHS's (2017) *Next Steps on the NHS Five Years Forward View* sets out a 10-point priority plan predominantly to address cost-effectiveness in the NHS to improve quality.

The Health and Social Care Act 2012 noted the role of the Care Quality Commission (CQC), which was originally established in 2009 to act as a regulator for health and social care in England. Their remit is to ensure that safe and high-quality services are provided to patients. Their aim is to ensure better joined-up care provision for everyone in hospital, in a care home and home settings. They assess and inspect health and social care provision and work to improve health and social care services with specific work around people affected under the Mental Health

Act. Glasper (2014: 110) highlighted that a new CQC inspection system gave a more focused inquiry into hospitals, care homes and other health and social care institutions. The focus is on five questions:

- Is it safe?
- Is it effective?
- Is it caring?
- Is it responsive to people's needs?
- Is it well-led?

The CQC fundamental standards relate to person-centred care, dignity and respect, consent, safety, safeguarding from abuse, food and drink, premises and equipment, governance, staffing, complaints, duty of candour and ratings display (www.cqc.org.uk). The Care Quality Commission (CQC) (2018) recently noted that the quality of care across England is mostly good and quality has improved overall, but there is too much variation and some services have deteriorated. Care providers are under pressure and there must be more local collaboration and joined-up care.

There are other quality frameworks presently in place to support the evidence required by the CQC. Power et al. (2012) identified the contribution of the Commissioning for Quality and Innovation (CQUIN) framework in raising the standards of health care based on a target system for providers with financial payments as rewards. The CQUIN (2018) 2017–2019 *Guidance* focus is on 13 targets:

- Improving the health of staff (1)
- Reducing serious infections (2)
- Improving the outcomes and experience of patients with mental health needs (3, 4 and 5)
- Enabling GPs to have better access to consultants to determine the best course of action for their patients and make it easier for GPs to access appointments for their patients (6 and 7)
- Improving patient experience from hospital to care home (8)
- Patients accessing advice and referral to services to prevent ill health related to tobacco and alcohol (9)
- Community services placing a greater emphasis on wound care leading to better patient and system outcomes (10)
- Empowering staff to help patients take more control of their own existing long-term conditions (11)
- Supporting patients to move through the urgent care services in a way that meets their clinical needs (12 and 13).

The NHS Safety Thermometer was one of the CQUIN schemes launched in 2012 to take a snapshot measure of common 'harms' in the NHS. There are five safety thermometers: Classic; Medication; Mental Health; Maternity; and Children and Young People.

Activity

Check out the website below for your speciality thermometer and explore the features for you and your speciliast team:

www.safetythermometer.nhs.uk

All of these demonstrate a desire to rebuild quality in the NHS, but also reflect some of the complexity of various health organisations and their standards currently.

Historically, during the 1970s and early 1980s, the concept of quality became more important in industry. Quality as a valued commodity began to be associated with the manufacturing industry, where products were inspected for their worth. Barr and Dowding (2016: 229) noted the development of quality from the 1960s to the twenty-first century (Table 13.1).

Table 13.1 Historical development of quality

	Traditional pre-1960	Technocratic 1960s and 1970s	TQM 1980s and 1990s	Contemporary health care quality – Service Improvement
Definition	La crème de la crème	Fitness for use Meeting requirements	Satisfying and delighting the customer	Clinical effectiveness Patient safety Patient experience
Who defines quality?	Everybody knows what it is	Experts	Customers	Triangulation of stakeholder views
Nature of quality	Attributes of product or service	Attributes of product or service	Process and outcomes	Systems, processes and outcomes
What produces good quality?	Good people and materials	Good people and materials	The right processes	The right systems and processes
Relationship to cost	Top quality is the most expensive	Quality can be found at all prices but improving quality implies raising costs	Quality is free	Public austerity affects care quality

However, this early emphasis on quality was rarely associated with the service industries and not particularly with health care. It was felt to be in business for the good of society, not profit, and thus closed to quality scrutiny. The British government launched the National Quality Campaign in 1984 for both private and public industries, with the NHS being strongly encouraged to put a quality control system in place. There was initial resistance and scepticism from professionals who felt that they already gave a quality service. From these initial developments, the NHS worked through concepts such as quality assurance, then moved through to the Total Quality Management concept (which focuses on meeting and satisfying the needs of customers), towards the idea of continuous process improvement. The latter idea focuses on an active journey of not only meeting customer needs but also 'delighting the customer'. Whether this phrase is appropriate in health service delivery is debatable, but at least it reflects that quality is not just about complacency and 'standing still'.

Past statutes introduced the National Performance Framework, and clinical governance and quality structures such as the newly renamed National Institute for Health and Care Excellence (NICE) which as the agency for establishing which overall treatments and interventions work best, has the remit of making sure clinicians know about them.

The Healthcare Quality Improvement Partnership (HQIP) (2015) used the Darzi definition of 'quality' (DH, 2008) which is seen as three dimensional:

- Clinical effectiveness: quality care is care which is delivered according to the best evidence as to what is clinically effective in improving an individual's health outcomes.
- Patient safety: quality care is care which is delivered so as to avoid all avoidable harm and risks to the individual's safety.
- Patient experience: quality care is care which looks to give the individual as positive an experience of receiving and recovering from the care as possible, including being treated according to what that individual wants or needs and with compassion, dignity and respect.

This definition has now been enshrined in legislation through the Health and Social Care Act 2012.

CONCEPTS AND DIMENSIONS OF QUALITY IN THE HEALTH SERVICE

Quality is a relative concept and although we all have some idea what is good and what is bad, identifying what is acceptable is not so straightforward. Quality could be about being effective and efficient. Drucker (1996 [1967]) defined efficiency simply as 'doing things right' and effectiveness as 'doing the right things right'. The questions to ask though are 'what is right?' and 'how do we know we are doing the right things right?' It may be very difficult to know what is right in emotional support, for example, so we can only 'best guess' initially and then later reflect on the outcomes to see how well the patient reacts. In other cases, we know that using an ABC approach to first aid is the right approach to use, based on evidence and research. The NHS (2017) noted that during 2017/18 CCGs and trusts would be expected to step up their work to get more value out of the NHS's growing, multi-billion pound investment in elective care. For GPs and CCGs this will mean tackling the clinical practice variation in referrals. For trusts this will mean tackling the variation in clinical quality and productivity revealed by the Getting it Right First Time (GIRFT) programme. CCGs and trusts will mean redesigning care pathways jointly to promote optimal patient care in line with the RightCare programme.

A model depicting the dimensions of quality may provide one approach to understanding quality for health professions. The Institute of Medicine (2001) identified the six dimensions of health care quality as:

1. Safety
2. Effectiveness
3. Equity
4. Efficiency
5. Timeliness
6. Patient centredness.

Other research has involved an exploration of which quality dimensions would be important to the health service. Interestingly Greaves et al. (2012) explored the 'cloud experience' of patients to unconventionally unearth how blogs and social media sites such as Twitter can be used to detect poor health care experiences in patients' own narratives. This development appears to be gaining momentum in recognising how the internet and social media have changed the lives of the population, thus giving them a more public voice. The early research work of Berry et al. (1988), using in-depth interviews with a number of 'customer' groups, concluded that the groups highlighted several dimensions of quality (Table 13.2). This expands quality dimensions from a non-expert basis and best practice and poor practice examples are provided.

Table 13.2 Dimensions of quality (Berry et al., 1988)

Quality Dimension	Best Practice	Poor Practice
Reliability	Good IT health information	Failure to contact service user if that was agreed
Responsiveness	Staff who can address issues that arise unexpectedly	Long waits without direct action/ no explanations from issues that arise unexpectedly
Competence	Skilled staff	Staff inadequately trained for tasks required

Quality Dimension	Best Practice	Poor Practice
Access	Ease of access to facilities or staff; good signposting and attention given to those with disabilities	Poor signposting/limited parking
Courtesy	Polite and helpful staff	Patronising and unhelpful staff
Communication	Staff who explain a diagnosis and alternative treatments/ interventions without jargon	Lack of information about what is happening or what could happen
Credibility	Staff you can trust and depend on	Staff who don't appear to have the full information about individuals
Security	A feeling of safeness/ confidentiality	Unlit access to facilities
Understanding	Staff who try to understand them as individuals	Staff who don't recognise a regular service user
Tangibles	Pleasing physical appearance of facilities	Poor/out of date equipment/ accommodation

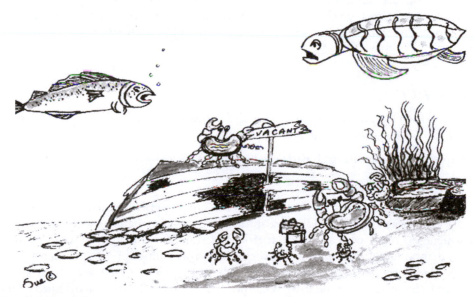

Source: Sue Saillet

The image above depicts the crab as an 'estate agent' trying to sell a dilapidated shipwreck to a turtle and fish which relates to the poor tangible dimension of quality.

QUALITY MODELS

CLINICAL GOVERNANCE

The notion that public services had a responsibility for monitoring and improving their provision, in the context of health care, was coined 'clinical governance'. It is defined as 'a system through which NHS organisations are accountable for continuously improving the quality of their services and safeguarding high standards of care by creating an environment in which excellence in clinical care will flourish' (Scally and Donaldson, 1998: 61; DH, 1998). Public Health England (2018) note that clinical governance encompasses quality assurance, quality improvement and risk and incident management.

STANDARDS, QUALITY ASSURANCE AND QUALITY IMPROVEMENT

The ability of the health service to assure quality is an important means of building public confidence but must be taken in light of what staff feel are important standards. The use of care or clinical pathways is one example of what patients/clients will expect and what commissioners will wish to build into their contracts.

Activity

Review the following NICE hypertension care pathway that you are perhaps familiar with and jot down your thoughts on the algorithm or flowchart.

https://pathways.nice.org.uk/pathways/hypertension

I think the hypertension flowchart shows a simple patient management and the ability to click to subfolders for more information on care management and specific treatment for those who are more at risk. The standards of care are well depicted in the diagram. In terms of the NHS, there can be difficulties in always reaching the standard required; it is important to identify how well a service measures up to these standards. So, what are standards? What do they mean for health practitioners? Barr and Dowding (2016: 242) state that standards must:

- describe the desired quality of performance
- have been agreed
- have been clearly written
- contain one major thought

- be measurable
- be concise
- be specific
- be achievable
- be clinically sound.

There are eight prerequisites for a successful standard:

- A philosophy
- The relevant skills and knowledge
- The authority to act
- Accountability
- The control of resources
- Organisational structure and management style
- The professional relationships
- The management of change.

Standard statements should be related, descriptive, free from bias, suitable for quantification, valid and reliable so that they are unambiguous. NICE provide national quality standards and clinical care pathway diagrams on a wide range of conditions and public health items.

Donabedian (2003: xiii) defined quality assurance as 'all actions taken to establish to protect, promote, and improve the quality in healthcare'. However, he notes that the term is misleading, offering up the term 'quality management' as an alternative but one that is not as widely used and well known as quality assurance. There is debate as to whether quality assurance concerns maintaining the health care quality and standards and whether Quality Improvement (QI) is a better term to focus on for raising standards. The World Health Organization (1983) identified the four main principles of quality assurance in health care as:

- professional performance (technical quality)
- resource use (efficiency)
- risk management
- patient satisfaction with the service provided.

Donabedian's (1966) early approach to quality evaluation has been regularly used within the NHS and serves as a reminder of the different domains that affect health care (see below).

- **Structure** The factors within the organisation that enable work to be carried out: these may be environmental facilities, equipment, staffing, educational facilities and management factors
- **Process** The performance or activity required to achieve the outcome, i.e. the care given to an individual, group or community
- **Outcome** The result of care and performance or the effect of care on an individual, group or community.

However, Keighley (1989) argued against the Donebedian approach and identified two elements of a quality standard: the technical performance and the expressive performance. Technical performance is something that the customer expects the NHS to deliver consistently. Good technical performance is achieved through knowledge that is required in training, in the use of supplies, the use of facilities, and most of all is dependent on the number of staff available to deliver the service. In contrast, expressive performance is concerned with staff attitudes – in their relationships and interactions with customers and with each other – and the way the staff deliver the service. This 'fits' well with the notion of 'non-technical skills' mentioned earlier, and the findings proposed by Berry et al. (1988), but it is also true to say that it is more difficult to define what constitutes 'good expressive performance', as this can be quite subjective to the individual giving or receiving it.

Activity

Think about your own clinical care delivery. Jot down how each of these aspects can be applied to your service.

CLINICAL AUDIT

NHS England (2018a) note the importance of the National Clinical Audit and Patient Outcomes Programme (NCAPOP) to improve outcomes for patients. Clinical audits can look at care nationwide or locally. Clinical audits attempt to do more than set standards and so assess and regularly monitor standards. The idea of measuring quality implies that there will be some benchmark of quality acceptability. The definition of a benchmark is 'a standard or point of reference against which metrics may be compared or assessed' (Sauro, 2018: 2).

NICE (2018) provide a framework for clinical audit which includes five stages:

1. Audit preparation
2. Identify population inclusion and exclusion criteria
3. Measure performance
4. Make improvements
5. Re-audit and sustain improvements.

NICE (2018) provide a quality standard improvement template which reflects an iterative model for audit. This audit template uses the three elements of Donebedian's quality framework of 'structure, process and outcome'.

Some examples in general practice relate to cervical screening, asthma and diabetic reviews and improving the annual check for those with learning disabilities, based on NICE quality standards. Clinical effectivess is really at the heart of standards, evidence-based practice and governance. On a broader health perspective,

---

Activity

Check out the NICE website for the template. It is complex, but you can see how this tool is used by many Trusts, GPs and commissioners for their quality improvement activity.

www.nice.org.uk/About/What-we-do/Into-practice/Audit-and-service-improvement

---

Key Performance Indicators (KPIs) are agreed between DH and NHS England and in the Public Health Outcomes Framework (PHOF). The 2018 *Integrated Urgent Care Key Performance Indicators and Quality Standards* published by NHS England makes interesting reading because of the recent concern about these services being able to cope, and the need for them to be redesigned to integrate between A&E departments, GP out-of-hours services, urgent care centres, NHS 111, and ambulance services (NHS England, 2018b).

Another quality monitoring aspect is the NHS financial and performance activity that is measured through the National Audit Office (NAO). It has the statutory role of scrutinising public spending for parliament. The NAO (2018) noted in a recent report that the NHS is well placed to get value for money from its investment in developing new care models reflecting a quality improvement culture within the NHS.

TOTAL QUALITY MANAGEMENT (TQM), LEAN AND SIX SIGMA MODELS

It is useful to explore overarching quality models that have been used in the health economy but previously been used in other industries to improve the business. Goetch and Davis (2014: 3) give the quality analogy of the three-legged stool model relating to:

- *People*: empowered staff, quality is expected not inspected
- *Processes*: cultural improvement, good enough is never good enough
- *Measures*: benchmarking, quality tools and target setting
- The 'seat' is then the customer focus.

They explore the continued importance of 'Total Quality' and the internal and external customer focus for survival which is linked to the TQM model. Total Quality Management is a business philosophy based on customer satisfaction and the notion of continuous improvement. TQM is a strategy aimed at the whole organisation in order that resources are better managed; people cooperate so that the organisation is more flexible and responsive to what are internal and external customers. It was

Deming (1986) who first introduced this quality model very successfully to manufacturing in Japan in the 1950s. One feature concerning the importance of 'customer focus' meant that organisations started to think very differently about their products and how they met with buyers' expectations. The notion of 'customers' as a feature within the health industry creates a difficulty. In business, customer growth is seen as an ideal and as healthy. If patients are considered customers in the NHS, their growth would infer a greater cost to an already stretched service. However, this aside, the use of 'customer' within the concept of quality has got a wider interpretation. Deming also proposed a Deming cycle of TQM which reflects four stages of improvement and change, i.e. Plan, Do, Check, Act (Figure 13.1).

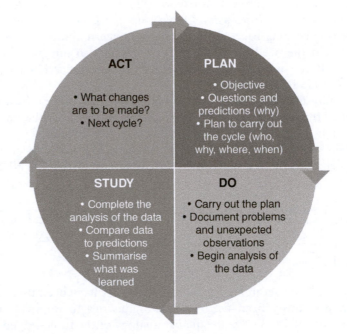

Figure 13.1   Plan, Do, Study, Act

Source: (Adapted from Deming 1986)

Mosadeghrad (2014) holds that TQM is not without its difficulties. His literature review research points to the following barriers: insufficient education and training, lack of employee involvement, lack of top management support, inadequate resources, deficient leadership, lack of a quality-oriented culture, poor communication, lack of a plan for change and employee resistance to change programmes. Mosadeghrad (2014) concludes that organisations need to better understand these quality barriers issues in their quality management focus.

Customers are individuals or groups of people who need a product or a service. The breadth of this definition means that customers can be our patients and clients, or *external customers*, as they are outside the organisation. In broader terms, external customers could also relate to any external agency that purchases a service from any health provider, such as an NHS Trust or one of the five regional teams associated with NHS England that support the commissioning of health services and education providers via the number of clinical commissioning groups (CCGs). There are also *internal customers* within an organisation, reflecting the interdependent relationships between organisational departments. All internal departments are affected by the quality of each other and no department/discipline works in isolation. If the X-Ray department did not come up with their services on time, then this would affect surgical and medical decisions. Similarly, if there was a poor catering service, medical and therapy staff may feel more disgruntled and this may influence the quality of interpersonal communications with patients. The LEAN model approach to quality focuses on the customer processes and aims to reduce the wasted or unnecessary processes – making them leaner – thereby improving the quality. If you think about it in health care processes, this is about the patient journey and the complexities involved in getting the patient to receive the right care appropriately. Patient journeys, however, are not linear by any means and the story below gives an example.

John developed head and neck cancer which was affected by the drug therapy for his ulcerative colitis. This was treated successfully but then his ulcerative colitis became worse and he had lower gastrointestinal surgery resulting in an ileostomy. Soon after this, an undetected upper gastrointestinal stomach cancer which was inoperable was discovered. John's journey in his last five years of life involved going from department to department across two hospitals, many consultants and health personnel, and a plethora of diagnostics. The fragmented approach to his journey left John and his family feeling frustrated with the poor communication and lack of joined-up services, and at times abandoned. John eventually died at home with his family beside him, which was his final choice. This journey of two years was traumatic at times and yet there was genuine care and compassion provided.

The LEAN methodology in health care involves five stages:

1. Define the population.
2. Map the value stream.
3. Reduce wastage.
4. Respond to what patients see as valuable.
5. Aim for perfection.

Six Sigma is a quality model related to TQM/LEAN which aims to improve the quality of processes by minimising and eventually removing errors and variations. It was introduced by Motorola in 1986 but was popularised by Jack Welch (who incorporated the strategy in his business processes at General Electric in the USA) and Bill Smith. Experts predict that Six Sigma will outshine TQM in due course. Six Sigma is more complicated than the overall TQM approach and has a basis of customer feedback with more accuracy and a results orientation. NHS England (2004) supports the NHS Modernisation Agency's (2004) document *10 High Impact*

Changes for Service Improvement and Delivery which provides examples of improvements for patient flow-through processes:

Change No. 1   Treat day surgery (rather than inpatient surgery) as the norm for elective surgery.

Change No. 2   Improve patient flow across the whole NHS system by improving access to key diagnostic tests.

Change No. 3   Manage variation in patient discharge thereby reducing length of stay.

Change No. 4   Manage variation in the patient admission process.

Change No. 5   Avoid unnecessary follow-ups for patients and provide necessary follow-ups in the right care setting.

Change No. 6   Increase the reliability of performing therapeutic interventions through a Care Bundle approach.

Change No.7   Apply a systematic approach to care for people with long-term conditions.

Change No. 8   Improve patient access by reducing the number of queues.

Change No. 9   Optimise patient flow through service bottlenecks using process templates.

Change No. 10   Redesign and extend roles in line with efficient patient pathways to attract and retain an effective workforce.

There are numerous and possibly contentious ways of identifying what overall quality means in the health service. We probably see health care quality models merging into an eclectic model communicated by government policy today, but depending on the audience one may enjoy more emphasis than the others.

PATIENT SAFETY AND HUMAN FACTORS

The poor state of care delivered at the Mid Staffordshire NHS Foundation Trust raised up a new approach to NHS quality after 2013. This new approach demonstrated the link between good care, safety and good leadership. McCaughan and Kaufman (2013) in their comprehensive review of patient safety knowledge noted the different 'patient safety' terminology:

- Harm – where health care negatively affects a patient's/client's health or quality of life; this may be due to errors or to those known possibilities such as surgical complications, adverse drug reactions or hospital acquired infections

- Errors or mistakes – due to faulty judgements, decisions or problem solving
- Slips and lapses – errors caused by a lack of attention or distraction
- Adverse events – unintended harm by medical management
- Patient safety incidents – i.e. unintended or unexpected incidents
- Near misses – i.e. potentially harmful but prevented
- 'Never' events – e.g. wrong limb amputation.

Adverse events can be related to primary, acute or tertiary care. Common adverse events may often be preventable. Some common examples may be:

- Development of pressure ulcers
- Chest infections
- Poor catheter care
- Medication errors
- 'Failure to rescue': unrecognised patient deterioration possibly resulting in cardiac arrest, suicide

Mollon (2014) analysed the concept of 'feeling safe during hospitalisation' using Walker and Avant's attributes, antecedents and consequences model. From the qualitative literature the analysis can be seen in Table 13.3. The conclusion was that more patient-centred care models and the creation of more positive environments were needed for patients to feel safe.

Table 13.3 Concept analysis of 'feeling safe' (Mollon, 2014)

Attributes	Antecedents	Consequences
Trust	Relationship	Control
Cared for	Environment	Hope
Presence	Suffering	Relaxed/calm
Knowledge		

The context of health care delivery and patient safety has over the years been challenged by the reduction of senior and more experienced staff available at weekends, evenings and nights in order to contain the staffing costs in unsocial hour payments. Moore (2014) notes the new strategy to transform hospital care for more consistent care 24/7. She notes the national research showing that patients admitted during the weekend have a significantly higher risk of dying within 30 days than those admitted on a Wednesday. This new approach means the 'manic Mondays' of ward rounds, discharges and requests for new diagnostics will be evened out over the week. This may also mean more extended and expanded practice with more experienced nurses taking the place of junior doctors in training during the unsocial periods. This will also influence the need to increase community health services to 24/7 provision, e.g. in the district nursing service, nursing and care homes. The difficulties with this are whether funding can be found for more health care practitioners.

Patient safety and medication prescription/administration are also significant. Around 1,800 patient prescriptions in three general practices across three primary care Trusts were examined in a retrospective case-note review, and Avery et al. (2012) noted that around one in 20 prescriptions contained a mild to moderate error and that one in 550 was viewed as serious, i.e. missing information on dosage or essential monitoring. Many factors were associated and more research is needed. McCaughan and Kaufman (2013: 51) identified three relevant models for health professionals assessing patient safety (see Table 13.4).

Table 13.4　Models of patient safety (after McCaughan and Kaufman, 2013)

Person Model (Person and Behaviour Characteristics)	System Model (Organisational Focus)	Human Factors (Combination of Person and System Models)
Individual characteristics: knowledge, skill and competence	Financial and environmental resources: staffing levels, administrative and managerial support and available equipment	The individual
Task complexity for individuals	Management priorities	The job
Team factors: leadership communication and supervision	Policies and standards	The organisation
	Culture of support or blame	Ergonometric and environmental technology to enhance better health care judgements

HUMAN FACTORS AND ROOT CAUSE ANALYSIS

The case of 37-year-old Elaine Bromiley, who died during a fairly minor surgical treatment in 2005, was investigated, and it was found that she was being treated by two experienced anaesthetists, two operating department practitioners, an ENT surgeon and two recovery nurses in an emergency situation. Emergency equipment was all at hand, including the tracheostomy kit that could have saved her life (Reid and Bromiley, 2012). The (2005) Harmer inquiry found that the surgical team were not neglectful, but that there was a lack of discussion between the team about the best course of action and confusion about the use of different pieces of equipment. It appears there was a lack of appreciation of human behaviour under the stressful situation and everyone lost sight of the escalating deterioration; the leadership and contribution of all in the team were poor. Elaine's husband, a pilot, has campaigned to understand the human factors and the absence of these non-technical skills that affected the emergency care needed for his wife. The similarities between the surgical context and aviation industry highlighted the need for more simulation training in the health industry. The UK Clinical Human Factors Group (CHFG) was set up. It is a broad coalition of health care professionals, managers and service users who have partnered with experts in human factors from health care and other high-risk industries to campaign for change in the NHS. The CHFG (2019) note that 'Human factors are organisational, individual, environmental, and job characteristics in ways that can impact safety'.

The role of human factors in medical care linked to patient safety is therefore seen as being different from the neglectfulness and incompetence of certain health care practitioners, which is often the worldview and subject of media attention when things go wrong in clinical care. The latter brings about a blame culture which can be unhelpful in moving the organisation to learn from past mistakes. Flin and Maran (2004) and White (2019) identified that in health care, cognitive, interpersonal and social non-technical skills are as important as technical skills. Cognitive skills include:

- Situation awareness
- Decision making
- Task management.

Interpersonal and social skills include:

- Leadership
- Followship
- Effective communication.

It is these non-technical skills that may affect health outcomes for patients when teams are under stress and do not perform at their most effective. This is also true where there is an authority or hierarchical difference in the multi-professional teams as well as between regulated and unregulated members of staff.

Accountability and having the confidence to speak up are essential at all levels of caregiving. Health care professionals need to engage all members of a team, at whatever level, to have a voice for the safety of patients. In 2004 the National Patient Safety Agency (NPSA) produced the 'Seven steps to patient safety' model (Table 13.5). Specific publications for mental health, primary care and general practice teams have also been produced. These are invaluable leadership issues for developing any team culture.

Table 13.5   Seven steps to patient safety for health care teams (NPSA, 2004)

Step 1: building a safety culture	Create a culture that is open and fair
Step 2: leading and supporting the practice team	Establishing a clear and strong focus on patient safety throughout your organisation
Step 3: integrating risk management activity	Developing systems and processes to manage your risks and identify and assess things that could go wrong
Step 4: promoting reporting	Ensuring staff can easily report incidents locally and nationally
Step 5: involving and communicating with patients and the public	Developing ways to communicate openly with and to listen to patients
Step 6: learning and sharing safety lessons	Encouraging staff to use root cause analysis to learn how and why incidents happen
Step 7: implementing solutions to prevent harm	Embed lessons through changes to practice, processes or systems

The role of patients and the public in monitoring the quality of their health services is not new but there is now an agenda to ensure their voices are heard more clearly. Shapiro et al. (2013), for instance, highlight the role of patients in the USA being more in control of checking on the quality of their surgical procedures. However, the public are often not well equipped to know how to determine what it is they should be checking when they are obviously concerned about their own health and pending treatment. Research has shown that coronary care nurses are more likely than any other health care professional to recognise, intercept and correct errors that are life threatening (Rothschild et al., 2006). Mansour (2014) notes that nursing education therefore has to address how to prepare students with knowledge and skills related to patient safety from early on in their courses. His quantitative research into student perceptions of patient safety is a useful start in raising awareness to influence practice, and he notes the value of the WHO's (2011) *Patient Safety Curriculum* which is globally recommended for embedding into all nurse education.

Moller (2013: 506) notes the importance of accountability and transparency in medical error reporting. Health service cultures must change from a blame culture where staff are reluctant to admit near misses or mistakes to a culture of fairness and understanding of the connection between human factors and system failures. She highlights a quote from a 2009 safety report:

To err is human – To delay is deadly.

Learning lessons from incidents, near misses and complaints is invaluable. Root Cause Analysis (RCA) is a structured process often used as a reactive method to identify causes after an adverse event has occurred, or as an investigative tool to identify causes after clinical audit findings demonstrate shortfalls in the quality of care. HQIP (2016) provides guidelines for RCA activities which reflect the techniques identified in problem solving including the often used 'Fishbone' model along with the Five Whys technique (see Chapter 8) .

Effective leadership, accountability and the quality of the organisational culture are therefore vital to maintain patient safety (McCaughan and Kaufman, 2013; Moller, 2013).

It appears then that there is consensus on what health care quality means and how it can be measured.

THE NHS OUTCOMES FRAMEWORK

The NHS Outcomes Framework (NHSOF) is a set of indicators developed by the Department of Health and Social Care to monitor the health outcomes of adults and children in England. The framework provides an overview of how the NHS is performing (NHS England, 2018c). Morbidity, mortality, survival potential, years of life lost, employment and critical incidents are measured annually. The framework is focused on improving health and reducing health inequalities through five domains:

- Preventing people from dying prematurely
- Enhancing quality of life for people with long-term conditions
- Helping people to recover from episodes of ill health or following injury
- Ensuring that people have a positive experience of care
- Treating and caring for people in a safe environment and protecting them from avoidable harm.

The Quality and Outcomes Framework (QOF) is a specific voluntary reward and incentive programme for GP practices in England, introduced in 2004.

Practices are rewarded for:

- their achievements in relation to how well the practice is organised
- how patients view their experience at the surgery
- the number of extra services offered, such as child health and maternity services
- how the practice manages the most prevalent chronic diseases such as asthma and diabetes.

The QOF is divided into clinical domains:

- Coronary heart disease
- Stroke
- Hypertension

- Diabetes mellitus
- Chronic obstructive pulmonary disease
- Epilepsy
- Hypothyroidism
- Cancer
- Mental health
- Asthma.

STAFF DEVELOPMENT

Ultimately, quality relies on well-trained and critical practitioners who are well motivated and enthusiastic about improving care continuously. Clinical governance, therefore, relies on professional regulation and lifelong learning. The importance of staff development is clear but it does depend on health organisations having the finances to deal with this. In NHS Trusts with high financial deficits, training budgets are the first to go. Therefore, the question of who funds staff development is an important issue as, ultimately, this aspect of quality underpins the health service clinical governance theme.

PROFESSIONAL DEVELOPMENT

The NMC's (2018c, 2018d, 2018e, 2018g) recent *Realising Professionalism: Standards for Education and Training* (including pre-registration and prescribing courses, student supervision and assessment) provides a new professional approach to allow for more flexibility and innovative routes to registration. Public safety is central to these standards and the NMC Quality Assurance Framework will be utised to approve and monitor this aspect of professional development. The new NMC (2018a) *Future Nurse: Standards of Proficiency for Registered Nurses* is structured under seven platforms and reflects the importance of leadership and quality:

- Being an accountable practitioner
- Promoting health and preventing ill health
- Assessing needs and planning care
- Providing and evaluating practice
- Leading and managing nursing care and working in teams
- Improving safety and quality of care
- Coordinating care.

All health care professionals are expected to acknowledge their own contribution to safety and quality of care by engaging in professional development activities within their sphere of work, e.g. the NMC's (2017a) *Revalidation* standards aim to provide a more robust nature to assuring quality care for those who are registered.

CONCLUSION

The main emphasis of this chapter has been to examine the concepts of quality and attempt to relate these to professional practice. An overview of quality in health care has been offered, and some of the historical developments and policy in quality have been highlighted – and then taken into the context of the contemporary health service, towards the concepts of clinical governance, clinical audit and patient safety. A number of quality models have been briefly explored. Finally, the importance of staff development has been examined to reflect the relevance for leaders of developing and motivating their teams towards self-mastery – for the benefit of patients/clients and improvements in care.

Summary of Key Points

This chapter has identified the importance of leadership and quality in the health service to meet the identified learning outcomes:

- **Identify the importance of quality in the health service for better patient outcomes** This was discussed in the context of present quality agendas through a variety of policy drivers.
- **Discuss the historical developments that led to the present quality agenda** The historical developments towards the present quality NHS agenda related to a number of quality gurus and their influence on the health service and health care delivery.
- **Discuss the importance of clinical governance and audit** These aspects of contemporary policy were explored and debated within the finite resources of health services.
- **Critically explore the principles of patient safety and the aspect of human factors associated with safe care.** This was discussed in the context of the remit of the Care Quality Commission, Health Outcomes Framework and National Audit Office.
- **Compare a variety of quality models to inform effective leadership for the continuous improvement of health care delivery** A number of models of quality including TQM, LEAN, Six Sigma and the NHS Outcomes Framework were examined within the context of current patient care delivery.
- **Relate the importance of leadership for professional learning and development** The notion of leadership in the context of clinical governance highlighted the requirement for registration, patient safety and planning for professional development.

ONLINE RESOURCES

For online resources, including SAGE journal articles, weblinks and videos, visit the book's website: https://study.sagepub.com/barr4e.

FURTHER READING

Parsley, K. and Corrigan, P. (1999) *Quality Improvement in Healthcare: Putting Evidence into Practice* (2nd edn). Gloucester: Stanley Thornes.
Peters, T. and Waterman, R. (1988) *In Search of Excellence*. London: HarperCollins.
Stephens, L. (2010) Improving the service: working together to promote normal birth, *British Journal of Midwifery, 18* (6): 348.

14 LEADERSHIP FOR CHANGE

Chapter Contents

Learning Outcomes

By the end of this chapter you will have had the opportunity to:

- Explore change theory
- Discuss the need for effective leadership throughout the change process
- Recognise effective change environments
- Debate the effects of change on individuals, groups and organisations
- Explore the value of Action Learning Sets in supporting change

INTRODUCTION

'... change is a constant in life – maybe the only constant there is – and sudden change is not unusual.'

(Paul O'Brien, 2015: 15)

This chapter will explain the process of change management and discuss the behaviours that might be seen in the organisation during change. Experience dictates that in many situations the process of change is not given enough attention to ensure that it is as successful and painless as possible. It may seem difficult, at times of change, to think about the future – particularly when there appears to be government-legislation-induced change after change. Few periods of history can be thought of as transforming but currently we appear to be living through one of those periods, particularly in health care. We are facing two major conflicting challenges: control of health care costs *and* the provision of quality care to all patients and clients. These two factors are fundamentally altering the health care delivery system and so impact on the ability to lead effectively during change.

DEFINING CHANGE

Although change appears constant and indeed a frequent event in health and health care, it is not always clear what it means. The BNET Business dictionary states that change is 'the coordination of a structured period transition from situation A to situation B to achieve lasting change within an organization' (www.change-management-coach.com). Change is no longer an irregular outing, an inconvenient upheaval to be undertaken once every ten years. Change is something we must learn to live with, structure and manage. Change is here to stay, and the winners will be those who cope with it (Bainbridge, 1996: 4). It is impossible to find a consistent definition of change; sometimes change is seen as being necessary, sometimes unnecessary, and at times one person believes that a change is necessary whereas another cannot see the point.

Activity

What does the above BNET definition mean to you?

How could it relate to a recent personal change you have encountered?

The first could imply that change is about *moving* – like a house or a job move from one place to another. Or it could be more complex and depend on how you perceive it. A recent personal change involved the installation/movement of a new printer in my home office. The benefit of taking time to read the information leaflets and examine various options has meant that there is not only an improved printing function but also that scanning and faxing are now possible – success! From simple to complex definitions it appears that there will be some form of movement along a continuum that could be either linear (Figure 14.1) or cyclical (Figure 14.2).

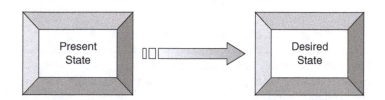

Figure 14.1   Linear continuum

However Freshwater (2014: 97) noted that 'change however, is not only an inevitablity, but is also a fundamental aspect of being human'. She also alludes to the fact that change does not always equate to improvement, and that the evidence and research for best practice for managing change appear to miss the *context* of how leaders facilitate a successful change, and focus instead on the *process* of managing change.

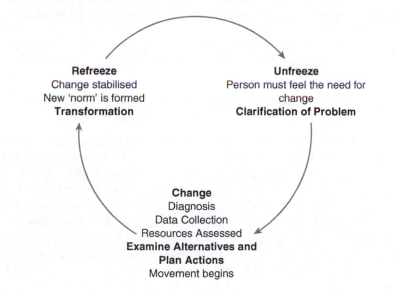

Figure 14.2   Cyclical process model: a combination of Lewin (1951) and Lippet et al. (1958)

LEADING CHANGE

There may be many examples of change in health care (Table 14.1). Some involve very large projects such as changing NHS Trust structures and thus cultures, and on the other side others are quite small, but all may have resonance with the health benefits for patients, clients and families. Ultimately these changes are about addressing *need*, especially in an era of 'information revolution' and aligned health technology.

Table 14.1   Some examples of changes in health care

- Advanced surgical, anaesthetic and medical treatments.
- Rapid response treatment for patients with suspected stroke along with early discharge rehabilitation services.
- Innovation of wireless point of care systems. Clinical information systems are individualised in the electronic patient record (EPR) and the longitudinal electronic health record (EHR). The use of personal digital assistants (PDAs) and voice-over Internet protocol (VoIP) is developing.
- Development of NHS 111 telephone line in the community.
- SMS/texting/social media services to reduce rates of defaulted appointments or enhance health education.
- How2trak software to improve wound care outcomes.
- Online booking for better general practice access; requesting repeat prescriptions, making a GP or specialist appointment.
- Development of skills such as Cognitive Behaviour Therapy (CBT), solution-focused, promotional and motivational guidance therapies to enhance mental health and well-being in adults and children.
- Setting up new local services to improve breastfeeding rates, reduce post-natal depression and address poverty and child protection issues through access to professional/peer support.
- Proton therapy.

This array of examples is just a mere few in the changing world of health care innovations. Some of these, however, put pressure on various patient through-put systems, but as with all change, there is a 'bedding-in' process that can be quite challenging. Throughout your career, if you get the opportunity to attend a professional conference, you will meet a range of new ideas, research, health industry products and services that have been recently developed that you may want to consider in your own field of practice. As we develop professionally we are charged with the notion of improving care through innovation. MacPheem and Suryaprakash (2012), through their project analysis research of 143 nurse leaders' year-long projects, concluded that first-line nurse leaders were well able to successfully manage projects beyond their traditional scope of responsibilities.

This highlights the nature of developing autonomy and responsibility in professional care, applicable to students and newly qualified personnel who often assume that their voices are not heard, and their opinions not wanted.

From the plethora of published material on issues of change management, many models might seem relevant in health and social care.

Ackerman (2004 [1997]) identified three types of change:

- **Developmental change** Planned or emergent incremental change focusing on the improvement of skills and processes
- **Transitional change** Planned and more radical organisational change (based on the work of Lewin, 1951; Kanter, 1983)
- **Transformational change** Radical organisational changes of structure, processes, culture and strategy based on learning and adaptation.

One widely recognised model of change, which is perhaps simplistic but well understood as in our first definition, is described by Lewin (1951), who suggests that there are three key stages to any change. These changes are:

- Unfreeze or unlock from the existing level of behaviour.
- Change the behaviour or move to a new level.
- Refreeze the behaviour at the new level.

Lewin's three-stage model can be applied to almost all change situations in order to analyse the success and failure of the whole process. In 1958 Lippet et al. suggested a three-phase model to enhance Lewin's model:

- The clarification or diagnosis of the problem
- The examination of alternatives and establishing a plan of action for the change
- The transformation of intentions into actions to bring about change.

These two models jointly create a useful cyclical process model that is applicable to the situation undergoing or requiring change. However, it should be noted that change in any health service is not always seen as being this simple.

THE LEADER AS AN INSTRUMENT OF CHANGE

In previous chapters, we discussed the benefits of knowing about your leadership/followership style (Chapter 1) and your problem-solving style (Chapter 2). Now we can take the perspective of the leader being an instrument of change. You, as a change leader, at any level, need to play to your strengths rather than your weaknesses/blind spots and use a reflective approach within your team when driving through change. It is important to remember that you are a role model and others will look to you for direction, motivation and commitment. The way you handle the process of change, the stress involved and the way you interact with others will determine the success or failure of the change project.

Some of the traditional change models such as Havelock (1973) and Rogers (1983) are useful and suggest comprehensive staged models for change and innovation (Table 14.2).

Table 14.2   Rogers' (1983) vs Havelock's (1973) models of change

Rogers' (1983: 20) Five Stage Diffusion of Innovation Model	Havelock's (1973) Six Stage Model
1. Knowledge	1. Build Relationship
2. Persuasion	2. Diagnose Problem
3. Decision	3. Acquire Resources
4. Implementation	4. Choose Solution
5. Confirmation	5. Gain Acceptance
	6. Stabilisation and Self-Renewal

Activity

Do you have any preference for one of these models?

I like Rogers' ideas because it highlights the fact that people involved with change need to be persuaded that the proposed change is necessary, and that this early stage must be successfully negotiated to ensure successful change. It also reinforces the importance of the leader in a changing situation. This can be anyone at any level within the organisation, but they must be aware of cultural beliefs, values and expectations when suggesting changes in their own organisation.

To ensure a successful change the present situation must be considered and information gathered to set the direction for improvement. More recent change models such as Galbraith's Star Model (2001), Denison's Model of Cultural Change (2009) and the RAPSIES model of change (Gopee and Galloway, 2017) reflect the complexity of change issues.

Galbraith's (2001) *star* model notes how change should 'fit' within several elements in the organisation and the interaction between all elements (www.jaygal braith.com/images/pdfs/StarModel.pdf). For example, changing the way tasks are carried out has implications for the organisational objectives, people, information, structures and rewards.

Denison's (2009) model is perhaps more advanced/comprehensive, acknowledging the importance of culture and stability as well as the internal and external influences in complex change environments. It has elements of an internal and external focus as well as the features of:

- strategic mission/goals
- adaptability
- consistency
- team involvement

These are worthy of exploration to understand the relevance in your own analysis of any improvement, change or innovation you wish to consider (Figure 14.3).

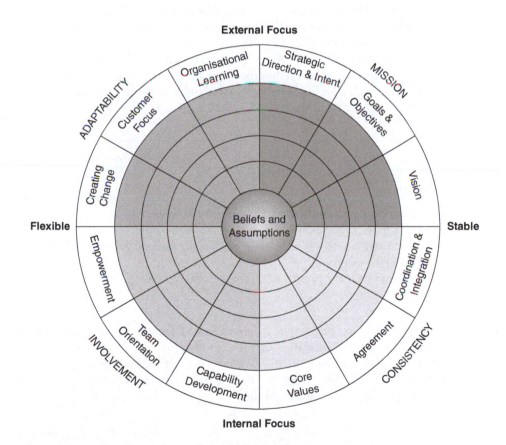

Figure 14.3   Denison's Model of Cultural Change (2009)

The seven-step RAPSIES model of change (Gopee and Galloway, 2017: 147) may be a useful 'step' framework for managing any change effectively.

The RAPSIES model focuses on the following steps:

- Recognising the need for an improvement in practice
- Analysing options for change-setting, identifying the people involved
- Preparing for change – identifying the change agent, the intended outcomes and the education required
- Strategies for the change process
- Implementing the change: piloting and timing
- Evaluation against intended outcomes
- Sustaining the change.

This change model gives more detail than Lewin's staged model and is a more democratic approach to change with a wide interpretation of where in the health industry this process may originate. So, for instance, a hospital porter who thinks there are too many patients waiting for hours on trolleys can provide a catalyst for change, as can a newly qualified health visitor who sees that there are conflicting health education messages for a 'back to sleep' policy from a paediatric orthopaedic department, or a health care assistant who is concerned that the speedy breakfast trolley routines in her ward do not allow enough time for more vulnerable older patients to be supported in helping them enjoy and eat their food.

Activity

These models are complex.

- If you are new to your health care profession, do you agree?
- What do you make of these for your own new leadership role?
- If you have experience as a health care professional, what do you make of these for your own leadership role?
- What action can you take to ensure you are considered a change leader?

It is useful to think of any new change in your clinical area and make notes about the wider aspects of change identified in these models; it may be that you would have liked more involvement or more development opportunities than have recently been promoted. On the other hand, we believe that RAPSIES offers a practical approach to change through to sustainability.

IMPACT OF GLOBALISATION

Gobbi (2017: 95) suggests that globalisation is a process that describes the way in which people and countries are increasingly connected and inter-independent. Globalisation across multinational industries such as pharmaceuticals involves great change. Interestingly, the migration of and movement of people between countries in supporting health care services is a key economic, political, social and cultural issue. There is active recruitment of doctors and nurses from across the world to support the NHS. This phenomenon must have an impact on some of the poorest countries' health systems. Global managers dealing in banking, global infection control and care provision face an arduous task of catalysing and steering change efforts as well as aligning extremely large and far-flung multinational corporations, and certainly do this amidst ethical concerns. Change interventions that work in one country do not always work in another, so health leaders must be aware of cultural beliefs, values and expectations when suggesting changes in their own organisation.

However, it must be said that global and even national research and development in health care delivery is important, and may trigger innovative ideas for developing, rather than directly importing, in a different context. The realm of global communication and telemedicine can have a positive effect on care provision, ensuring that effective data protection and patient confidentiality are in place.

Activity

- Have you read any of the recent clinical literature concerning your own specialism from abroad such as Europe, the USA, Australia or Asia?
- You may have dismissed this because it was 'irrelevant or foreign'. Reflect on the relevant assumptions you held.

Time is always a problem for busy health care professionals working in practice and keeping up to date with literature and evidence. Bullen et al. (2014) note the challenge of conducting and integrating research into clinical practice and the difficulty of time constraints for practitioners engaging in research.

Having attended a few global and national conferences as well as procuring an RN licence abroad, the bigger picture is helpful, and I now appreciate there is much to learn from a broader global perspective. Health-related experience abroad helps us with the 'helicopter view of our own practice' and can allow us to proceed to plan for innovative changes. I remember being surprised by seeing whiteboards over patients' beds in the USA where nurses wrote and agreed the 'simple daily collaborative care plans/goals' (this would follow a daily nursing health assessment). This felt 'patient agreed and centred' but was challenging for me against the backdrop of a reserved British and NHS culture. However, I thought the alternative might be that UK patients/families were often unaware of any informal/formal daily assessment and plans for the day/weeks. So now I would question the notion of how we really involve patient and public communication in all health contexts. In retrospect, the USA and UK health cultures are so very different, but I now believe a more open and transparent care partnership really is the way forward, and that opening myself to global evidence-based health care can advance medical and care innovation and change.

RESPONSE TO CHANGE

Kramer (1974) identified a phenomenon described as the 'Reality Shock' that was seen to occur when a student nurse becomes a registered nurse. A conflict between the student nurse's expectations of the role and its reality in the work setting emerged. The four phases of role transition from student to professional identified in Chapter 11 are:

1. The honeymoon phase
2. The shock phase
3. The recovery phase
4. The resolution phase.

While Kramer's work related to a nursing scenario, and may be considered dated, these findings are the well-known stages expected of any project change. It is natural that when a change is proposed there will be some reaction to the event. The point where the need for change becomes a desire to change is accepted as being pivotal and thus the start of the movement process. If we take as an example the changes to moving and handling procedures, it was during the 1990s that the great risks of poor moving and handling practices in clinical care were identified. The RCN initiated change for professional groups amid little or no debate with external organisations. Due to the lack of involvement of care organisations, acceptance of change was not easy; there was no clear starting point and it is difficult to identify when or even if the 'need for change' became a 'desire for change'.

Reactions to change are often surprising to change leaders because of the wide spectrum of emotions involved. Kübler-Ross (1970) identified ten potential reactions to bereavement. While her work examined the reactions to death and dying, the emotional features can be applied to all change – as those who experience the change are being drawn away from their comfort zone into an unknown area.

There are many reasons why resistance to change occurs, and leaders need to try and anticipate these and understand them as natural phenomena. Kotter and Schlesinger (1979) identified four key reasons:

- **Self interest** People resist change if they perceive that they may lose out in some way. This could be as simple as a loss of power or input in decision making. There are many individuals who simply resent being told what to do. Similarly, staff tend to think that their own approach is the best with sayings such as 'this is how it has always been done so why change' and 'if it ain't broke, don't fix it'.
- **Misunderstanding and lack of trust** Strangely, efforts to create safer working systems can be negatively received and not trusted. It is vital that the leader engenders enthusiasm for the proposed change, letting all the team know what is happening at each stage in order to combat this element and take on board their individual issues into the change plan.

- **Low tolerance to change** Some people are concerned with stability and security and find change daunting. (See cartoon for different assessment of a situation).
- **Different assessments or expectations** There are often different perceptions of the change process held by the people involved and the costs of that change will be higher or lower for different groups. Indeed, the cost of the proposed change must be considered in influencing the outcome. The force-field analysis plays a large part in determining where change is needed, and the cost of that change will lead to success. Conflict is seen when the benefits of a proposed change are biased towards one group's needs at the expense of another group. So, if the change is seen to benefit only the organisational management structure but add further work for the workforce there is likely to be little cooperation with the process.

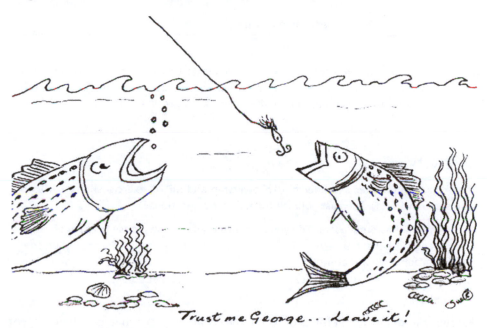

Trust me George... Leave it!

Source: Sue Saillet

LEADING THE TEAM THROUGH CHANGE

Leaders need to assess everyone's willingness to take change on board. There will be some people in the team who, inherently, do not like any sort of change and will demonstrate a low tolerance to any new initiatives. Within some areas of the health service there has been constant change over recent years and team members may exhibit signs of change fatigue in these rapidly developing areas due to constant patterns of change. However, there may be many levels of change makers and change resisters; within any team, there will be individuals who react to change in many ways (Table 14.3).

Table 14.3 Types of individuals (adapted from Rogers and Shoemaker, 1971)

Innovator	Love change and thrive on it.
Early Adopter	Readily accepts the change but may need a little more persuading
Early Majority	Prefer status quo but will accept the change
Later Majority	Resists change and only accepts the change after others have
Laggards	Openly antagonistic

This might seem quite a simplistic view and tends to categorise individual team members in relation to how they may react to change at one point in time rather than seeing individuals as changing as the process progresses.

Activity

Think back to Chapter 2 (Leadership/Followership and MBTI® exercises) to see if you can spot any trends. Then ask yourself the following questions:

- Which behavioural pattern do you most often adopt in response to change?
- Does your behaviour always fit this pattern or does it change depending on the situation or your maturity?

Knowing about different kinds of reaction to change means that as a change agent you can look for the resistors to change; they will be recognised by statements such as:

- 'We tried that before.'
- 'No one else does that.'
- 'It will never work.'
- 'We have always done it this way.'
- 'When I was the student, this is what we were taught, why change?'

These are all negative statements and to be a successful change leader you need to recognise them as such and work to help the resistor accept the need for change.

You will not be surprised to know that your attitude towards change depends on several factors; the situation you find yourself in has a great part to play together with whether you see the change as having a positive influence on your employment position. You might think of other factors that have influenced you in the past and made you behave like a laggard rather than an early adopter. It is now prudent to explore the effects of successful and unsuccessful change and the ways in which a leader can affect outcomes.

SUCCESSFUL VS UNSUCCESSFUL CHANGE

In health care provision, the need for change has never been greater, both in practice and management systems. The effective leader will recognise that change brings with it several feelings, including a sense of achievement, loss, pride and stress. It is important that you understand the change development process because leaders must be able to give a rationale for it and communicate an understandable plan to those who must manage the change and incorporate it into their lives (Porter-O'Grady and Malloch, 2018). Effective leaders will embrace change and lead health care delivery forward; they will exhibit exceptional planning skills and be flexible in adapting to the change they have directly initiated.

As previously discussed, the feelings generated when change is imminent are like those experienced during bereavement or loss (Table 14.2). Unplanned change may be accidental or change by drift (Marquis and Huston, 2006: 171) – this is particularly noticeable when the *change is imposed* and a selection of obstructive behaviours may be seen. By contrast, during a change that is expected, rehearsed and informed, the behaviours exhibited are more complimentary and positive in their manner. Planned change occurs because of an intended effort by the change agent. As a leader, you will need to be that change agent and make efforts in planning change carefully. Initiating and coordinating change requires well-developed leadership and management skills. Dye (2006 [2000]) goes as far as to say that one of the most fundamental values that differentiates effective leaders from average ones is the desire to 'make a difference'.

UNPLANNED CHANGE

Activity

Try to remember a time in your life that involved unnecessary or unplanned change.

- Why did you think it was unnecessary?
- Did it follow Lewin's or Lippet et al.'s model?
- What could have been done to make the change more acceptable?

A colleague told me about her shift patterns at work, in a local GP practice, being changed overnight and without any consultation. When she spoke to her manager, she was told that her contract allowed this to happen and that there was no need for consultation. My colleague was not happy and felt that she had to find new employment as there was no way the employers were going to change their minds. Following her resignation, channels of negotiation were opened, and an agreement was reached. Clearly when this situation is related to Lewin's model one can see that there was no opportunity for 'unfreezing', whereby the situation is recognised as requiring change, but the managers went straight to the 'change' element with very little success. Had the situation been handled differently, with discussion and information being offered throughout, there may not have been as much resistance to the change, thereby leading to greater success.

All too often leaders of change have a plan but do not share it or encourage input from others. They might not see the importance of effective communication. For example, if the plan/change is seen as short term, the leader can become short-sighted; if it is someone else's idea and is not 'owned' by the leader, communication can be weak. Whatever the situation we must all recognise that change occurs and so we must be able to plan to manage that change. NHS England (2018d) are currently examining the way forward through their Sustainable Improvement Team; they are asking for contributions from health care providers in relation to all aspects of provision. Figure 14.4 depicts the effects on people when change is not handled well, and very few people know what is happening, why it is happening, or how long the change will take, so it is vital that we all contribute to the discussions so that the NHS develops to better meet the UK's needs.

All change cannot be contained, directed or managed. Unplanned change will continue to happen in a haphazard way, but planned change will be targeted and purposeful. When managers make decisions that appear to be unrelated to current work practices it can be unsettling for the workforce. The uncertainty of the whole process means that decisions may be based on unspoken, sometimes unconscious assumptions about the organisation, its environment and future (Mintzberg, 1989), so resistance may be high. The common mistakes made when change is difficult or unsuccessful are:

- Inappropriate timescales
- Unclear aims
- Inadequate resources
- Ignoring knock-on effects
- Contamination in trying to change too many things at once
- Hijacking – where someone who may wish to settle an old score tries to sabotage the new project
- Incorrect diagnosis – limited force-field analysis or a knee-jerk reaction to solving the problem
- Lack of ownership.

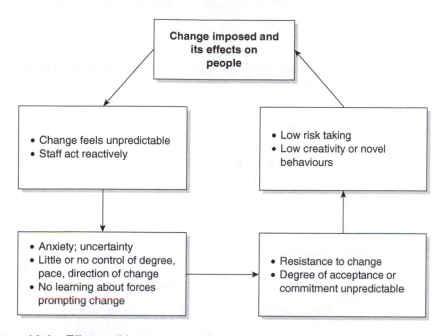

Figure 14.4   Effects of imposed change

PLANNED CHANGE

Planned change is well thought out, timely and necessary. The rhetoric of planned change features all the positive aspects of informing the workforce of what is happening and why. It is a reasoned and well-thought-out activity which will have a positive benefit for care delivery. The change might be thought to be well planned but there may be pockets of the workforce who have a less rosy view of it. Figure 14.5 depicts the effects on people when the change is handled well, and everyone knows what is happening, why it is happening, and how long the change will take.

Kotter and Schlesinger (1979) described a broader range of strategies a leader of change might consider, facilitating a more successful process. These are:

- Education and persuasion
- Participation and involvement
- Facilitation and support
- Negotiation and agreement
- Manipulation and co-option
- Implicit or explicit coercion
- Review and monitoring.

Activity

Can you think of a well-planned change in your practice area? Jot down which elements within Figure 14.5 were successful.

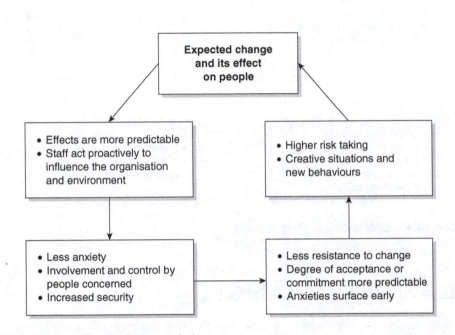

Figure 14.5   Effects of planned change

You might have thought of many instances where change was discussed and started well but hit difficulties, and the whole process became confused due to slippage or various interpretations of people's expectations. In hindsight you may have thought that those leading the change could have managed the change approach better.

The diagram in Figure 14.6 depicts the notion that integrating all elements of change strategies is useful for successful change and no one strategy would achieve effective change alone.

EDUCATION AND PERSUASION

One of the most frequently used ways of minimising resistance to change is through educating people about the need for change. Education is vital during the 'unfreezing' stage of the change process. However, persuasion is required within the approach. There are a variety of approaches to education and persuasion that might be of help:

- The legal argument
- The ethical argument
- The financial argument
- The evidence argument
- Meeting professional standards.

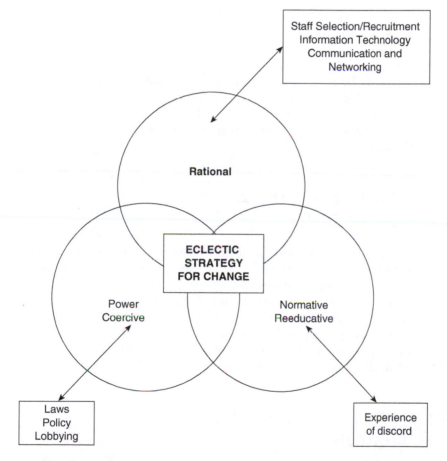

Figure 14.6 Strategies for change

PARTICIPATION AND INVOLVEMENT

It is important that staff, carers and those receiving care are involved in the decision-making process.

FACILITATION AND SUPPORT

If negative feelings towards the change are exhibited, then it is important to consider the empathetic and sympathetic approaches of facilitation. Training is usually seen as a good start to the support process, moving on to co-working and effective supervision during the change. Skilled facilitators should spend time preparing as well as understanding the factual content of the change.

NEGOTIATION AND AGREEMENT

As part of acceptance of the new methods and behaviours there may be issues for group agreement. To reach a consensus and agreement, it may be necessary to negotiate the way forward in small steps to allow the 'later majority, laggards and rejecters' to reach an acceptable outcome. However, you reach the desired outcome you – as leader – must ensure that undue pressure is not placed on any single individual.

MANIPULATION AND CO-OPTION

If the change process is not working, it may be necessary to resort to a more subversive method to manipulate people to agree. Co-opting a hesitant member of staff to assist in the process may give them ownership and can be very effective in getting them 'on side'. Once this has been achieved they may bring others with them, thereby assisting in the smooth running of the process. Should you have a group member who is strongly opposed to the change, they may try to hijack the outcome and affect the dynamics of the group; the infiltration of a key supportive individual might assist in changing the views of that person.

IMPLICIT OR EXPLICIT COERCION

When all else fails, creating a power base where the change leader could offer some sort of reward for adhering to the change or punishment for resisting it can be resorted to. Some care organisations resort to considering disciplinary actions if the change is not implemented. This can only be considered as a last resort. It must be remembered that if punishment is the driving force behind the change then there is a very real possibility that once these threats are removed the resisting group will go back to their old ways.

REVIEW AND MONITORING

As with all changes there must be an evaluative period to conclude. The change should be measured and related to how well it has been accepted and adopted. The review needs to be ongoing in order to ensure that the old practices are not reverted to.

Activity

Have you been involved in a change situation where there was resistance to a change?

- Consider the way this resistance was overcome.
- Make notes on the effect the change had on the group.

I can remember a time when we wanted to introduce 'pre-operative visiting' for all our patients so that they would know what to expect in the anaesthetic room. We did not want to tell the patients about the details of surgery in case of raising anxieties. At the time, it was felt that all patients would want to know what was going to happen to them in the anaesthetic; they were shown photographs of the anaesthetic environment, briefly told about the monitoring equipment to be used, and any questions they wanted to ask were answered. Clearly, for one anxious patient this was too much information and he declined the operation. Following this episode, the surgeon forbade the anaesthetic nursing staff from going near his patients. We had to write a script so that the surgeon could see what his patients were being told, but for a while we only went to see the patients if requested. The change had been implemented without full communication with all involved, but fortunately a compromise was reached which served the needs of all concerned.

PROJECT MANAGEMENT

The activity of planning a project for change is a vital skill for experienced health care professional leaders. Project management can be defined as the discipline of planning, organising, securing and managing resources to bring about the achievement of objectives within a project. There are various models for project management, depending on the industry involved. Within health care the use of models ranging from the very simple, e.g. Plan, Do, Check, Act (Chapter 13), to quite complex ones, e.g. Prince2, is prevalent. In Prince2 there are clear procedures for roles and tight management of resources. The overall corporate management oversees the starting up, initiation, controlling of stages, managing boundaries, and project closure as separate entities.

In the early stages of your career, once qualified, you may be asked to lead out on a practice innovation or service improvement. You may well then link this request with change management and initially consider a simple approach to a project management activity. Buttrick (2005) noted the stages of project management are:

- Initiating
- Planning
- Executing
- Monitoring
- Closing.

It is important, in all these stages, to communicate with a wide group of stakeholders for success to occur and become more externally as well as internally focused. Initially you will need to liaise and network with patients, colleagues and interested parties – in both an informal and a formal manner prior to perhaps writing a report proposing your ideas for the project to gain support from senior colleagues. These activities require several management tools, some of which may be new and some quite challenging. One of the first useful activities is to examine the project issue using PEST (Political, Economic, Social and Technological) and SWOT (Strengths, Weaknesses, Opportunities and Threats) analyses with various stakeholders.

PEST ANALYSIS

Upton and Brooks (1995) note various perspectives related to change management which help in trying to see the need for change. These perspectives can be viewed as:

1. Very broad trends at a national and international level
2. Regional and localised changes that affect patterns of service delivery
3. The leader as an instrument of change.

The first two perspectives are very important in understanding why change may be necessary, but the third is vital if you are to lead change effectively. Without this understanding it would be very difficult for you as a leader or manager to ensure that what you are doing fits with prevailing trends in society and health care delivery.

POLITICAL CONTEXT

Brexit discussions are ongoing but there are elements that need to be clarified, e.g. what happens to EHIC? Will it still be possible to claim monies if hospitalised in an EU country? Recent policy changes concerning NHS Trusts and community-led services in a market health economy continue to focus on quality, performance standards and patient power. Public accountability, while still allowing for local decision making, remains on the agenda, but a reduction in the bureaucracy of health service management is planned. All these changes are purported to squeeze more out of the NHS while devolving accountability and responsibility away from central government to a level closer to the patient.

ECONOMIC CONTEXT

Most of the developed world's governments are looking at ways in which they can contain health care expenditure by rationalising or prioritising treatments, setting ceilings on procedure costs, and achieving cost improvements. There are attempts to integrate cost, quality and outcome to aid decision making by policy makers and planners.

SOCIAL CONTEXT

As the population lives longer, the cost of care is increasing for the vulnerable and chronically ill. This, alongside global mobility from countries with poorer health care provision, is out of line with other demographic factors. There are also higher consumer expectations about the breadth and quality of services that are received. In addition, there is greater public sophistication in terms of understanding and choosing what is needed or wanted. All these factors add to the overall cost of health and social care.

TECHNOLOGICAL CONTEXT

Discoveries in the fields of health care interventions, medicine and total health systems continue to reshape the NHS and look likely to accelerate. Of course, this aspect is harder to predict but potentially may have the greatest impact on health care delivery. Overall, it requires a high degree of flexibility and ability to respond quickly and effectively to change within the service.

SWOT ANALYSIS

This tool was discussed in Chapter 2 for personal development. Although the originator is unknown, it is useful in all project management in its assistance in reviewing the internal environment of the local organisation.

Activity

Considering your own clinical team, populate the SWOT grid below.

Strengths	Weaknesses
Opportunities	Threats

You might have considered as strengths your team's commitment to high-quality patient care and that you have a full complement of staff; under weaknesses you may identify occasional team conflict around duty rostering. The opportunity for clinical updates for both students and staff may be recorded and threats may come from the amalgamation of services across acute and primary care.

PLANNING FOR CHANGE

Once the broad view of the internal and external environments has been explored, the impact of the project needs to be seen in the context of the strength of the drivers for change. Lewin's (1951) force-field analysis is another useful tool to review the sustainability of any change envisaged.

Using a force-field analysis that includes both hard (quantitative) and soft (qualitative) factors, it is possible to depict how significant the proposed change might be and predict its success. An example of a part analysis might be seen when a new 12-hour working shift pattern is suggested (Figure 14.7).

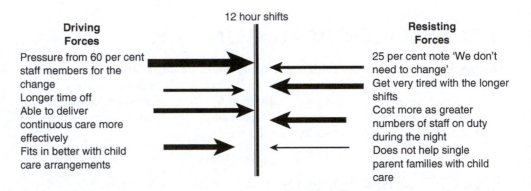

Figure 14.7   Force-field analysis for change related to implementing a 12-hour shift pattern

You can see from the strength of the arrows that some of the forces are much stronger than others, so that the overall need for change appears to be the stronger argument and it would therefore be useful to continue to plan for change. This change must be planned effectively and initially should be considered as a pilot project – with an evaluation date to see whether the change should continue.

Often the results of such an exercise demonstrate that the proposed change is not quite as strongly required as first thought. It also helps to identify the restraining factors, so that appropriate strategies might be considered, but it is important to gather together a project team if you can so that you get a good picture of the current situation. This will help the team develop a sense of ownership of the proposed change.

Activity

Think of a situation, within your clinical area, where a change may be necessary and draw up a force-field analysis of the need for that change. You might have found this relatively easy.

- Did it give the results you expected?
- Did it highlight the need for the proposed change?

You could ask some of the following questions to indicate how ready for change the workplace team is:

1. How ingrained are the various forces?
2. Which ones are the most open to reduction?
3. What influence can we use to help overcome difficulties or constraints?
4. Are there things we need to find out in order to get a clearer picture of the local influences?

It is therefore prudent to consider the following when driving through a change in the workplace: direction, time scales, communication, resources, making change real and job security (Table 14.4).

The GANTT chart, developed by Henry Laurence Gantt in the 1910s, is used to illustrate a schedule of activity, usually against a timeline. We probably do not realise that we use them in everyday life, for example when planning for a holiday or shopping for Christmas. There are many examples of GANTT charts on the internet; Google the term and surf around the wide variation offered – most work on an Excel application principle which may be the easiest method for starting.

Table 14.4 Considerations for driving through change

Direction	Everyone clearly understands what is happening. There is a sense of purpose.
Timescales	Clear and relevant – may be achieved by using a GANTT chart.
Communication	If ineffectual then there are clear grounds for rumour, innuendo and gossip. Gets rid of hidden agendas.
Consultation	Staff need to be informed and involved at every stage of the change.
Resources	Time, money, people, materials – where will they come from and how will they be paid for? Increasingly, employers rely on goodwill that may lead to employee resentment.

(Continued)

Table 14.4 (Continued)

Making change real	Involve yourself and behave in ways consistent with the change you are trying to bring about.
Job security	During organisational mergers and reconfigurations, people need to know their place in the new structure. They will not commit to change if their personal place is not secured.

ACTION LEARNING SETS

More and more, action-learning sets are utilised to facilitate change in the health service, although they can be seen as taking valuable resources in a time-strapped health service environment (Malloch and Porter-O'Grady, 2005: 153). Action learning sets help individuals see the need for change and bring their own personal relationship into the change process. Action learning is seen in the context of learning and reflection, supported by colleagues, with the purpose of change. It is based on the following principles of team working:

- Meeting regularly
- Consistent membership
- Addressing members' problem tasks
- Sharing, support, questioning
- Group success
- Review
- Facilitation.

In order for action learning to succeed, there is a need to agree the following ground rules:

- Confidentiality
- Commitment and continuity of attendance
- Clarity of objectives
- Constructive challenge
- Work as a group of peers
- Recognise individual strengths/limitations
- The role of the facilitator is clearly defined.

Scenarios for change are set up and the facilitator assumes a questioning stance. The whole group engages with helping individuals face their change difficulty. The elements in Figure 14.8 could be potential frameworks to ensure all those involved recognise the change issues and have ownership of that process.

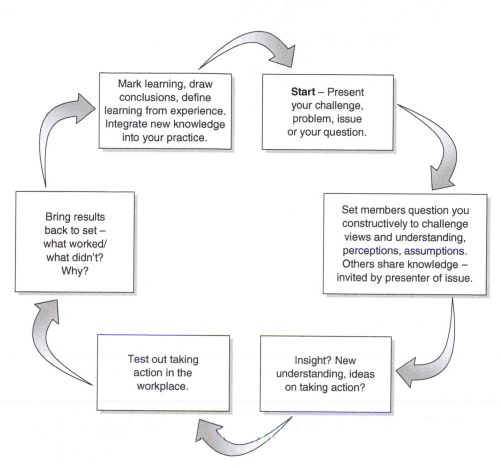

Figure 14.8 Action learning model
Source: Revans, 2011

Rayner et al. (2002) identify that action learning offers a unique opportunity to develop leadership skills in a safe, non-threatening situation. The ability of leaders or facilitators to analyse problems, gain personal confidence and identify solutions for change for the benefit of clinical effectiveness is paramount. Douglas and Machin (2004) emphasised the value of action learning sets for interdisciplinary collaboration in their grounded theory research in mental health.

The skills, knowledge and experience of the individuals whose responsibility it is to bring about change are varied and complex. It is vital that they consider the intricacies of people's response to change and how that might make the path to change difficult, full of barriers and pitfalls. Good preparation and planning of the process and involvement of interested parties at all stages helps to ensure appropriate support, encouragement and action, thus increasing the potential for successful change.

THE LEARNING ZONE

More and more, learning zones are being used within business and health care (Foundation of Nursing Studies (FoNS), 2018). The purpose of these is to highlight the learning opportunities for all health care students and enable everyone to contribute to ongoing discussion.

Remember the skills, knowledge and experience of the individuals whose responsibility it is to bring about change are varied and complex. It is vital that they consider the intricacies of people's response to change and how that might make the path to change difficult, full of barriers and pitfalls. Good preparation and planning of the process and involvement of interested parties at all stages helps to ensure appropriate support, encouragement and action, thereby increasing the potential for successful change.

CONCLUDING THOUGHTS

Malloch and Porter-O'Grady (2005: 180) state:

> Like any other pursuit, leadership is a journey. The only difference with regard to leadership is that leadership is a journey with no permanent destination.

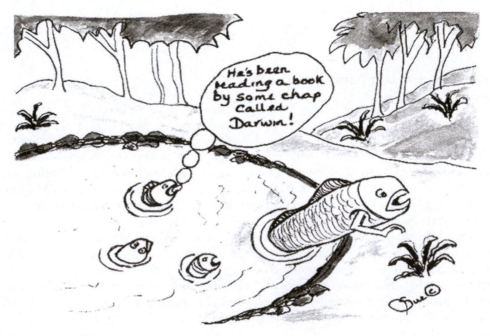

Source: Sue Saillet

This book has demonstrated how we might embark on that journey, support actions with theory, and successfully arrive at our individual and collective destinations. The leadership role reflects the journey of life, as the cartoon depicts the learning journey has just begun, and as such is confined not only to our professional role but also to how we conduct ourselves in the community.

It is, therefore, prudent to consider ways in which each of us can develop as potential leaders in the world of today and for tomorrow. Changes are occurring on a scale as important as those of the Industrial Revolution, and the health service needs to anticipate and respond to those changes. Education and training are vital to the plethora of changes (Health Education England (Lord Wills), 2015).

The speed of economic, political, social and technological change in today's world has implications for changing health services that are 'fit for purpose'. It is easy to look back to some glorious era, say, when the NHS was 'born', and believe that with a few adjustments we can go back to this health service where people were only too glad to be able to get their glasses provided by the NHS. The health services of the future will need to be very different and this requires leaders to push these developments through. Leaders need to have an 'eye' for the future and some literature evidence has tried to capture the notion of 'future building' exercises. This is seen as more than just crystal ball gazing, now being a management discipline that is adapting to the needs of the current political and financial environment.

Activity

A leader has a role in ensuring the success of any change in the workplace by supporting participants in that change and challenging them to extend their practice:

- Consider how you would support your colleagues while developing your leadership role.
- List the attributes you feel are necessary to ensure you complete this role effectively.
- Consider which attributes you feel are strong in your leadership style.
- List and suggest how you can address the weaknesses you identified.

You may have considered several requisites highlighted when you completed the leadership/followership styles questionnaire (Chapter 2). Essentially you need to demonstrate awareness regarding the enhancement and developing leadership roles within your team and develop the professional respect of colleagues together with the necessary expertise and experience to carry out the role. There are many other examples you might have identified. It is important to remember that when leading, effective goal setting must be applied and communicated so that everyone involved knows what is expected of them and can fulfil their potential. You may think of your role in terms of a flowchart like the one depicted in Figure 14.9, either cyclical or linear, so ensuring that all participants are 'kept in the loop'.

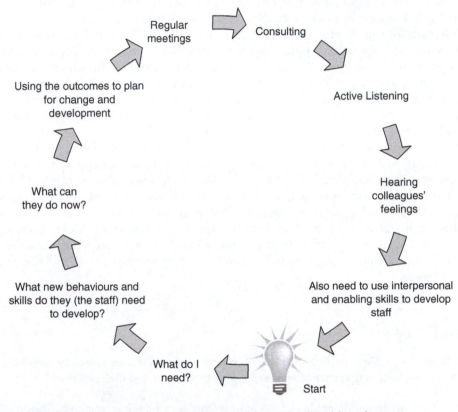

Figure 14.9   Forward planning and developing a leadership role

Activity

Drawing on all the concepts discussed within this book we can attempt to look to the future. Consider the changing role of the health care leader.

- How would you design the basic competencies of the leader to reflect the needs of the twenty-first century in a technology healing context?
- What knowledge would be essential for the processes of rework?
- What protective skills would be necessary for the leader?
- What would you leave behind that would not compromise the future value of health care provision?

Letting go of the past is a difficult exercise and requires careful analysis of what should be retained and what might be given up. If we consider the basic competencies of the health care leader we recognise that there is a need for better communication skills, so that everyone in the organisation knows what is happening and why. Similarly, there may be a case for changing work priorities; in the past, evidence suggested that 'holism' was the way forward rather than task orientation. It would be interesting to debate whether the constant demands put on health care services mean this notion of holistic care is something of a luxury. Ask the following questions to evaluate how you perform as a leader personally and as a leader within your clinical environment (Table 14.5):

Table 14.5 Doing well: self vs team

For me personally:	How well am I doing?	For my clinical area:	How well are we doing?
	How do I compare with highly effective leaders – how should I be doing?		How do we compare with similar clinical areas – how well should we be doing?
	What more should I aim to achieve to make it happen next year?		What more should the clinical area do to make it happen?
	What must I do to make it happen?		What must the clinical area do to make it happen?
	What is my timetable for action and how shall I monitor progress?		What should the clinical area's timetable for action be and how should progress be monitored?

It is vital that effective health care leaders in the future take cognisance of the theories related to leadership. This book has attempted to demonstrate how this can be done in a variety of situations; it offers some solutions and ways in which you can apply theory to practice in a variety of health care settings. In the words of Nelson Mandela:

It is better to lead from behind and to put others in front, especially when you celebrate victory when nice things occur. You take the front line when there is danger. Then people will appreciate your leadership.

Source: http://nelsonmandelas.com/nelson-mandela-quotes

Summary of Key Points

This chapter has explored a variety of strategies that can lead to successful change. These are:

- **Explore change theory** Several definitions, theories, models and perspectives have been utilised to reflect the breadth of theory underpinning the concept of change.

(Continued)

(Continued)

- **Discuss the need for effective leadership throughout the change process** The importance of leadership to shape change and lead people through the process of change was explored and there were a number of strategies proposed for effective leadership in this area.
- **Recognise effective change environments** Planned and unplanned change outcomes were discussed and the implications for success and difficulties were explored.
- **Debate the effects of change on individuals, groups and organisations** The varieties of effects of change on health care teams and individuals were debated and the impact on improving and changing care for patients and clients was highlighted.
- **Explore the value of Action Learning Sets in supporting change** This model of change was linked to the notion of team learning, problem solving and reflection using a facilitative approach.

ONLINE RESOURCES

For online resources, including SAGE journal articles, weblinks and videos, visit the book's website: https://study.sagepub.com/barr4e.

FURTHER READING

Baulcomb, J.S. (2003) Management of change through force-field analysis, *Journal of Nursing Management*, 11: 275–80.

Butler, L. and Leach, N. (2011) *Action Learning for Change: A Practical Guide for Managers*. Cirencester: Management Books 2000 Ltd.

Davies, C., Finlay, L. and Bullman, A. (2000) *Changing Practice in Health and Social Care*. London: Sage/Open University.

Gerrish, K. (2000) Still fumbling along? A comparative study of newly qualified nurses' perception of the transition from student to qualified nurse, *Journal of Advanced Nursing*, 32 (2): 473–80.

Paton, R. and McCalman, J. (2000) *Change Management: A Guide to Effective Implementation* (2nd edn). London: Sage.

REFERENCES

Academy of Medical Royal Colleges (2008) *A Clinician's Guide to Record Standards – Part 1: Why Standardise the Structure and Content of Medical Records?* NHS Digital and Health Information Policy Directorate.

Ackerman, L. (2004[1997]) 'Change in Development, Transition or Transformation: The Question of Change in Organisations', in D. Van Eynde, J. Hoy and D. Van Eynde (eds), *Organisation Development Classics*. San Francisco, CA: Jossey-Bass.

Ackoff, R.L. (1993[1981]) 'The Art and Science of Mess Management', in C. Maby and B. Mayonwhite (eds), *Managing Change* (2nd edn). London: Sage, pp. 47–54.

Ackoff, R.L. and Greenburg, D. (2008) *Turning Learning Right Side Up*. Mahwah, NJ: Pearson/ Prentice Hall.

Adair, J. (2006) *How to Grow Leaders*. London: Kogan Page.

Adair, J. (2010) *Develop Your Leadership Skills*. London: Kogan Page.

Agor, W.H. (1986) Intuition: the new management tool, *Nursing Success Today*, 1: 23–4.

Akerjordet, K. and Severinsson, E. (2010) The state of the science of emotional intelligence related to nursing leadership: an integrative review, *Nursing Management*, 18 (4): 363–82.

Almost, J. (2006) Conflict within nursing work environments: concept analysis, *Journal of Advanced Nursing*, 53 (4): 444–53.

Alvesson, M. and Spicer, A. (eds) (2010) *Metaphors We Lead By: Understanding Leadership in the Real World*. Abingdon: Routledge.

Ames, H.M.R., Glenton, C. and Lewin, S. (2017) Parents' and informal caregivers' views and experiences of communication about routine childhood vaccination: a synthesis of qualitative evidence (Art. No.: CD011787). *Cochrane Database of Systematic Reviews*, http://dx.doi.org/10.1002/14651858.CD011787.pub2

Andrews, M. (2017) Some reflections on transcultural nursing's contribution when cultures clash, *Journal of Transcultural Nursing*, 28 (4): 625.

Anonson, J., Walker, M.E., Arries, E., Maposa, S., Telford, P. and Berry, L. (2014) Qualities of exemplary nurse leaders' perspectives of frontline nurses, *Journal of Nursing Management*, 22: 127–36.

Ansoff, H.I. (1987) *Corporate Strategy* (revised edn). London: Penguin Books.

Aronowitz, A. (2009) *Human Trafficking, Human Misery: The Global Trade in Human Beings*. Westport, CT: Praegar.

Armstrong, M. (1990) *How to be a Better Manager* (3rd edn). London: Kogan Page.

Assanova, M. and McGuire, M. (2009) *Applicability Analysis of the Emotional Intelligence Theory*. Available at http://citeseerx.ist.psu.edu/viewdoc/summary?doi=10.1.1.472.8431 (accessed 31 July 2018).

Avery, A.J., Barber, N., Ghaleb, M., Franklin, B.D., Armstrong, S., Crowe, S., Dhillon, S., Freyer, H., Howad, R., Pezzolesi, C., Serumaga, B., Swanwick, G. and Talabi, O. (2012) *Investigating the Prevalence and Causes of Prescribing Errors in General Practice*. Available at www.gmc-uk.org/about/what-we-do-and-why/data-and-research/research-and-insight-archive/investigating-the-prevalence-and-causes-of-prescribing-errors-in-general-practice (accessed 9 January 2019).

Bainbridge, C. (1996) *Designing for Change: A Practical Guide for Business Transformation*. New York: John Wiley.

Baker, R. (2003) *A Review of Deaths of Patients at Gosport War Memorial Hospital*. Leicester: Department of Health Sciences, University of Leicester..

Bandler, R. and Grindler, J. (1990) *Frogs into Princes: Introduction to Neurolinguistic Programming*. London: Eden Grove Editions.

Bar, M.A., Leurer, M.K., Warshawski, S. and Itzhaki, M. (2018) The role of personal resilience and personality traits of healthcare students on their attitudes towards interprofessional collaboration, *Nurse Education Today*, 61: 36–42.

Bar-On, R. (1997) *Bar-On Emotional Quotient Inventory: Technical Manual*. Toronto, Canada: Multi-Health Systems.

Barr, H. (2002) *Interprofessional Education Today, Yesterday and Tomorrow: A Review*. London: LTSN HS&P.

Barr, J. (2007) 'Ethics in Primary Care', in G. Hawley (ed.), *Ethics in Clinical Practice: An Interprofessional Approach*. Harlow: Pearson.

Barr, J. and Dowding, L. (2012) *Leadership in Healthcare*, 2nd edition. London: SAGE.

Barr, J. and Dowding, L. (2016) *Leadership in Health Care* (3rd edn). London: Sage.

Barzey, S. (2005) Dealing with difficult people and situations, *Nursing Times*, 101 (16): 62–3.

Bass, B. (1985) *Leadership and Performance Beyond Expectations*. New York: Free Press.

Bass, B. and Avolio, B.J. (1990) Developing transformational leadership: 1992 and beyond, *Journal of European Industrial Training*, 14: 21–7.

BBC (2012) 'Which is the world's biggest employer?'. Available at www.bbc.co.uk/news/magazine-17429786 (accessed 25 February 2018).

Beauchamp, T.L. and Childress, J.F. (2013) *Principles of Biomedical Ethics* (7th edn). New York: Oxford University Press.

Belbin, M. (2000) *Beyond the Team*. London: Routledge.

Belbin, R.M. (2011) *The Coming Shape of Organization: Management Teams*. New York: Routledge.

Belbin, R.M. (2015) *Beyond the Team*. London: Routledge. Available at www.belbin.com/media/1336/belbin-for-students.pdf (accessed 11 July 2018).

Bender, M., Connelly, C. and Brown, C. (2013) Interdisciplinary collaboration: the role of the clinical leader, *Journal of Nursing Management*, 21: 165–74.

Benner, P. (1984) *From Novice to Expert – Excellence and Power in Clinical Nursing Practice*. Reading, MA: Addison Wesley.

Benner, P. and Tanner, C. (1987) Clinical decision making: how expert nurses use intuition, *American Journal of Nursing*, 87 (1): 23–31.

Bennett, M. (1986) A development approach to training for intercultural sensitivity, *International Journal of Relations*, 10: 179–96.

Bennis, W.G. (1999) The leadership advantage, *Leader to Leader*, 12 (Spring).

Bennis, W.G. and Nanus, B. (2004) *Leaders: Strategies for Taking Charge* (2nd edn). New York: HarperCollins.

Bennis, W.G., Parikh, J. and Leesom, R. (1994) *Beyond Leadership: Balancing Economics, Ethics and Ecology*. London: Blackwell.

Bergman, E. (2014) Managing conflict in clinical health care with diminished reliance on third party intervention forging an ethical and legal mandate for effective physician–patient communication, *Cardozo Journal of Conflict Resolution*, 15: 473–9.

Berry, L., Zeithaml, V. and Parasuraman, A. (1988) The service quality puzzle, *Business Horizon*, Sept.–Oct.: 35–43, in M. Moullin (2002) *Delivering Excellence in Health and Social Care*. Buckingham: Open University Press.

Berwick, D. (2013) *A Promise to Learn – A Commitment to Act: Improving the Safety of Patients in England*. London: Department of Health.

Blackpool Teaching Hospitals (2015) 'Blackpool NHS Trust grows its own staff'. Available at www.bfwh.nhs.uk/blackpool-nhs-trust-grows-its-own-staff/ (accessed 6 August 2018).

Blake, R.R. and McCanse, A.A. (1991) *Leadership Dilemmas – Grid Solutions*. Houston, TX: Gulf.

Blake, R.R. and Mouton, J.S. (1985) *The Managerial Grid 111*. Houston, TX: Gulf.

Bolam v Friern Hospital Management Committee [1957] 2 All ER 118 [1957].

Borrill, C., West, M., Shapiro, D. and Rees, A. (2000) Team-working and effectiveness in the NHS, *British Journal of Health Care Management*, 6: 364–71.

Borton, T. (1970) *Reach, Touch and Teach*. London: Hutchinson.

Boylan, O. and Loughrey, C. (2007) Developing emotional intelligence in GP trainers and registrars, *Education for Primary Care*, 18 (6): 745–8.

Bradbury-Jones, C., Sambrook, S. and Irvine, F. (2007) Power and empowerment in nursing: a fourth theoretical approach, *Journal of Advanced Nursing*, 62 (2): 258–66.

Brake, T. (1997) *The Global Leader: Critical Factor for Creating the World Class Organisation*. Chicago, IL: Irwin Professional Publishing.

Buchanan, D. and Badham, R. (2008) *Power, Politics and Organizational Change: Winning the Turf Game* (2nd edn). London: Sage.

Buchanan, D. and Huczynski, A. (2017) *Organizational Behaviour* (9th edn). Harlow: Pearson.

Buck, D. and Jabbal, J. (2014) Tackling poverty: Making more of the NHS in England. Available at www.kingsfund.org.uk/sites/default/files/field/field_publication_file/tackling-poverty-research-paper-jrf-kingsfund-nov14.pdf (accessed 5 August 2018).

Buckenham, M.A. (1988) Student nurse perception of the staff nurse role, *Journal of Advanced Nursing*, 13: 662–70.

Buckingham, C. and Adams, A. (2000) Clarifying clinical decision making: interpreting nursing intuition, heurists and medical diagnosis, *Journal of Advanced Nursing*, 32 (4): 990–8.

Bucknall, T. (2000) Critical care nurses' decision-making activities in the natural setting, *Journal of Clinical Nursing*, 9 (1): 25–36.

Bullen, T., Maher, K., Rosenberg, J.P. and Smith, B. (2014) Establishing research in a palliative care clinical setting: perceived barriers and implemented strategies, *Applied Nursing Research*, 27: 78–83.

Burns, J.M. (2010) *Leadership*. New York: Harper Perennial Modern Classics.

Busquets, M. and Caïs, J. (2017) Informed consent: a study of patients with life-threatening illnesses, *Nursing Ethics*, 24 (4): 430–40.

Butler, K.M. and Hardin-Pierce, M. (2005) Leadership strategies to enhance the transition from nursing student role to professional nurse, *Nurse Leadership Forum*, Spring, 9 (3): 110–17.

Buttrick, R. (2005) *The Project Workout*. (3rd edn). Harlow: Pearson Education.

Cable, D.M. and Parsons, C.K. (2001) Socialisation tactics and person–organisation fit, *Personnel Psychology*, 54 (1): 1–24.

Cardwell, M., Clark, L. and Meldrum, C. (1996) *Psychology for A-Level*. London: Collins Educational.

Care Act 2014, c.23. Available at www.legislation.gov.uk/ukpga/2014/23/contents/enacted (accessed 9 January 2019).

Care Quality Commission (2018) *The state of health and adult social care in England 2017/18*. Newcastle upon Tyne: CQC.

Carlyle, T. (1841) *On Heroes and Hero Worship and Heroic in History*. Boston, MA: Adams.

Carnes, K., Cottrell, D. and Layton, M.C. (2004) *Management Insights: Discovering the Truths to Management Success*. Dallas, TX: Cornerstone Leadership Institute.

Carter, C.M. (2016) *The Complete Guide to Generation Alpha, The Children of Millenials*. Available at www.forbes.com/sites/christinecarter/2016/12/21/the-complete-guide-to-generation-alpha-the-children-of-millennials/#1278cf0f3623 (accessed 26 January 2019)

Cemi, T., Curtis, G.J. and Colmar, S.H. (2012) Cognitive-experiential self theory and conflict-handling styles, *International Journal of Conflict Management*, 23 (4): 362–81.

Centre for the Advancement of Interprofessional Education (CAIPE) (1997) Interprofessional education: a definition, *CAIPE Bulletin* 13.

Chan, J.C.Y., Sit, E.N.M. and Lau, W.M. (2014) Conflict management styles, emotional intelligence and implicit theories of personality of nursing students: a cross sectional study, *Nurse Education Today*, 34: 934–9.

Chang Y-S., Coxon K., Portela, A., Furuta, M. and Bick, D. (2018) Interventions to support effective communication between maternity care staff and women in labour: a mixed-methods systematic review, *Midwifery*, 59: 4–16.

Children Act 1989, c.41. Available at www.legislation.gov.uk/ukpga/1989/41/contents (accessed 9 January 2019)

Children Act 2004, c.31. Available at www.legislation.gov.uk/ukpga/2004/31/contents (accessed 9 January 2019)

Children and Families Act 2014, c.6. Available at www.legislation.gov.uk/ukpga/2014/6/contents/enacted (accessed 9 January 2019)

Children and Social Work Act 2017, c.16. Available at www.legislation.gov.uk/ukpga/2017/16/contents/enacted (accessed 9 January 2019)

Children and Young Persons Act 2008, c.23. Available at www.legislation.gov.uk/ukpga/2008/23/pdfs/ukpga_20080023_en.pdf (accessed 9 January 2019)

Chugh, D. and Brief, A.P. (2008) '1964 Was Not That Long Ago: A Story of Gateways and Pathways', in A.P. Brief (ed.), *Diversity at Work*. Cambridge: Cambridge University Press.

Clawson, J. (2013) *Level Three Leadership: Getting Below the Surface* (5th edn). London: Pearson.

Clinical Human Factors Group (CHFG) (2019) *What are Clinical Human Factors?* Available at https://chfg.org/what-are-clinical-human-factors (accessed 29 Janaury 2019).

Collins, J. (2001) Level 5 leadership: the triumph of humility and fierce resolve, *Harvard Business Review*, January: 67–76.

Commissioning for Quality and Innovation (CQUIN) (2018): *Guidance*. London: NHS.

Commissioning for Quality and Innovation (CQUIN)(2018) *Guidance for 2017–2019*. London: NHS England.

Cooke, H. (2006) Scapegoating and the unpopular nurse, *Nurse Education Today*, 27: 177–84.

Cooper, R.K. & Q-Metrics (1996–1997) *EQ Map: Intepretation Guide*. San Francisco, CA: AIT & Essi Systems.

Cooper, S., Kinsman, L., Buykx, P., McConnell-Henry, T., Endacott, R. and Scholes, J. (2010) Managing the deteriorating patient in a simulated environment: nursing students' knowledge, skill and situation awareness, *Journal of Clinical Nursing*, 19 (15–16): 2309–18.

Coulter, A. (2011) *Engaging Patients in Healthcare*. Maidenhead: Open University Press/McGraw Hill.

Covey, S. (2004) *The Seven Habits of Highly Effective People: Powerful Lessons in Personal Change* (15th anniversary edn). London: Simon and Schuster.

Cox, C. (2010) Legal responsibility and accountability, *Nursing Management*, 17 (3): 18–20.

Crainer, S. (1996) *Key Management Ideas*. London: Pitman.

Cummings, J. (2012) 'Compassion in Practice'. Available at www.england.nhs.uk/wp-content/uploads/2012/12/compassion-in-practice.pdf (accessed 2 April 2018).

Cunningham, I. (1986) 'Leadership development : Mapping the field' (unpublished paper), Ashridge Management College, Berkhamstead.

Cyert, R.M. and March, J.G. (1963) *A Behavioural Theory of the Firm*. London: Prentice Hall.

Dackert, I. (2010) The impact of team climate for innovation on wellbeing and stress in elderly care, *Journal of Nursing Management*, 18: 302–10.

Daft, R.L. (2015) *Organizational Theory and Design*. Boston: Centage.

Daft, R.L. (2017) *The Leadership Experience* (6th edn). India: Centage.

Damasio, A.R. (1994) *Descartes' Error*. New York: G. P. Putnam's Sons.

Daniels, N. and Sabin, J. (2002) *Setting Limits Fairly: Can We Learn to Share Scarce Resources?* Oxford: Oxford University Press.

Darzi, A. (2018) *The Lord Darzi Review of Health and Care Interim Report*. London: Institute for Public Policy Research.

de Bono, E. (1990) *Lateral Thinking: Creativity Step by Step*. New York: HarperCollins.

De Dreu, C.K.W. and Weingart, L.R. (2003) Task versus relationship conflict, team performance, and team member satisfaction: a meta-analysis. *Journal of Applied Psychology*, 88, 741–9.

Deming, W.E. (1986) *Out of the Crisis*. Cambridge: Cambridge University Press. Available from: http://asq.org/learn-about-quality/project-planning-tools/overview/pdca-cycle.html (accessed 20 November 2018).

Denison, D.R. (2009) *Denison Model*. Available at www.denisonconsulting.com/knowledge-center/model (accessed 11 May 2015).

Department for Education (2010) Haringey local safeguarding children board serious case review 'child a' November 2008. Available at www.gov.uk/government/publications/haringey-local-safeguarding-children-board-first-serious-case-review-child-a (accessed 28 February 2018).

Department of Health (DH) (1974) *Health and Safety at Work Act*. London: HMSO. Available at www.legislation.gov.uk/ukpga/1974/37/section/2 (accessed 28 February 2018).

Department of Health (DH) (1998) *A First-Class Service: Quality in the New NHS Health Services*. London: HMSO.

Department of Health (DH) (1999) *The Management of Health and Safety at Work Regulations*. Available at www.legislation.gov.uk/uksi/1999/3242/contents/made (accessed 28 February 2018).

Department of Health (DH) (2000) *An Organisation with Memory*. London: Department of Health.

Department of Health (DH) (2002) *Learning from Bristol: The Department of Health's Response to the Report of the Public Inquiry in Children's Health Surgery at the Bristol Royal Infirmary 1984–1995* (Kennedy Report). London: HMSO.

Department of Health (DH) (2003) *Confidentiality: NHS Code of Practice*. London: Department of Health.

Department of Health (DH) (2004) *The NHS Knowledge and Skills Framework (NHS KSF) and the Development Review Process*. London: HMSO.

Department of Health (DH) (2005a) *Safety, Health and Welfare at Work Act 2005*. Available at: https://www.hsa.ie/eng/Legislation/Acts/Safety_Health_and_Welfare_at_Work/SI_No_10_of_2005.pdf (accessed 26 January 2019).

Department of Health (DH) (2007) *Capacity and Capability: Building the Workforce*. London: HMSO.

Department of Health (DH) (2008) *High Quality Care for All: NHS Next Stage Review, Final Report* (Darzi). London: HMSO.

Department of Health (DH) (2014) *Post-Legislative Assessment of The Health and Social Care Act*. London: HMSO.

Department of Health (DH) (2015) *No Secrets: Guidance on Developing and Implementing Multi-Agency Policies and Procedures to Protect Vulnerable Adults from Abuse*. London: Department of Health.

Department of Health (DH) (2017) *Promoting professionalism, reforming regulation: A paper for consultation*. Available at www.gov.uk/government/consultations/promoting-professionalism-reforming-regulation (accessed 31 May 2018).

Department of Health and Social Care (DHSC) (2015) *The NHS Constitution: The NHS Belongs to Us All*. Available at https://assets.publishing.service.gov.uk/government/uploads/system/uploads/attachment_data/file/480482/NHS_Constitution_WEB.pdf (accessed 6 August 2018).

DePree, M. (2004[1987]) *Leadership is an Art*. New York: Doubleday.

Dilts, R. (2006) *Sleight of Mouth*. Capitola, CA: Meta Publications.

Disability Discrimination Act 1995, c.50. Available at www.legislation.gov.uk/ukpga/1995/50/contents (accessed 9 January 2019)

Disability Discrimination Act 2005, c.13. Available at www.legislation.gov.uk/ukpga/2005/13/contents (accessed 9 January 2019)

Doherty, C. and Doherty, W. (2005) Patients' preferences for involvement in clinical decision-making in secondary care and the factors that influence their preferences, *Journal of Nursing Management*, 13 (2): 119–27.

Doherty, T.L., Horne, T. and Wootton, S. (2014) *Managing Public Services – Implementing Change: A Thoughtful Approach to the Practice of Management* (2nd edn) London: Routledge.

Donabedian, A. (1966) Criteria and standards for quality assessment and monitoring, *Quality Review Bulletin*, 2 (3): 99–100.

Donabedian, A. (2003) *An Introduction to Quality Assurance in Healthcare*. New York: Oxford University Press.

Donahue, M.P. (2011) *Nursing: The Finest Art* (3rd edn). St Louis, MO: Mosby.

Douglas, S. and Machin, T. (2004) A model for setting up interdisciplinary collaborative working in groups: lessons from an experience of action learning. *Journal of Psychiatric and Mental Health Nursing*. 11(2):189–93.

Dowding, L. and Barr, J. (2002) *Managing in Health Care: A Guide for Nurses, Midwives and Health Visitors*. London: Pearson Education.

Doyle, C., Lennox, L. and Bell, D. (2013) A systematic review of evidence on the links between patient experience and clinical safety and effectiveness, *BMJ Open 3*, e001570. Available at http://dx.doi.org/10.1136/bmjopen-2012-001570.

Driscoll, J. (2007) *Practising Clinical Supervision: A Reflective Approach for Healthcare Professionals*. Philadelphia, PA: Balliere Tindall, Elsevier. Available at www.nottingham.ac.uk/nmp/sonet/rlos/placs/critical_reflection/models/driscoll.html (accessed 26 January 2019).

Drucker, P.F. (1996[1967]) 'The Effective Executive', in H. Flanagan and P. Spurgeon (eds), *Public Sector Managerial Effectiveness*. Milton Keynes: Open University Press.

Drucker, P.F. (1989) *The Practice of Management*. London: Heinemann.

Dye, C.F. (2006[2000]) 'Leadership in Healthcare: Values at the Top', in B.L. Marquis and C.J. Huston (eds), *Leadership Roles and Management Functions in Nursing: Theory and Application*. Philadelphia, PA: Lippincott Williams & Wilkins.

Early Intervention Foundation (2014) *Early Intervention in Domestic Violence and Abuse*. Available at www.eif.org.uk/files/pdf/early-intervention-in-domestic-violence-and-abuse-full-report.pdf (accessed 29 January 2019).

Egan, G. (2013) *The Skilled Helper* (10th revised international edn). London: Cengage Learning Inc.

Ellis, P. and Bach, S. (2015) *Leadership, Management and Team Working in Nursing* (2nd edn). London/Exeter: SAGE/Learning Matters.

English Oxford Living Dictionaries (2018) Available at https://en.oxforddictionaries.com/definition/emotional_intelligence (accessed 5 April 2018).

Equality Act 2010, c.15. Available at www.legislation.gov.uk/ukpga/2010/15/contents (accessed 9 January 2019)

Erickson, M.H. (2002) 'The Seminars of Milton H. Erickson'. Presentation to the San Diego Society of Clinical Hypnotherapy No. 1 (Seminars of Milton H. Erickson). Phoenix, AZ: The Milton H. Erickson Foundation Press.

Espenshade, T. and Radford, A.W. (2009) *No Longer Separate, Not Yet Equal: Race and Class in Elite College Admission and Campus Life* (2nd edn). Woodstock, UK: Princeton University Press.

Etzioni, A. (ed.) (1969) *The Semi-Professions and their Organization*. London: Collier-Macmillan.

Farrell, G. (2001) From tall poppies to squashed weeds: why don't nurses pull together more?, *Journal of Advanced Nursing*, 35 (1): 26–33.

Fayol, H. (1925) *General and Industrial Management*. London: Pitman and Sons.

Female Genital Mutilation Act 2003, c.31. Available at www.legislation.gov.uk/ukpga/2003/31/contents (accessed 9 January 2019)

Fenton, K. (2012) 'What is Clinical Leadership?', *Nursing Times*. Available at www.nursing-times.net/clinical-archive/leadership/what-is-clinical-leadership/5045399.article (accessed 9 October 2018).

Fiedler, F.E. (1967) *A Theory of Leadership Effectiveness*. New York: McGraw-Hill.

Fleming, N. (2010) *VARK: A Guide to Learning Styles*. Available at www.vark-learn.com/home (accessed 11 July 2018).

Fletcher, L. and Buka, P. (1999) *A Legal Framework for Caring*. London: Macmillan.

Flin, R. and Maran, N. (2004) Identifying and training non-technical skills for teams in acute medicine, *Quality and Safety in Health Care*, 13 (1): i80–4.

Flynn, J.R. (2009) *What Is Intelligence? Beyond the Flynn Effect* (expanded paperback edn). Cambridge: Cambridge University Press.

Foot, K. (2016) *Collaborating against Human Trafficking: Cross-sector Challenges and Practices*. Maryland, USA: Rowman and Littlefield.

Ford, J. (2006) Discourses of leadership: gender, identity and contradiction in a UK public sector organisation, *Leadership*, 2 (1): 77–99.

Forsyth, D.R. (2010) *Group Dynamics* (5th edn). Belmont, CA: Wadsworth Cengage Learning.

Foucault, M. (1995) *Discipline and Punish: The Birth of the Prison*. New York: Vantage.

Foundation of Nursing Studies (FoNS) (2018) *The Learning Zone*. Available at www.fons.org/learning-zone/learning-zone (accessed 21 July 2018).

Francis, R. (2013) *Report of the Mid-Staffordshire NHS Foundation Trust Public Inquiry: Executive Summary*. Chaired by Robert Francis QC. Available at http://cdn.basw.co.uk/upload/basw_121924-10.pdf (accessed 6 March 2018).

Franke, R.H. and Kaul, J.D. (1978) The Hawthorne Experiments: first statistical interpretation. *American Sociological Review*, 43 (5): 623–43.

Freidson, E. (1970) *Profession of Medicine: A Study of the Sociology of Applied Knowledge*. Chicago, IL: University of Chicago Press.

French, W.L. and Bell, C.H. (1990) *Organization Development: Behavioural Science Interventions for Organization Improvement* (4th edn). London: Prentice Hall.

Freshwater, D. (2014) Board editorial: the challenge of global leadership: managing change, leading movement, *Journal of Research in Nursing*, *19* (2): 93–7.

Freud, S. (1911) *Interpretation of Dreams* (3rd edn) (trans. A.A. Brill). New York: Plain Label Books.

Frew, D.R. (1977) Leadership and followership, *Personnel Journal*, *54* (2): 90–7.

Fry, S and Johnstone, M. (2008) *Ethics in Nursing Practice: A Guide to Ethical Decision-making*. Geneva: International Council of Nurses.

Full Gospel Businessman's Training (2014) Available at www.fgbt.org/Leadership-Principles/the-6-c-s-of-decision-making.html (accessed 11 April 2018).

Galbraith, J.R. (2001) *Designing Organisations: An Executive Guide to Strategy, Structure and Process* (2nd rev. edn). San Francisco, CA: Jossey-Bass.

Gardner, H. (1983) *Frames of Mind*. New York. Basic Books.

Gardner, H. (1990) *Leading Minds*. London: Harper Collins.

General Medical Council (GMC) (2013) *Leadership and Management for All Doctors*. London: GMC.

General Medical Council (GMC) (2014) *Good Medical Practice*. London: GMC.

General Medical Council (GMC) (2017) *Registration and Licensing*. Available at www.gmc-uk.org/doctors/index.asp (accessed 24 October 2001).

George, B. (2003) *Authentic Leadership: Rediscovering the Secrets to Creating Lasting Value*. San Fransisco, CA: Jossey-Bass.

Gibbs, G. (1988) *Learning by Doing: A Guide to Teaching and Learning Methods*. Oxford: Further Education Unit, Oxford Polytechnic.

Gibson, J.L., Martin, D.K. and Singer, P.A. (2005) Priority setting in hospitals: fairness, inclusiveness, and the problem of institutional power differences, *Social Science & Medicine*, 61: 2355–62.

Giger, J.N. and Davidhizar, R.E. (2004) *Transcultural Nursing, Assessment and Intervention* (4th edn). Baltimore, MD: Mosby.

Gilbert, T. (1995) Nursing: empowerment and the problem of power, *Journal of Advanced Nursing*, *21* (5): 865–71.

Gilligan, C. (1977) In a different voice: women's conceptions of self and of morality. *Harvard Educational Review*, *47* (4): 481–517.

Giuliani, R.W. (2002) *Leadership*. New York: Hyperion.

Glasper, A. (2014) CQC develops new criteria for quality and safety of care, *British Journal of Nursing*, *23* (2): 110–11.

Gobbi, M. (2017) 'Global Issues for Nursing Leadership', in R. Taylor and B. Webster-Henderson (eds), *The Essentials of Nursing Leadership*. London: Sage.

Goetch, D.L. and Davis, S. (2014) *Quality Management for Organizational Excellence: Introduction to Total Quality*. (7th edn). Harlow: Pearson Education.

Goldman, S. and Kahnweiller, W.M. (2000) A collaborator profile for executives for non-profit organisation, *Non-profit Management and Leadership*, 10: 435–50.

Goleman, D. (1995) *Emotional Intelligence*. New York: Bantam.

Goleman, D. (2018) Available at www.danielgoleman.info/topics/emotional-intelligence/ (accessed 4 April 2018).

Goodwin, D. (2014) 'Decision-making and accountability: differences of distribution, *Sociology of Health & Illness*, 36 (1): 44–59.

Gopee, N. and Galloway, J. (2017) *Leadership and Management in Healthcare* (3rd edn). London: Sage.

Greaves, F., Ramirez-Cano, D., Millett, C., Darzi, A. and Donaldson, L. (2012) Harnessing the cloud of patient experience: using social media to detect poor quality healthcare, *British Medical Journal Quality and Safety*, doi:10.1136/bmjqs-2012-001527.

Green, C. (2012) Nursing intuition: a valid form of knowledge, *Nursing Philosophy*, 13 (2): 98–111.

Greenhalgh, T., Robert, G., Bate, P., Kyriakidou, O., Macfarlane, F. and Peacock, R. (2004) *How to Spread Good Ideas: A Systematic Review of the Literature on Diffusion, Dissemination and Sustainability of Innovations in Health Service Delivery and Organisation*. London: NCCSDU.

Greenleaf, R.K. (1977) *Servant Leadership: A Journey in the Nature of Legitimate Power and Greatness*. New York: Paulist.

Greenleaf, R.K. (1998) *Power of Servant Leadership*. San Francisco, CA: Berrett-Koehler.

Griffith, B.A. and Dunham, E.B. (2015) *Working in Teams: Moving from High Potential to High Performance*. London: Sage.

Griffith, K. (2009) *The Religious Aspects of Nursing Care*. Available at https://nursing.ubc. ca/sites/nursing.ubc.ca/files/documents/ReligiousAspectsofNursingCareEEdition.pdf (accessed 13 March 2018).

Griffith, K. (2014) Respecting a patient's wish to refuse life-sustaining treatment, *British Journal of Nursing*, 23 (6): 332–3.

Griffiths, S. (2014) Perspective: global challenges for public health: dilemmas for leadership, *Journal of Research in Nursing*, 19 (2): 163–6.

Grohar-Murray, M.E. and DiCroce, H.R. (2002) *Leadership and Management in Nursing* (3rd edn). London: Prentice Hall.

Grohar-Murray, M.E., DiCroce, H.R. and Langan, J.C. (2010) *Leadership and Management in Nursing* (4th edn). London: Prentice Hall.

Grossman, S. and Valiga, T.M. (2016) *The New Leadership Challenge: Creating the Future of Nursing* (5th edn). Philadelphia, PA: FA Davis.

Gulick, L. (1937) 'Notes on the Theory of the Organisation', in L. Gulick and L. Urwick (eds), *Papers on the Science of Administration*. New York: Institute of Public Administration.

Haddad, A.M. (1992) Ethical problems in home health care, *Journal of Nursing Administration*, 22 (3): 46–51.

Hague, G., Malos, E. and Dear, W. (1996) *Multi-agency Work and Domestic Violence: A National Study of Inter-Agency Initiatives*. Bristol: Policy Press.

Handy, C.B. (1985) *Understanding Organisations* (3rd edn). Oxford: Oxford University Press.

Handy, C.B. (1993) *Understanding Organisations* (4th edn). Oxford: Oxford University Press.

Hardy, R. (2018) 'Ashya's Miracle', *Daily Mail*, 3 March, pp.10–11.

Hargie, O. (2017) *Skilled Interpersonal Communication* (6th edn) Abingdon: Routledge.

Hargie, O. and Tourish, D. (eds) (2009) *Auditing Organizational Communication: A Handbook of Research, Theory and Practice*. Hove: Routledge.

Harmer, M. (2005) *The Case of Elaine Bromiley*. Available at https://emcrit.org/wp-content/uploads/ElaineBromileyAnonymousReport.pdf (accessed 29 January 2019).

Harris, G. (2015) *Paramedic Carreer Framework* (3rd edn). Available at www.collegeofpara medics.co.uk/publications/post-reg-career-framework (accessed 26 January 2019).

Hartley, P. (1997) *Group Communication*. London: Routledge.

Hartman, R.L. and Crume, A.L. (2014) Educating nursing students in team conflict communication, *Journal of Nursing Education and Practice*, 4 (11): 107–18.

Haslam, S.A., Reicher, S.D. and Platow, M.J. (2013) *The New Psychology of Leadership: Identity, Influence and Power*. Hove: Psychology Press.

Havelock, R.G. (1973) *The Change Agent's Guide to Innovation in Education*. Englewood Cliffs, NJ: Educational Technology.

Hawley, G. (2007) *Ethics in Clinical Practice: An Interprofessional Approach*. Harlow: Pearson.

Health and Care Professions Council (HCPC) (2016) *Standards of Conduct, Performance and Ethics*. London: HCPC. Available at www.hcpc-uk.org/publications/standards/index.asp?id=38 (accessed 9 February 2019).

Health and Care Professions Council (HCPC) (2017a) *Standards of Continuing Professional Development*. Available at www.hcpc-uk.org/standards/standards-of-continuing-profes-sional-development (accessed 9 February 2019).

Health and Care Professions Council (HCPC) (2017b) *Continuing Professional Development and Your Registration*. London: HCPC.

Health and Care Professions Council (HCPC) (2017c) *Promoting Professionalism, Reforming Regulation. A Paper for Consultation*. Response to DH Consultation Document. Available at www.hcpc-uk.org/aboutus/consultations/external/index.asp?id=231 (accessed 9 February 2019).

Health and Social Care Act 2012, c7. Available at www.legislation.gov.uk/ukpga/2012/7/contents/enacted (accessed 9 January 2019).

Health and Social Care (Health and Safety) Act (2015) Available at www.legislation.gov.uk/ukpga/2015/28/pdfs/ukpga_20150028_en.pdf (accessed 8th Feb 2019).

Health Education England (Lord Willis) (2015) *Raising the Bar*. London: HEE.

Healthcare Quality Improvement Partnership (HQIP) (2015) *A Guide to Quality Improvement Methods*. London: HQIP.

Healthcare Quality Improvement Partnership (HQIP) (2016) *Using Root Cause Analysis Techniques in Clinical Audit* London: HQIP.

Hein, S. (2003) *History and Definition of Emotional Intelligence*. Available at www.eqi.org/history.htm (accessed 11 July 2018).

Helman, C. (2007) *Culture, Health and Illness* (5th edn). London: Hodder Arnold.

Herring, J. (2012) *Medical Law and Ethics*. Oxford: Oxford University Press.

Hersey, P. and Blanchard, K. (1977) *Management of Organisational Behaviour: Utilising Human Resources* (3rd edn). Englewood Cliffs, NJ: Prentice Hall.

Herzberg, F. (1966) *Work and the Nature of Man*. London: Staples Press.

Hewison, A. and Stanton, A. (2003) From conflict to collaboration? Contrasts and convergence in the development of nursing and management theory (2), *Journal of Nursing Management*, 11 (1): 15–24.

Hibbert, J.H. and Peters, E. (2003) Supporting informed consumer health care decisions: data presentation approaches that facilitate the use of information in choice, *Annual Review of Public Health*, 24: 413–33.

HM Government (2013) *Working Together to Safeguard Children: A Guide to Inter-agency Working to Safeguard and Promote the Welfare of Children*. London: DfE.

HM Government (2018) *Working Together to Safeguard Children: A Guide to Interagency Working to Safeguard and Promote the Welfare of Children*. London: DfE.

Hodge, M.A. (2017) The impact of the clinical nurse leader (CNL) on quality patient outcomes, *The South Carolina Nurse*, 24(10): 10. Available at www.scnurses.org (accessed 28 November 2017).

Hofsted, G. (1980) *Culture's Consequences*. Beverley Hills: Sage, in The Open University (1985) *International Perspectives Unit 16, Block V*, 'Wider Perspectives, Managing in Organisations'. Milton Keynes: Open University Press.

Hogan, R. and Hogan, J. (2007) *Hogan Personality Inventory Manual* (3rd edn). Tulsa, OK: Hogan Assessment Systems.

Honey, P. (2001) *Improve your People Skills* (2nd edn). London: The Chartered Institute of Personnel and Development.

Honey, P. and Mumford, A. (1982) *The Manual of Learning Styles*. Maidenhead: Peter Honey.

Horsburgh, M., Lamdin, R. and Williamson, E. (2001) Multiprofessional learning: the attitudes of medical, nursing and pharmacy students to shared learning, *Medical Education*, *35* (9): 876–83.

Howarth, M. and Haigh, C. (2007) The myth of patient centrality in integrated care: the case of back pain services, *Journal of Integrated Care*, 7 (11 July). Available at www.ncbi.nlm.nih.gov/pmc/articles/PMC1919416/pdf/ijic2007–200727.pdf (accessed 1 June 2011).

Howatson-Jones, I.L. (2004) The servant leader, *Nursing Management*, *11* (3): 20–4.

Huber, D. (2014) *Leadership and Nursing Care Management* (5th edn). St Louis, MO: Elsevier Saunders.

Human Rights Act 1998, c.42. Available at www.legislation.gov.uk/ukpga/1998/42/contents (accessed 9 January 2019)

Humphries, J. (1998) *Managing Successful Teams: How to Get the Results You Want by Working Effectively with Others*. Oxford: How To Books.

Hursthouse, R. (1999) *On Virtue Ethics*. Oxford: Oxford University Press.

Iles, V. and Sutherland, K. (2001) *Organisational Change: Managing Change in the NHS*. London: The National Co-ordinating Centre for NHS Service Delivery, Organization, Research and Development.

Information Governance Alliance/DH (2016) *Records Management Code of Practice for Health and Social Care 2016*. Available at https://digital.nhs.uk/data-and-information/looking-after-information/data-security-and-information-governance/codes-of-practice-for-handling-information-in-health-and-care/records-management-code-of-practice-for-health-and-social-care-2016 (accessed on 5 August 2018).

Ishikawa, K. (1985) *What is Total Quality Control?* Englewood Cliffs, NJ: Prentice Hall.

Issigonis, A. (n.d.) Available at www.bainyquote.com/authors/alec_issigonis (accessed 29 January 2019).

Jackson, S.E. (1996) *The Consequences of Diversity in Multidisciplinary Work Teams*, cited in M.A. West (1996) *Handbook of Work Group Psychology*. Chichester: Wiley & Sons, pp. 53–75.

Janis, I.L. (1982) *Groupthink* (2nd edn). Boston, MA: Houghton Mifflin.

Jay, A. (2014) *Independent Inquiry into Child Sexual Exploitation in Rotherham (1997 – 2013)* (Jay Report). Available at www.rotherham.gov.uk/downloads/file/1407/independent_inquiry_cse_in_rotherham (accessed 15 May 2018).

Jeffrey, A.D. (2013) *The Art of Nursing Leadership*. Available at www.nurseleader.com/article/S1541-4612(12)00254-6/fulltext (accessed 29 October 2017).

Johns, C. (1995) Framing learning through reflection within Karper's fundamental ways of knowing in nursing, *Journal of Advanced Nursing*, 22 (2): 226–34.

Johnson, J.E. and Garvin W.S. (2017) Advanced practice nurses: developing a business plan for an independent ambulatory clinical practice, *Nursing Economics*, *35* (3):126–40.

Johnson, G. and Scholes, K. (1989) *Exploring Corporate Strategy*. London: Prentice Hall.

Joint Emergency Services Interoperability Principles (JESIP) (2018a) *Joint Decision Model*. Available at https://jesip.org.uk/joint-decision-model (accessed 7 June 2018).

Joint Emergency Services Interoperability Principles (JESIP) (2018b) *Working Together Saving Lives*. Available at https://jesip.org.uk/home (accessed 7 June 2018).

Kagawa-Singer, M. and Chung, R. (1994) A paradigm of culturally based care in ethnic minority populations, *Journal of Community Psychology*, 22 (3): 192–208.

Kampadoo, K., Sanghera, J. and Battanaik, B. (2016) *Trafficking and Prostitution Reconsidered: New Perspectives on Migration, Sex Work and Human Rights* (2nd edn). Oxford: Routledge.

Kanter, R.M. (1983) *The Change Masters*. London: George Allen.

Kanter, R.M. (1991) 'Change Master Skills: What It Takes To Be Creative', in J. Henry and D. Walker (eds), *Managing Innovation*. London: Sage/Open University.

Kanter, R.M. (1993) *Men and Women of the Corporation* (2nd edn). New York: Basic Books.

Katz, R.L. (1955) Skills of an effective administrator, *Harvard Business Review*, 33 (1): 33–42.

Keighley, T. (1989) Developments in quality assurance, *Senior Nurse*, 9: 7–10.

Kelley, R.E. (1992) *The Power of Followship*. London: Bantam/Dell.

Kelly-Heidenthal, P. (2004) *Essentials of Nursing Leadership and Management*. New York: Thomson Delmar Learning.

Kennedy, I. (2001) *The Report of the Public Inquiry into Children's Heart Surgery at the Bristol Royal Infirmary 1984–1995; Learning from Bristol* (presented July 2001). Available at https://webarchive.nationalarchives.gov.uk/20090811143822/http://www.bristol-inquiry.org.uk/final_report/the_report.pdf (accessed 21 January 2019).

Kennedy, I. (2013) *Review of the Response of Heart of England NHS Foundation Trust to Concerns about Mr Ian Paterson's Surgical Practice; Lessons to be Learned; and Recommendations*. Available at www.heartofengland.nhs.uk/wp-content/uploads/Kennedy-Report-Final.pdf (accessed 28 February 2018).

Keogh, B. (2013) *Review into the Quality of Care and Treatment Provided by 14 Hospital Trusts in England: Overview Report*. London: HMSO.

Keogh, B. (2017) Professor Sir Bruce Keogh: Keynote speech to Expo 2017. Available at www.youtube.com/watch?v=3zT0uDBcork (accessed 12 February 2019).

Kerslake, Lord (2018) *The Kerslake Report: An independent review into the preparedness for, and emergency response to, the Manchester Arena attack on 22nd May 2017*. Available at www.jesip.org.uk/uploads/media/Documents%20Products/Kerslake_Report_Manchester_Are.pdf (accessed 26 January 2019).

Kets de Vries, M.F.R. and Mead, C. (1992) 'The Development of the Global Leader within the Multinational Corporation', in V. Pucik, N.M. Tichy and C.K. Barnett (eds), *Globalizing Management, Creating and Leading the Competitive Organization*. New York: Wiley.

Kilner, T. (2004) Desirable attributes of the ambulance technician, paramedic, and clinical supervisor: findings from a Delphi study, *Emergency Medicine Journal*, 21: 374–8.

King, I.M. (1981) *A Theory for Nursing: Systems, Concepts, Process*. New York: Delmar.

Kingsley, C. (1863) *The Water-Babies*. London: Macmillan & Co.

Kipling, R. (2018[1902]) 'The Elephant's Child', in R. Kipling, *Just So Stories for Little Children*. Oxford: Usborne Publishing Ltd.

Kite, N. and Kay, F. (2012) *Understanding Emotional Intelligence: Strategies for Boosting your EQ and Using It in the Workplace*. London: Kogan Page.

Kjellström, S., Avby, G., Arekoug-Josefsson, K. and Andersson Bäck, M. (2017) Work motivation among healthcare professionals: a study of well functioning primary healthcare centers in Sweden, *Journal of Health Organization and Management*, 31 (4): 487–502.

Klagsbrun, J. (2011) *Listening and Focusing: Holistic Health Care Tools for Nurses*. Available at www.focusing.org/klagsbrun.html (accessed 2 April 2018).

Kopf, E.W. (1916) Florence Nightingale as statistician, *Publications of the American Statistical Association*, 15 (116): 388–404.

Kotter, J.P. (2008) *A Sense of Urgency*. Boston, MA: Harvard Business Press.

Kotter, J.P. and Schlesinger, L.A. (1979) Choosing strategies for change, *Harvard Business Review*, March/April, cited in J. Hayes (2002) *The Theory and Practice of Change Management*. Basingstoke: Palgrave.

Kouzes, J.M. and Posner, B.Z. (2007) *The Leadership Challenge* (4th edn). San Francisco, CA: Jossey-Bass.

Kramer, M. (1974) *Reality Shock: Why Nurses Leave Nursing*. St Louis, MO: Mosby.

Kübler-Ross, E. (1970) *On Death and Dying*. London: Tavistock Publications.

Laming, W.H. (2009) *The Protection of Children in England: A Progress Report*. Available at www.gov.uk/government/publications/the-protection-of-children-in-england-a-progress-report (accessed 22 July 2018).

Lancaster, J. (1999) *Nursing Issues in Leading and Managing Change*. Charlottesville, VA: Mosby.

Landsberg, M. (2003) *The Tao of Motivation: Inspire Yourself and Others*. London: Profile.

Laschinger, H.K.S. (2010) Towards a comprehensive theory of nurse/patient empowerment applying Kanter's empowerment theory to patient care, *Journal of Nursing Management*, *18* (1): 4–13.

Laurenson, M. and Brockelhurst, H. (2011) Interprofessionalism, personalization and care provision, *British Journal of Community Nursing*, 16 (4): 184–90.

Lave, J. and Wenger, E. (1991) *Situated Learning: Legitimate Peripheral Participation*. Cambridge: Cambridge University Press.

Laverack, G. (2005) *Public Health: Power and Professional Practice*. London: Palgrave Macmillan.

Leavitt, H.J. (1965) 'Applied Organisational Change in Industry: Structural, Technological and Humanistic Approaches', in J.G. March (ed.), *Handbook of Organisations*. Chicago, IL: Rand McNally.

Leavitt, H.J. (1978) *Managerial Psychology* (4th edn). Chicago, IL: University of Chicago Press.

Leavitt, H.J. (2005) *Top Down: Why Hierarchies Are Here to Stay and How To Manage Them More Effectively*. Boston, MA: Harvard Business School Press.

Lee, H.J. (2017) How emotional intelligence relates to job satisfaction and burnout in public service jobs. *International Review of Administrative Sciences*. Available at http://journals.sagepub.com/doi/pdf/10.1177/0020852316670489 (accessed 4 April 2018).

Leininger, M. (1997) Transcultural nursing research to transform nursing education and practice: 40 years image, *Journal of Nursing Scholarship*, 29: 341–7.

Leininger, M.M. and McFarland, M.R. (2006) *Culture, Care, Diversity and Universality: A Worldwide Theory for Nursing* (2nd edn). Sudbury, MA: Jones & Bartlett.

Lewin, K. (1951) *Field Theory in Social Sciences*. New York: Harper & Row.

Lewin, K., Lippitt, R. and White, R.K. (1939) Patterns of aggressive behaviour in experimentally created social climates, *Journal of Social Psychology*, 10: 271–99.

Linstead, S., Fulop, L. and Lilley, S. (2004) *Management and Organization: A Critical Reader*. Basingstoke: Palgrave Macmillan.

Lippet, R., Watson, J. and Wesley, B. (1958) *The Theory of Planned Change*. New York: Harcourt Brace Jovanovich.

Littlejohn, P. (2012) The missing link: using emotional intelligence to reduce workplace stress and workplace violence in our nursing and other health care professions, *Journal of Professional Nursing*, 28 (6): 360–8.

Lobel, S.A. (1990) Global leadership competencies: managing to a different drumbeat, *Human Resource Management*, 29 (1): 39–47.

Lucas, S. (1999) *The Passionate Organisation*. New York: American Management Association.

Luft, J. and Ingham, H. (1955) '"The Johari Window": a graphic model of interpersonal awareness'. *Proceedings of the Western Training Laboratory in Group Development*. Los Angeles: UCLA.

Lynn, R. (2008) *The Global Bell Curve: Race, IQ, and Inequality Worldwide*. Augusta, GA: Washington Summit Publishers.

MacDonald, I., Burke, C. and Stewart, K. (2016) *Systems Leadership: Creating Positive Organisations*. Oxford: Routledge.

MacPheem, M. and Suryaprakash, N. (2012) First-line nurse leaders health-care change management initiatives', *Journal of Nursing Management*, 20: 249–59.

Malby, R. (1994) *The Challenges for Nursing and Midwifery in the 21st Century: A Briefing Document*. Leeds: University of Leeds.

Malloch, K. and Porter, O'Grady T. (2005) *The Quantum Leader*. MA: Jones and Bartlett Publishers.

Manley, K. and Titchen, A. (2017) Facilitation skills: the catalyst for increased effectiveness in consultant practice and clinical systems leadership, *Educational Action Research*, 25 (2): 256–79.

Mann, R.D. (1959) A review of the relationship between personality and performance in small groups, *Psychological Bulletin*, 66 (4): 241–70.

Mansour, M. (2014) Factor analysis of nursing students' perception of patient safety education, *Nurse Education Today*. Available at http://dx.doi.org/10.1016/j.nedt.2014.04.020 (accessed 28 August 2014).

Markham, G. (2005) Gender in leadership, *Nursing Management*, 3 (1): 18–19.

Markham, S.K. and Aiman-Smith, L. (2001) Product champions: truths, myths and management, *Research Technology Management*, 44 (3): 44–50.

Marquis, B.L. and Huston, C.L. (2006) *Leadership Roles and Management Functions in Nursing: Theory and Application* (5th edn). Philadelphia, PA: Lippincott.

Marquis, B.L. and Huston, C.L. (2017) *Leadership Roles and Management Functions in Nursing: Theory and Application* (9th international edn). Philadelphia, PA: Wolters Kluwer.

Marriner Tomey, A. (2008) *Guide to Nursing Management and Leadership* (8th edn). St Louis, MO: Mosby.

Martin, C.A. (2003) Transitional timelines, *Nursing Management (USA)*, 34 (4): 25–6, 28.

Martin, V. (2001) Service planning and governance, *Nursing Management*, 8 (3): 33–7.

Maslow, A. (1987) *Motivation and Personality* (3rd edn). Harlow: Addison Wesley.

Mathieu, J.E., Maynard, T.S., Rapp, T. and Gilson, L. (2008) Team effectiveness 1997–2007: A review of recent advancements and a glimpse into the future, *Journal of Management*, 34 (3): 410–76.

Maxwell, J.C. (1999) *The 21 Indispensable Qualities of a Leader*. Nashville, TN: Thomas Nelson.

Mayer, J.D. and Salovey, P. (1993) The intelligence of emotional intelligence, *Intelligence*, 17: 433–42.

Mayer, J.D., DiPaolo, M.T. and Salovey, P. (1990) Perceiving affective content in ambiguous visual stimuli: a component of emotional intelligence, *Journal of Personality Assessment*, 54: 772–81.

Mayer, J.D., Salovey, P., Caruso, D.R. and Sitarenios, G. (2001) Emotional intelligence as a standard intelligence, *Emotion*, 1: 232–42.

McAlpine, A. (2000) *The New Machiavelli: The Art of Politics in Business*. New York: Wiley.

McCallum, J., Duffy, K., Hastie, E., Ness, V. and Price, L. (2013) Developing nursing students' decision-making skills: are early warning scoring systems helpful?, *Nurse Education in Practice*, 13 (1): 1–3.

McCaughan, D. and Kaufman, G. (2013) 'Patient safety: threats and solutions', *Nursing Standard*, 27 (44): 48–55.

McClelland, D.C. (1984) *Human Motivation*. New Jersey: Longman Higher Education.

McCrae, N. (2011) Whither nursing models? The value of nursing theory in the context of evidence-based practice and multidisciplinary care, *Journal of Advanced Nursing*, 68 (1): 222–9.

McCrindle, M. (2018) *What comes after Generation Z? Introducing Generation Alpha.* Available at https://mccrindle.com.au/insights/blogarchive/what-comes-after-generation-z-introducing-generation-alpha (accessed 25 January 2019).

McCutcheon, H. and Pincombe, J. (2001) Intuition: an important tool in the practice of nursing, *Journal of Advanced Nursing*, 35 (3): 342–8.

McDowell, J. (1979) Virtue and reason. *The Monist*, 62 (3): 331–50.

McElhaney, R. (1996) Conflict management in nursing administration, *Nursing Management*, 24: 65–6, cited in P.E.B. Valentine (2001) A gender perspective on conflict management strategies of nurses, *Journal of Nursing Scholarship*, 33 (1): 69–74.

McGregor, D. (1987) *The Human Side of Enterprise*. London: Penguin.

McMullen, B. (2003) Emotional intelligence, *BMJ Career Focus*, 326: 7381.

McNeese-Smith, D.K. and Crook, M. (2003) Nursing values and a changing nurse workforce: values, age, and job stages, *Journal of Nursing Administration*, 33 (5): 260–70.

Mendes, A. (2015) Cultural competence: part of good personalised dementia care, *Nursing and Residential Care*, 17 (6): 338–41.

Mental Capacity Act 2005, c.9. Available at www.legislation.gov.uk/ukpga/2005/9/contents (accessed 9 January 2019)

Mental Health Units (Use of Force) Act 2018. Available at www.legislation.gov.uk/ukpga/2018/27/enacted (accessed 21 February 2019).

Miller, W.R. and Rollnick, S. (2002) *Motivational Interviewing: Preparing People to Change.* London: Guilford.

Miner, J.B. (2005) *Organisational Behaviour 1: Essential Theories of Motivation and Leadership.* New York: M.E. Sharpe.

Mintzberg, H. (1989) *Mintzberg on Management: Inside Our Strange World of Organizations.* New York: Free Press.

Mintzberg, H. (1998) '5 Ps for Strategy', in H. Mintzberg, J. Quinn and S. Ghoshal (eds), *The Strategy Process* (revised European edn). Englewood Cliffs, NJ: Prentice Hall.

Mintzberg, H., Lampel, J., Quinn, J.B. and Ghoshal, S. (2003) *The Strategy Process: Concepts, Context, Cases* (2nd edn). New York: Prentice Hall/Financial Times Management.

Moller, J. (2013) Leadership accountability and patient safety, *Journal of Gynaecology and Neonatal Nurses (AWHONN)*, 42 (5): 506–7.

Mollon, D. (2014) Feeling safe during an inpatient hospitalization: a concept analysis, *Journal of Advanced Nursing*, 70 (8): 1727–37.

Moore, A. (2014) Seven-day challenge, *Nursing Standard*, 28 (29): 20–2.

Moran, R.T. and Riesenberger, J.R. (1994) *The Global Challenge: Building the New Worldwide Enterprise*. London: McGraw-Hill.

Morgan, J. and Vardy, F. (2009) Diversity in the workplace, *American Economic Review*, 99 (1): 472–85.

Mosadeghrad, A.M. (2014) Why TQM programmes fail? A pathology approach, *TQM Journal*, 26 (2): 160–87.

Mubarak, F. and Noor, A. (2018) Effect of authentic leadership on employee creativity in project-based organizations with the mediating roles of work engagement and psychological empowerment, *Cogent Business and Management*. Available at www.tandfonline.com/doi/abs/10.1080/23311975.2018.1429348 (accessed 8 February 2018).

Muir Gray, J.A. (2007) *How to Get Better Value Health Care.* Oxford: Offox.

Muir, N. (2004) Clinical decision-making: theory and practice, *Nursing Standard, 18* (36): 47–52.

Mukamel, D.B., Cai, S. and Temkin-Greener, H. (2009) Cost implications of organising nursing home workforce in teams, *Health Services Research, 44:* 1309–25.

Mullaly, S. (2001) Leadership and politics, *Nursing Management, 8* (4): 21–7.

Mullins, L.J. (2016) *Management and Organisational Behaviour* (11th edn). New York: FT Publishing International.

Mumford, A. (1997) *How to Manage Your Learning Environment.* London. Peter Honey Publications.

Myers-Briggs, I. (1995) *Gifts Differing: Understanding Personality Type.* Palo Alto, CA: Davies-Black Publishing.

National Audit Office (2016) *Managing the Supply of NHS Clinical Staff in England.* London: NAO.

National Audit Office (2018) *Developing New Care Models through NHS Vanguards.* London: NAO.

National Health Service Clinical Commissioners (NHSCC) (2015) *Local Solutions to National Challenges.* London: NHS.

National Information Board (NIB) (2014) *Personalised Health and Care 2020: A Framework for Action.* Available at www.gov.uk/government/publications/personalised-health-and-care-2020 (accessed on 28 February 2018).

National Institute for Health and Care Excellence (NICE) (2012) *Patient Experience in Adult NHS Services: Improving the Experience of Care for People Using Adult NHS Services.* CG138. Available at www.nice.org.uk/Guidance/CG138 (accessed 21 January 2019).

National Institute for Health and Care Excellence. (NICE) (2018) *Audit and Service Improvement.* Available at www.nice.org.uk/about/what-we-do/into-practice/audit-and-service-improvement (accessed 6 August 2018).

National Nursing Research Unit (NNRU) (2012) Intentional rounding: what is the evidence?, *Policy+ Evidence, Issues and Opinions in Healthcare, 35.*

National Nursing Research Unit (NNRU) (2013) Does NHS Staff Wellbeing Affect Patient Experience of Care?, *Policy Plus,* 39. London: Kings College.

National Patient Safety Agency (NPSA) (2004) *Seven Steps to Patient Safety.* London: NHS.

National Professional Qualification for Headship (NPQH) (2005) *Securing the Commitment of Others to the Vision (D1.2) in National College for School Leadership.* London: NPQH.

Nelson, S., Wild, D. and Szczepura, A. (2009) Innovation in residential care homes: an inreach nursing team project, *Primary Health Care, 19* (1): 31–4.

NHS Clinical Commissioners (2015) *About CCGs.* Available at www.nhscc.org/ccgs/ (accessed 26 July 2018).

NHS Employers (2018) *Gender in the NHS Infographic.* Available at www.nhsemployers.org/case-studies-and-resources/2018/05/gender-in-the-nhs-infographic (accessed 25 January 2019).

NHS England (2004) 10 High Impact Changes for Services Improvement. Available at www.england.nhs.uk/improvement-hub/publication/10-high-impact-changes-for-service-improvement-and-delivery/ (accessed 10 August 2018).

NHS England (2014) *Five Year Forward View.* Available at www.england.nhs.uk/wp-content/uploads/2014/10/5yfv-web.pdf (accessed 8 March 2018).

NHS England (2016) *Leading Change, Adding Value.* Available at www.england.nhs.uk/wp-content/uploads/2016/05/nursing-framework.pdf (accessed 29 March 2018).

NHS England (2017) *Next Steps on the NHS Five Year Forward View*. Available at www.england.nhs.uk/wp-content/uploads/2017/03/NEXT-STEPS-ON-THE-NHS-FIVE-YEAR-FORWARD-VIEW.pdf (accessed 8 March 2018).

NHS England (2018a) *Clinical Audit*. Available at www.england.nhs.uk/clinaudit/ (accessed 10 August 2018).

NHS England (2018b) *Integrated Urgent Care Key Performance Indicators and Quality Standards 2018*. Available at www.england.nhs.uk/publication/integrated-urgent-care-key-performance-indicators-and-quality-standards-2018/ (accessed 10 August 2018).

NHS England (2018c) *NHS Outcomes Framework Indicators*, May 2018 release. Available at https://digital.nhs.uk/data-and-information/publications/clinical-indicators/nhs-outcomes-framework/current (accessed 10 August 2018).

NHS England (2018d) *Your Right to Work and Practise in the UK*. Available at www.england.nhs.uk/gp/gpfv/workforce/building-the-general-practice-workforce/international-gp-recruitment/your-right-to-work-and-practice-in-the-uk/ (accessed 13 August 2018).

NHS Improvement (2016) *Evidence from NHS Improvement on Clinical Staff Shortages: A Workforce Analysis*. London: NHS Improvement. Available at www.gov.uk/government/uploads/system/uploads/attachment_data/file/500288/Clinical_workforce_report.pdf (accessed 15 March 2018).

NHS Improvement/NHS England (2016) *Freedom to Speak Up Review Report*. Available at http://webarchive.nationalarchives.gov.uk/20150218150512/http://freedomtospeakup.org.uk/the-report/ Chaired by Sir Robert Francis QC (accessed 15 October 2017).

NHS Jobs (2014) Available at www.jobs.nhs.uk/about_nhs.html (accessed 22 July 2018).

NHS Leadership Academy (2011) *Leadership Framework*. Coventry: NHS Institute for Innovation and Improvement.

NHS Leadership Academy (2012) Available at www.leadershipacademy.nhs.uk/wp-content/uploads/2012/11/NHSLeadership-Framework-LeadershipFrameworkSelfAssessmentTool.pdf (accessed 3 March 2018).

NHS Modernisation Agency (2004) *10 High Impact Changes for Service Improvement and Delivery: Guide for Leaders*. Available at www.england.nhs.uk/improvement-hub/publication/10-high-impact-changes-for-service-improvement-and-delivery/ (accessed 13 July 2018).

Nibblelink, C. and Brewer, B. (2018) Decision-making in nursing practice: an integrative literature review, *Journal of Clinical Nursing*, 27: 917–28.

Nightingale, F. (1867) Letter to the Editor, *Macmillans Magazine*. In M. Baly (1991) *As Miss Nightingale Said …* London: Scutari Press.

Noddings, N. (2013) *Caring: A Feminine Approach to Ethics and Moral Education* (2nd edn). Oakland: University of California Press.

Northcott, J. (1991) *Britain in 2010: The PSI Report*. London: Policy Studies Institute.

Northouse, P.G. (2016) *Leadership: Theory and Practice* (7th edn). London: Sage.

Nuffield Trust (2018) *The NHS Workforce in Numbers*. Available at www.nuffieldtrust.org.uk/resource/the-nhs-workforce-in-numbers (accessed 14 March 2018).

Nursing and Midwifery Council (NMC) (2006) Preceptorship Guidelines. Circular 21/2006. London: NMC.

Nursing and Midwifery Council (NMC) (2009) *Standards for Competence for Registered Midwives*. London: NMC.

Nursing and Midwifery Council (NMC) (2010) *Midwives' Rules and Standards*. London: NMC.

Nursing and Midwifery Council (NMC) (2014) *Standards for Competence for Registered Midwives*. London: NMC.

Nursing and Midwifery Council (NMC) (2015) *The Code: Professional standards of practice and behaviour for Nurses, and Midwives*. London: NMC.

Nursing and Midwifery Council (NMC) (2017a) *Revalidation: How to revalidate with the NMC*. London: NMC.

Nursing and Midwifery Council (NMC) (2017b) *Enabling Professionalism in Nursing and Midwifery Practice*. London: NMC.

Nursing and Midwifery Council (NMC) (2017c) *Report on English Language Consultation Document*. London: NMC.

Nursing and Midwifery Council (NMC) (2017d) *Raising Concerns: Guidance for Nurses and Midwives*. London: NMC.

Nursing and Midwifery Council (NMC) (2018a) *Future Nurse: Standards of Proficiency for Registered Nurses*. London: NMC.

Nursing and Midwifery Council (NMC) (2018b) *The Code: Professional Standards of Practice and Behaviour for Nurses, Midwives and Nursing Associates*. London: NMC.

Nursing and Midwifery Council (NMC) (2018c) *Realising Professionalism: Standards for Education and Training Part 1: Standards Framework for Nursing and Midwifery Education*. London: NMC.

Nursing and Midwifery Council (NMC) (2018d) *Realising Professionalism: Standards for Education and Training Part 2: Standards for Student Supervision and Assessment*. London: NMC.

Nursing and Midwifery Council (NMC) (2018e) *Realising Professionalism: Standards for Education and Training Part 3: Standards for Pre-Registraining Programmes*. London: NMC.

Nursing and Midwifery Council (NMC) (2018f) *Standards of Proficiency for Nursing Associates*. London: NMC.

Nursing and Midwifery Council (NMC) (2018g) *Realising Professionalism: Standards for Education and Training: Standards for Pre-Registration Nursing Associates Programmes*. London: NMC.

O'Brien, P. (2015) *Great Decisions, Perfect Timing: Cultivating Intuitive Intelligence*. Portland, OR: Divination Foundation Press.

Orchard, C.A. (2010) Persistent isolationist or collaborator? The nurse's role in interprofessional collaborative practice, *Journal of Nursing Management*, 18: 248–57.

Osland, J.S., Bird, A., Mendenhall, M.E. and Osland, A. (2006) 'Developing Global Leadership Capabilities and Global Mindset: A Review', in G.K. Sthal and I. Bjorkman (eds), *Handbook of Research in International Human Resource Management*. Cheltenham: Edward Elgar, pp. 197–22.

Ouchi, W. (1981) *Theory Z: How American Business Can Meet the Japanese Challenge*. Harlow: Addison Wesley.

Owen, J. (2009) *How to Lead* (2nd edn). London: Pearson.

Palfrey, C. (2000) *Key Concepts in Health Care Policy and Planning*. London: Macmillan.

Pau, A. and Croucher, R. (2003) Emotional intelligence and perceived stress in dental undergraduates, *Journal of Dental Education*, 67: 1023–8.

Pearson, A., Borbasi, S., Fitzgerald, M., Kowanko, I. and Walsh, K. (1997) 'Evidence based nursing: an examination of nursing within the international evidence-based health care practice movement', RCNA Discussion Document No. 1, *Nursing Review*. Sydney: RCNA.

Pecanac, K.E. and Schwarze, M.L. (2018) Conflict in the intensive care unit: nursing advocacy and surgical agency, *Nursing Ethics*, 25 (1): 69–79. Available at http://journals.sagepub.com/doi/pdf/10.1177/0969733016638144 (accessed 11 April 2018).

Peters, T. and Waterman, R.H. (2004) *In Search of Excellence*. London: Profile.

Petri, L (2010) Concept analysis of interdisciplinary collaboration, *Nursing Forum*, 4 (2): 72–82.

Phillips, C., Esterman, A. and Kenny, A. (2015) The theory of organisational socialisation and its potential for improving transition experienced for new graduate nursing, *Nurse Education Today*, 35 (1): 118–24.

Pollard, K.C., Thomas, J. and Miers, M. (2010) *Understanding Interprofessional Working in Health and Social Care: Theory and Practice*. London: Palgrave Macmillan.

Pondy, L.R. (1992) Reflections on organisational conflict, *Journal of Organizational Behaviour*, 13 (3): 257–61.

Porter, M. (1985) *Competitive Advantage: Creating and Sustaining Superior Performance*. New York: The Free Press.

Porter-O'Grady and Malloch, K., T. (2018) *Quantum Leadership* (5th edn). London: Jones and Bartlett.

Porter O' Grady, T. and Mallock, K. (2018) *Quantum Leadership: Creating Sustainable Value in Health Care*, 5th edition. Burlington, MA: Jones and Bartlett Learning.

Power, M., Stewart, K. and Brotherton, A. (2012) What is the NHS Safety Thermometer?, *Clinical Risk*, 18 (5): 163–9.

Public Health England (2018) Clinical Governance. Available at www.gov.uk/government/publications/newborn-hearing-screening-programme-nhsp-operational-guidance/4-clinical-governance (accessed 6 November 2018).

Public Policy Exchange (2016) *Preparing for the Impact of Brexit on the NHS: Challenges in Funding, Recruitment and Research*. Available at www.publicpolicyexchange.co.uk/events/GI13-PPE3 (accessed 28 November 2017).

Pucik, V., Tichy, N.M. and Barnett C.K. (eds) (1992) *Globalizing Management, Creating and Leading the Competitive Organization*. New York: Wiley.

Pyzdek, T. and Keller, P. (2014) *The Six Sigma Handbook* (4th edn). London: McGraw-Hill.

Race Relations Act 1965, c.73. Available at www.parliament.uk/about/living-heritage/transformingsociety/private-lives/relationships/collections1/race-relations-act-1965/race-relations-act-1965 (accessed 9 January 2019)

Radcliffe, S. (2012) *Leadership: Plain and Simple*. (2nd edn). Harlow: Pearson.

Rafferty, A. (1993) *Leading Questions: A Discussion Paper on the Issues of Nurse Leadership*. London: King's Fund.

Rahim, M.A. (1983) A measure of styles of handling interpersonal conflict, *Academy of Management Journal*, 26: 368–75.

Rahim, M.A. (2011) *Managing Conflict in Organizations*. Piscataway, NJ: Transaction.

Rankin, B. (2013) Emotional intelligence: enhancing values-based practice and compassionate care in nursing, *Journal of Advanced Nursing*, 69 (12): 2717–25.

Rayner, D., Chisholm, H. and Appleby, H. (2002) Developing leadership through action learning, *Nursing Standard*, 16 (29): 37–9.

Reeves, S., MacMillan, K. and van Soren, M. (2010) Leadership of interprofessional health and social care teams: a socio-historical analysis, *Journal of Nursing Management*, 18 (3): 258–64.

Regan, S., Laschinger, H.K.S. and Wong, C.A. (2016) The influence of empowerment, authentic leadership and professional practice environments on nurses' perceived interprofessional collaboration, *Journal of Nursing Management*, 24: E54–E61.

Reid, J. and Bromiley, M. (2012) Clinical human factors: the need to speak up to improve patient safety, *Nursing Standard*, 26 (35): 35–40.

Revans, R. (2011) *ABC of Action Learning*. Farnham: Gower

Rhinesmith, S.H. (1993) A managers' guide to globalisation: six keys to success in a changing world, *Human Resource Development Quarterly*, 6 (3): 323–7.

Ringrose, D. (2013) Development of an organizational excellent framework, *The TQM Journal*, 25 (4): 441–52.

Rippon, S. (2001) Nurturing nursing leadership – How does your garden grow?, *Nursing Management*, 8 (7): 11–15.

Robertson, C. (1997) *The Wordsworth Dictionary of Quotations*. London: Wordsworth.

Robinson, S. and Griffiths, P. (2009) *Scoping Review: Preceptorship for Newly Qualified Nurses: Impacts, Facilitators and Constraints*. London: King's Fund National Nursing Research Unit.

Robotham, A. and Frost, M. (2005) *Health Visiting Specialist Community Public Health Nursing* (2nd edn). London: Elsevier.

Rock, D. (2008) SCARF: a brain-based model for collaborating with and influencing others, *NeuroLeadership Journal*, 1: 44–52.

Rock, D., Tang, Y. and Dixon, P. (2009) Neuroscience of engagement, *NeuroLeadership Journal*, 2: 1–9.

Rogers, E. and Shoemaker, F. (1971) *Communication of Innovations: A Cross-cultural Report*. New York: Free Press.

Rogers, E.M. (1983) *Diffusion of Innovations* (3rd edn). New York: Free Press.

Ronda-Perez, E. and La Parra, D. (2016) Eradicating human trafficking: a social and public health policy priority, *Epidemiology and Psychiatric Science*, 25: 347–8.

Roper, N., Logan, W.W. and Tierney, A. (1980) *The Elements of Nursing*. London: Churchill Livingstone.

Roper, N., Logan, W.W. and Tierney, A. (2000) *The Roper, Logan & Tierney Model of Nursing: Based on Activities of Living*. Edinburgh: Elsevier Health Services.

Rosener, J. (1990) Ways women lead, *Harvard Business Review*, cited in G. Markham (1996), Gender in leadership, *Nursing Management*, 3 (1): 18–19.

Rothschild, J.M., Hurley, A.C., Landrigan, C.P., Cronin, J.W., Martell-Waldrop, K., Foskett, C., Burdick, E., Czeisler, C.A. and Bates, D.W. (2006) Recovery from medical errors: the critical care nursing safety net, *Joint Commission Journal on Quality and Patient Safety*, 32 (2): 63–72.

Royal College of Nursing (RCN) (2005) *Working with Care: Improving Working Relationships in Healthcare*. London: RCN.

Royal College of Nursing (RCN) (2017) *Record Keeping: The Facts*. London: RCN.

Rushmer, R. (2005) Blurred boundaries damage inter-professional working, *Nurse Researcher*, 12 (3): 74–85.

Sadler, P. (2003) *Leadership MBA Masterclass* (2nd edn). London: Kogan Page.

Safeguarding Vulnerable Groups Act 2006, c.47. Available at www.legislation.gov.uk/ukpga/2006/47/contents (accessed 9 January 2019)

Salovey, P. and Mayer, J.D. (1990) Emotional intelligence, *Imagination, Cognition and Personality*, 9: 185–211.

Salovey, P., Bracket, M.A. and Mayer, J. (2004) *Emotional Intelligence: Key Readings on the Mayer and Salovey Model*. Port Chester, NY: National Professional Resources Inc.

Salzman, M.B. (2018) *Psychology of Culture*. Honolulu, HI: Springer.

Sardar, Z. and Van Loon, B. (1997) *Cultural Studies for Beginners*. London: Icon.

Sauro, J. (2018) *Benchmarking the User Experience*. Denver, CO: MeasuringU Press.

Scally, G. and Donaldson, L. (1998) Clinical governance and the drive for quality improvement in the new NHS in England, *British Medical Journal*, 317: 61–5.

Schein, E.H. (1985) *Organizational Culture and Leadership*. San Francisco, CA: Jossey-Bass.

Schein, E.H. (1992) 'Coming to a New Awareness of Organizational Culture', in G. Salaman (ed.), *Human Resource Strategies*. London: Sage.

Schein, E.H. (2017) *Organisational Culture and Leadership* (5th edn). Hoboken, NJ: Wiley.

Schmalenburg, C. and Kramer, M. (1979) *Coping with Reality Shock*. Wakefield, MA: Nursing Resources.

Schön, D. (1987) *Educating the Reflective Practitioner: Towards a New Design for Teaching and Learning in the Professions*. San Francisco, CA: Jossey-Bass.

Schweitzer, A. (n.d.) Available at www.brainyquote.com/quotes/albert_schweitzer_121165 (accessed 20 January 2019).

Scott, I. (1998) Challenging the future, *Nursing Management*, 4 (9): 18–21.

Scrivener, R., Hand, T. and Hooper, R. (2011) Accountability and responsibility: principle of nursing practice B, *Nursing Standard*, 25 (29): 35–6.

Seacole, M. (2005 [1857]) *Wonderful Adventures of Mrs. Seacole in Many Lands*. London: Penguin Classics.

Seligman, M.E.P. (2011) *Authentic Happiness: Using the New Positive Psychology to Realise Your Potential for Lasting Fulfilment*. New York: Atria.

Senge, P. (1990) *The Fifth Discipline: The Art and Practice of the Learning Organisation*. New York: Doubleday.

Senge, P., Hamilton, H. and Kania, J. (2015) *The Dawn of System Leadership*. Stanford Social Innovation Review. Available at https://ssir.org/articles/entry/the_dawn_of_system_leadership (accessed 8 February 2018).

Shannon, C.E. and Weaver, W. (1954) *The Mathematical Theory of Communication*. Urbana-Champaign, IL: University of Illinois Press.

Shanta, L. and Connolly, M. (2013) Using King's Interacting Systems Theory to link emotional intelligence and nursing practice, *Journal of Professional Nursing*, 29(3): 174–80.

Shapiro, F., Punwani, N. and Urman, R. (2013) 'Putting the patient into Patient Safety Checklists', *AORN Journal*, 98 (4): 413.

Shorten, A. and Wallace, M. (1997) Evidence based practice: the future is clear, *Australian Nursing Journal*, 4 (6): 22–4, cited in B.J. Taylor (2000) *Reflective Practice: A Guide for Nurses and Midwives*. Buckingham: Open University Press.

Simon, H.A. (1964[1960]) 'The Corporation: Will It Be Managed by Machines?', in H. Leavitt and L.R. Pondy (eds), *Readings in Managerial Psychology*. Chicago: University of Chicago Press.

Simon, H.A. (1977) *The New Science of Management Decision* (revised edn). London: Prentice Hall.

Simon, H.A. (1980) Cognitive science: the newest science of the artificial, *Cognitive Science*, 4: 33–46.

Simon, H.A. (1994) 'Administrative behaviour: how organisations can be understood in terms of decision processes'. Conference Presentation, 11 March, Department of Computer Science, Roskilde University.

Smith, P. (2011) *The Emotional Labour of Nursing Revisited: Can Nurses Still Care?* (2nd edn). Basingstoke: Palgrave Macmillan.

Snape, D., Kirkham J., Preston J., Popay, J., Britten, N., Collins, M., Froggatt, K., Gibson, A., Lobban, F., Wyatt, K. and Jacoby, A. (2014) Exploring areas of consensus and conflict around values underpinning public involvement in health and social care research: a modified Delphi study, *British Medical Journal Open*, 4 (1): e00427.

Snell, M. (2009) 'Factors that Increase the Incidence of Groupthink in Hospitals: The Perception of Nurses and Managers'. DBA dissertation, Arizona ProQuest LLC.

Snow, J. (2001) Looking beyond nursing for clues to effective leadership, *Journal of Nursing Administration*, 31 (9): 440–3.

Sommerfeldt, S.A. (2013) Articulating nursing in an interprofessional world, *Nurse Education in Practice*, 13: 519–23.

Song, S (2017, Spring) 'Multiculturalism', *The Stanford Encyclopedia of Philosophy*, Edward N. Zalta (ed.). Available at https://plato.stanford.edu/archives/spr2017/entries/multicultur alism (accessed 15 February 2018).

Stanley, D. (2010) Multigenerational workforce issues and their implications for leadership in nursing, *Journal of Nursing Management*, 18: 846–52.

Starns, P. (2000) *Nurses at War: Women in the Frontline 1939–45*. Stroud: Sutton.

Steffaleno, A. and Carlson, E. (2010) Providing direct care nurses research and evidence-based practice information: an essential component of nursing leadership, *Journal of Nursing Management*, 18 (1): 84–9.

Stewart, I.M. (1918) Popular fallacies about nursing education, *The Modern Hospital*, 18 (1), cited in M.P. Donahue (2011) *Nursing – The Finest Art*. St Louis, MO: Mosby.

Stoddart, K., Ciccu-Moore, R., Grant, F., Niven, B.A., Paterson, H. and Wallace, A. (2014) Care comfort rounds, *Nursing Management*, 20 (9): 18–23.

Stogdill, R. (1974) *Handbook of Leadership: A Survey of Theory and Research*. New York: Free Press.

Storey, J. and Holti, R. (2013) *Towards a New Model of Leadership for the NHS*. London: NHS Leadership Academy and Open University Business School.

Stott, K. (1992) *Making Management Work*. London: Prentice Hall.

Stott, K. and Walker, A. (1995) *Making Management Work: A Practical Approach*. London: Prentice Hall.

Studer Group (2007) Best practices: Sacred Heart Hospital, Pensicola, Florida. Hourly rounding supplement. Gulf Breeze, cited in *Policy+*, National Nursing Research Unit, King's College London, Issue 35, April 2012.

Sullivan, E.J. and Garland, G. (2010) *Practical Leadership and Management in Nursing* (2nd edn). Harlow: Pearson.

Sullivan, E.J. and Garland, G. (2013) *Practical Leadership and Management in Healthcare: For Nurses and Allied Health Professionals*. London: Pearson.

Tang, C.J., Zhou, W.T., Chan, S.W-C and Liaw, S Y. (2018) Interprofessional collaboration between junior doctors and nurses in the general ward setting: a qualitative exploratory study, *Journal of Nursing Management*, 26: 11–18.

Tannenbaum, R. and Schmidt, W.H. (1958) How to choose a leadership pattern, *Harvard Business Review*, 36: 95–101.

Tappen, R., Weiss, S. and Whitehead, D. (2009[2004]) 'Tools for Leadership and Management Problem Solving', in D. Whitehead, S. Weiss and R. Tappen (eds), *Essentials of Nursing Leadership and Management* (5th edn). Philadelphia, PA: FA Davis.

Taylor, B.J. (2010) *Reflective Practice for Health Care Professionals: A Practical Guide* (3rd edn). Maidenhead: Open University Press.

Taylor, F.W. (1947) *Scientific Management*. New York: Harper & Row.

The Health Foundation (2013) *Quality improvement made simple*. London: The Health Foundation.

The Health Foundation (2015) *Person-centred Care Made Simple*. Available at www.health. org.uk/sites/default/files/PersonCentredCareMadeSimple.pdf (accessed 25 January 2019).

The Health Foundation (2016) *Briefing: NHS Finances outside the EU*. London: The Health Foundation.

The Institute of Medicine (IoM) (2001) *Crossing the Quality Chasm*. London: IoM.

The King's Fund (2010) *The Future of Leadership and Management in the NHS: No More Heroes*. London: King's Fund.

The King's Fund (2011) *The Future of Leadership and Management in the NHS: No More Heroes*. Available at www.kingsfund.org.uk/sites/default/files/future-of-leadership-and-management-nhs-may-2011-kings-fund.pdf (accessed 8 February 2018).

The King's Fund (2012a) *Hospital Pathways Programme: Lessons Learned*. Available at www.kingsfund.org.uk/publications/articles/hospital-pathways-programme-lessons-learned (accessed 1 March 2018).

The King's Fund (2012b) *Will Hourly Rounds Help Nurses to Concentrate More on Caring?* London: King's Fund.

The King's Fund (2013) *Why Aren't There More Women Leaders in the NHS?* Available at www.kingsfund.org.uk/blog/2013/07/why-aren%E2%80%99t-there-more-women-leaders-nhs (accessed 13 March 2018).

The King's Fund (2015) *The Practice of System Leadership: Being Comfortable with Chaos*. Available at www.kingsfund.org.uk/sites/default/files/field/field_publication_file/System-leadership-Kings-Fund-May-2015.pdf (accessed 28 February 2018).

The King's Fund (2016) *Five Big Issues for Health and Social Care after Brexit Vote*. Available at www.kingsfund.org.uk/publications/articles/brexit-and-nhs (accessed 17 January 2018).

The King's Fund (2018) *How Is the NHS Performing 2018?* Available at www.kingsfund.org.uk/publications/how-nhs-performing-march-2018#health-care-surveys (accessed 4 June 2018).

The Lord Laming Report (2009) *The Protection of Children in England: A Progress Report*. Available at http://dera.ioe.ac.uk/8646/1/12_03_09_children.pdf (accessed 9 March 2018).

The Open University (1996) P679 – Planning and Managing Change. Milton Keynes: Open University Press.

The United Nations (2000) Available at www.un.org/millenniumgoals (accessed 20 February 2019).

ThisWay Global (2017) *7 Biggest Diversity Issues in the Workplace*. Available at www.thisway-global.com/blog/diversity/top-diversity-issues-in-the-workplace (accessed 8 January 2018).

Thomas, K.W. (1976) 'Conflict and Conflict Management', in M.D. Dunnette (ed.), *Handbook of Industrial and Organisational Psychology*. Chicago, IL: Rand McNally.

Thomas, K.W. (1977) Towards multidimensional values in teaching: the example of conflict behaviours, *Academy of Management Review*, July: 487.

Thompson, P. and Hyrkas, K. (2014) Global nursing leadership (editorial), *Journal of Nursing Management*, 22 (1): 1–3.

Thorndike, E.L. (1932) *The Fundamentals of Learning*. New York: Teachers College Press.

Thornton, C. (2016) *Group and Team Coaching: The Secret Life of Groups* (Essential Coaching Skills and Knowledge) (2nd edn). London: Routledge.

Tjosvold, D. (2008) The conflict-positive organization: it depends upon us, *Journal of Organizational Behaviour*, 29: 19–28. Available at https://onlinelibrary.wiley.com/doi/abs/10.1002/job.473 (accessed 11 April 2018).

Tuckman, B.C. and Jensen, M.A. (1977) Stages of small group development revisited, *Group and Organization Studies*, 2 (4): 419–27.

Tuckman, B.W. (1965) Developmental sequence in small groups, *Psychological Bulletin*, 63: 384–99.

Tylor, E.B. (1997[1871]) 'Primitive Cultures', in Z. Sardar and B. Van Loon (eds), *Cultural Studies for Beginners*. London: Icon.

UNISON (2011) *Duty of Care Handbook*. London: UNISON.

University of Salford (2009) *Salford Student Becomes First Deaf Male Nurse*. Available at http://staff.salford.ac.uk/newsitem/1247 (accessed 2 November 2017).

Upton, T. and Brooks, B. (NAHAT) (1995) *Managing Change in the NHS*. London: Kogan Page.

Urisman, T., Garcia, A. and Harris, H.W. (2018) Impact of surgical intensive care unit interdisciplinary rounds on interprofessional collaboration and quality of care: mixed qualitative–quantitative study, *Intensive and Critical Care Nursing*, 44: 18–23.

Valentine, P.E.B. (2001) A gender perspective on conflict management strategies of nurses, *Journal of Nursing Scholarship*, *33* (1): 69–74.

Van Aken, J.E. and Berends, H. (2018) *Problem-solving in Organizations: A Methodological Handbook for Business and Management Students* (3rd edn). Cambridge: Cambridge University Press.

Van Seters, D.A. and Field, R.H.G. (1990) The evolution of leadership theory, *Journal of Organisational Change Management*, *3*: 3.

VanGundy, A.B. (1988) *Techniques of Structured Problem Solving* (2nd edn). London: Van Nostrand Reinhold.

Vitello-Cicciu, J.M. (2002) Exploring emotional intelligence: implications for nurse leaders, *JONA*, *32* (4): 203–9.

Vroom, V.H. (1964) *Work and Motivation*. New York: Wiley.

Vroom, V.H. and Jago, A.G. (1988) *The New Leadership*. Englewood Cliffs, NJ: Prentice Hall.

Vroom, V.H. and Yetton, P.W. (1973) *Leadership and Decision Making*. Pittsburgh: University of Pittsburgh.

Waite, R. and McKinney, N.S. (2014) Enhancing conflict competency, *The Association of Black Nursing Faculty Journal*, *25* (4): 123–8.

Walker, L.O. and Avant, K.C. (2010) *Strategies for Theory Construction in Nursing* (5th edn). Englewood Cliffs, NJ: Prentice Hall.

Walmsley, J., Reynolds, J., Shakespeare, P. and Woolfe, R. (1997) *Health, Welfare and Practice: Reflecting on Relationship*. London: Sage/Open University.

Waterlow, J. (2005) *The Waterlow Pressure Prevention Manual*. Available at judy-waterlow. co.uk (accessed 1 March 2018).

Weaver, H. (2013) *Determined and Dedicated*. Available at www.nursingtimes.net (accessed 2 November 2017).

Weberg, D. (2012) Complexity leadership: a healthcare imperative, *Nursing Forum*, *47* (14): 68–77.

Weightman, J. (1999) *Introducing Organisational Behaviour*. Harlow: Addison Wesley Longman.

Weightman, J. (2004) *Managing People* (2nd edn). London: Chartered Institute of Personnel Development.

Weisbord, M. (1976) Organisational diagnosis: six places to look with or without a theory, *Group and Organisational Studies*, *1*: 430–47, in V. Iles and K. Sutherland (2001) *Organisational Change: Managing Change in the NHS*. London: The National Co-ordinating Centre for NHS Service Delivery, Organisation, Research and Development.

Weitz, R., Brinkerhoft, D., White, L.K. and Ortega, S.T. (2011) *Essentials of Sociology* (9th edn). Boston, MA: Wadsworth Cengage Learning.

West M.A. (2012) *Effective Teamwork: Practical Lessons from Organizational Research* (3rd edn). Chichester: Blackwell.

West, M., Eskert, R., Collins, R. and Chowla, R. (2017) *Caring to Change: How Compassionate Leadership Can Stimulate Innovation in Health Care*. London: The King's Fund. Available at www.kingsfund.org.uk/sites/default/files/field/field_publication_file/Caring_to_change_Kings_Fund_May_2017.pdf (accessed 1 March 2018).

White, N. (2012) Understanding the role of non-technical skills in patient safety, *Nursing Standard*, *26* (26): 43–8.

White, R.K. and Lippitt, R. (2006[1960]) 'Autocracy and Democracy: An Experimental Inquiry', in B.L. Marquis and C.J. Huston (eds), *Leadership Roles and Management Functions in Nursing: Theory and Application* (5th edn). Philadelphia, PA: Lippincott.

Whitehead, D., Weiss, S. and Tappen, R. (2009) *Essentials of Nursing Leadership and Management* (5th edn). Philadelphia, PA: F.A. Davis Company.

Wickware, C. (2018) GPs to face new rationing programme for surgery referrals, *PULSE*, 29 May. Available at www.pulsetoday.co.uk/news/commissioning/commissioning-topics/refer-rals/gps-to-face-new-rationing-programme-for-surgery-referrals/20036794.article (accessed 3 August 2018).

Wilkinson, G. and Miers, M. (1999) *Power and Nursing Practice*. London: Macmillan.

Wong, C.S. and Law, K.S. (2002) The effects of leader and follower emotional intelligence on performance and attitude: an exploratory study, *The Leadership Quarterly*, 13: 243–68.

Wood, J.T. (2012) *Gendered Lives: Communication, Gender and Culture* (10th edn). Cincinnati, OH: Wadsworth.

Wordnik (n.d) Available at www.wordnik.com/words/intuition (accessed 29 January 2019).

World Health Organization (WHO) (1983) *The Principles of Quality Assurance*. Copenhagen: WHO (report on a WHO meeting).

World Health Organization (2011) *Patient Safety Curriculum Guide: Multi-professional Edition*. Available at http://whqlibdoc.who.int/publications/2011/9789241501958_eng.pdf (accessed 18 September 2014).

World Health Organization (WHO) (2008) *Primary Health Care: Now More Than Ever*. Geneva: WHO.

World Health Organization (WHO) (2010) *Framework for Action on Interprofessional Education and Collaborative Practice*. Available at http://apps.who.int/iris/bitstream/handle/10665/70185/WHO_HRH_HPN_10.3_eng.pdf;jsessionid=89363BA99F70973961F71D46CD2D2BA2?sequence=1 (accessed 26 July 2018).

Wright, T. (2000) The phantom menace, *Nursing Management*, 6 (5): 5.

Xyrichis, A. and Ream, E. (2008) Teamwork: a concept analysis, *Journal of Advanced Nursing*, 61 (2): 232–41.

Young, M. (2016) *Seniority, Strength, and Serendipity: What Makes a Good Lead Developer?* Available at https://capgemini.github.io/learning/seniority-serendipity/ (accessed 1 October 2017).

Yukl, G., Goron, A. and Taber, T. (2002) A hierarchical taxonomy of leadership behaviour. Integrating a half century of behaviour research, *Journal of Leadership and Organizational Studies*, 9 (1): 15–32.

Zaccaro, S.J., Kemp, C. and Bader, P. (2004) 'Leader Traits and Attributes'. In J. Antonakis, A.T. Cianciolo and R.J. Sternberg (eds), *The Nature of Leadership*. Thousand Oaks, CA: Sage,. pp. 101–24.

Zydziunaite, V., Suominen, T., Astedt-Kurki, P. and Lepaite, D. (2010) Ethical dilemmas concerning decision making within healthcare leadership: a systematic literature review, *Medicina* (Kaunas), 46 (9): 596–603.

INDEX

Note: Tables and figures are indicated by page numbers in bold print.